W9-DCV-732

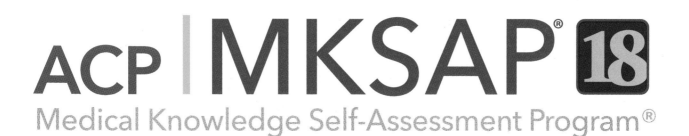

ACP | MKSAP® 18

Medical Knowledge Self-Assessment Program®

Gastroenterology and Hepatology

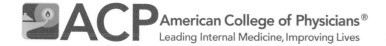

ACP American College of Physicians®
Leading Internal Medicine, Improving Lives

Welcome to the Gastroenterology and Hepatology Section of MKSAP 18!

In these pages, you will find updated information on gastroesophageal reflux disease, Barrett esophagus, *Helicobacter pylori* infection, gastrointestinal complications of NSAIDS, celiac disease, inflammatory bowel disease, liver disease, gallbladder disease, and other clinical challenges. All of these topics are uniquely focused on the needs of generalists and subspecialists *outside* of gastroenterology and hepatology.

The core content of MKSAP 18 has been developed as in previous editions—all essential information that is newly researched and written in 11 topic areas of internal medicine—created by dozens of leading generalists and subspecialists and guided by certification and recertification requirements, emerging knowledge in the field, and user feedback. MKSAP 18 also contains 1200 all-new peer-reviewed, psychometrically validated, multiple-choice questions (MCQs) for self-assessment and study, including 96 in Gastroenterology and Hepatology. MKSAP 18 continues to include *High Value Care* (HVC) recommendations, based on the concept of balancing clinical benefit with costs and harms, with associated MCQs illustrating these principles and HVC Key Points called out in the text. Internists practicing in the hospital setting can easily find comprehensive *Hospitalist*-focused content and MCQs, specially designated in blue and with the H symbol.

If you purchased MKSAP 18 Complete, you also have access to MKSAP 18 Digital, with additional tools allowing you to customize your learning experience. MKSAP Digital includes regular text updates with new, practice-changing information, 200 new self-assessment questions, and enhanced custom-quiz options. MKSAP Complete also includes more than 1200 electronic, adaptive learning-enhanced flashcards for quick review of important concepts, as well as an updated and enhanced version of Virtual Dx, MKSAP's image-based self-assessment tool. As before, MKSAP 18 Digital is optimized for use on your mobile devices, with iOS- and Android-based apps allowing you to sync between your apps and online account and submit for CME credits and MOC points online.

Please visit us at the MKSAP Resource Site (mksap.acponline.org) to find out how we can help you study, earn CME credit and MOC points, and stay up to date.

On behalf of the many internists who have offered their time and expertise to create the content for MKSAP 18 and the editorial staff who work to bring this material to you in the best possible way, we are honored that you have chosen to use MKSAP 18 and appreciate any feedback about the program you may have. Please feel free to send any comments to mksap_editors@acponline.org.

Sincerely,

Patrick C. Alguire, MD, FACP
Editor-in-Chief
Senior Vice President Emeritus
Medical Education Division
American College of Physicians

Gastroenterology and Hepatology

Committee

John Poterucha, MD, Section Editor[1]
Professor of Medicine
Division of Gastroenterology and Hepatology
Mayo Clinic College of Medicine
Rochester, Minnesota

Seth A. Gross, MD[2]
Chief of Gastroenterology
Tisch Hospital
Associate Professor of Medicine
NYU Langone Medical Center
New York, New York

Sonia S. Kupfer, MD[1]
Assistant Professor of Medicine
Section of Gastroenterology, Hepatology, and Nutrition
Department of Medicine
University of Chicago
Chicago, Illinois

Michael D. Leise, MD[2]
Associate Professor of Medicine
Division of Gastroenterology and Hepatology
Mayo Clinic College of Medicine
Rochester, Minnesota

Michele Lewis, MD, MMSc, FACP[2]
Assistant Professor of Medicine
Division of Gastroenterology and Hepatology
Director, Internal Medicine Residency Program
Mayo Clinic Florida
Jacksonville, Florida

Roman Perri, MD[1]
Assistant Professor of Medicine
Division of Gastroenterology, Hepatology, and Nutrition
Vanderbilt University Medical Center
Nashville, Tennessee

Richard J. Saad, MD, MS[2]
Associate Professor of Medicine
Michigan Medicine
University of Michigan
Ann Arbor, Michigan

Seth Sweetser, MD[2]
Associate Professor of Medicine
Division of Gastroenterology and Hepatology
Department of Medicine
Mayo Clinic College of Medicine
Rochester, Minnesota

Editor-in-Chief

Patrick C. Alguire, MD, FACP[2]
Senior Vice President Emeritus, Medical Education
American College of Physicians
Philadelphia, Pennsylvania

Deputy Editor

Denise M. Dupras, MD, PhD, FACP[1]
Associate Program Director
Department of Internal Medicine
Associate Professor of Medicine
Mayo Clinic College of Medicine
Rochester, Minnesota

Gastroenterology and Hepatology Reviewers

Sushil K. Ahlawat, MD, FACP[1]
Monjur Ahmed, MBBS, FACP[1]
Benedict E. Aimua, MBBS, FACP[1]
Tulay Aksoy, MD, FACP[1]
Victor Ankoma-Sey, MD, FACP[2]
Jamie Barkin, MD, MACP[2]
Michael J. Blecker, MD, FACP[1]
David E. Bobman, MD, FACP[1]
Henry C. Bodenheimer Jr., MD, FACP[2]
Fernando F. Stancampiano, MD, FACP[1]

Hospital Medicine Gastroenterology and Hepatology Reviewers

Adam Garber, MD, FACP[2]
Lokesh Kumar Jha, MBBS, FACP[1]

Gastroenterology and Hepatology ACP Editorial Staff

Julia Nawrocki, Digital Content Associate/Editor, Self-Assessment and Educational Programs
Margaret Wells, Director, Self-Assessment and Educational Programs
Becky Krumm, Managing Editor, Self-Assessment and Educational Programs

ACP Principal Staff

Davoren Chick, MD, FACP[2]
Senior Vice President, Medical Education

Patrick C. Alguire, MD, FACP[2]
Senior Vice President Emeritus, Medical Education

Sean McKinney[1]
Vice President, Medical Education

Margaret Wells[1]
Director, Self-Assessment and Educational Programs

Becky Krumm[1]
Managing Editor

Valerie Dangovetsky[1]
Administrator

Ellen McDonald, PhD[1]
Senior Staff Editor

Megan Zborowski[1]
Senior Staff Editor

Randy Hendrickson[1]
Production Administrator/Editor

Julia Nawrocki[1]
Digital Content Associate/Editor

Linnea Donnarumma[1]
Staff Editor

Chuck Emig[1]
Staff Editor

Jackie Twomey[1]
Staff Editor

Joysa Winter[1]
Staff Editor

Kimberly Kerns[1]
Administrative Coordinator

---

1. Has no relationships with any entity producing, marketing, reselling, or distributing health care goods or services consumed by, or used on, patients.

2. Has disclosed relationship(s) with any entity producing, marketing, reselling, or distributing health care goods or services consumed by, or used on, patients.

Disclosure of relationships with any entity producing, marketing, reselling, or distributing health care goods or services consumed by, or used on, patients.

Patrick C. Alguire, MD, FACP
Royalties
UpToDate

Victor Ankoma-Sey, MD, FACP
Employment
Liver Associates of Texas, P.A.
Speakers Bureau
AbbVie, Bristol-Myers Squibb Co., Gilead Sciences Inc., Janssen, Merck, Salix Pharmaceuticals

Jamie Barkin, MD, MACP
Research grants/Contracts
EndoChoice Inc.
Consultantship
AbbVie

Henry C. Bodenheimer, Jr., MD, FACP
Employment
Northwell Health
Honoraria
Intercept Pharmaceuticals Inc.
Consultantship
Intercept Pharmaceuticals Inc., Takeda Pharmaceutical Co. Ltd.
Stock Options/Holdings
Biogen, Catalyst, Celgene, CorMedix Inc., CVS Health, Dexcom Inc., Gilead Sciences Inc., GlaxoSmithKline plc, Invivo, Johnson & Johnson, Mallinckrodt plc, Medtronic plc, NeoGenomics Inc., Sanofi, United Therapeutics Corp.

Davoren Chick, MD, FACP
Royalties
Wolters Kluwer Publishing
Consultantship
EBSCO Health's DynaMed Plus
Other: Owner and sole proprietor of Coding 101 LLC; research consultant (spouse) for Vedanta Biosciences Inc.

Adam Garber, MD, FACP
Stock Options/Holdings
GE

Seth A. Gross, MD
Consultantship
Cook Group, CDx Diagnostics, Given Imaging, Olympus
Stock Options/Holdings
CSA Medical Inc.

Michael D. Leise, MD
Research Grants/Contracts
Gilead Sciences Inc., Merck
Royalties
UpToDate

Michele Lewis, MD, MMSc, FACP
Honoraria
UpToDate

Richard Saad, MD, MS
Consultantship
Allergan plc, Ironwood Pharmaceuticals Inc., Salix Pharmaceuticals, Synergy Pharmaceuticals Inc., Quest Diagnostics
Research Grants/Contracts
Prometheus Laboratories Inc. (Principal Investigator), Salix Pharmaceuticals

Seth Sweetser, MD
Research Grants/Contracts
Exact Sciences Corp.

Acknowledgments

The American College of Physicians (ACP) gratefully acknowledges the special contributions to the development and production of the 18th edition of the Medical Knowledge Self-Assessment Program® (MKSAP® 18) made by the following people:

Graphic Design: Barry Moshinski (Director, Graphic Services), Michael Ripca (Graphics Technical Administrator), and Jennifer Gropper (Graphic Designer).

Production/Systems: Dan Hoffmann (Director, Information Technology), Scott Hurd (Manager, Content Systems), Neil Kohl (Senior Architect), and Chris Patterson (Senior Architect).

MKSAP 18 Digital: Under the direction of Steven Spadt (Senior Vice President, Technology), the digital version of MKSAP 18 was developed within the ACP's Digital Products and Services Department, led by Brian Sweigard (Director, Digital Products and Services). Other members of the team included Dan Barron (Senior Web Application Developer/Architect), Chris Forrest (Senior Software Developer/Design Lead), Kathleen Hoover (Senior Web Developer), Kara Regis (Manager, User Interface Design and Development), Brad Lord (Senior Web Application Developer), and John McKnight (Senior Web Developer).

The College also wishes to acknowledge that many other persons, too numerous to mention, have contributed to the production of this program. Without their dedicated efforts, this program would not have been possible.

MKSAP Resource Site (mksap.acponline.org)

The MKSAP Resource Site (mksap.acponline.org) is a continually updated site that provides links to MKSAP 18 online answer sheets for print subscribers; access to MKSAP 18 Digital; Board Basics® e-book access instructions; information on Continuing Medical Education (CME), Maintenance of Certification (MOC), and international Continuing Professional Development (CPD) and MOC; errata; and other new information.

International MOC/CPD

For information and instructions on submission of international MOC/CPD, please go to the MKSAP Resource Site (mksap.acponline.org).

Continuing Medical Education

The American College of Physicians is accredited by the Accreditation Council for Continuing Medical Education (ACCME) to provide continuing medical education for physicians.

The American College of Physicians designates this enduring material, MKSAP 18, for a maximum of 275 *AMA PRA Category 1 Credits*™. Physicians should claim only the credit commensurate with the extent of their participation in the activity.

Up to 22 *AMA PRA Category 1 Credits*™ are available from July 31, 2018, to July 31, 2021, for the MKSAP 18 Gastroentrology and Hepatology section.

Learning Objectives

The learning objectives of MKSAP 18 are to:

- Close gaps between actual care in your practice and preferred standards of care, based on best evidence
- Diagnose disease states that are less common and sometimes overlooked and confusing
- Improve management of comorbid conditions that can complicate patient care
- Determine when to refer patients for surgery or care by subspecialists
- Pass the ABIM Certification Examination
- Pass the ABIM Maintenance of Certification Examination

Target Audience

- General internists and primary care physicians
- Subspecialists who need to remain up to date in internal medicine
- Residents preparing for the certifying examination in internal medicine
- Physicians preparing for maintenance of certification in internal medicine (recertification)

ABIM Maintenance of Certification

Check the MKSAP Resource Site (mksap.acponline.org) for the latest information on how MKSAP tests can be used to apply to the American Board of Internal Medicine (ABIM) for Maintenance of Certification (MOC) points following completion of the CME activity.

Successful completion of the CME activity, which includes participation in the evaluation component, enables the participant to earn up to 275 medical knowledge MOC points in the ABIM's MOC program. It is the CME activity provider's responsibility to submit participant completion information to ACCME for the purpose of granting MOC credit.

Earn Instantaneous CME Credits or MOC Points Online

Print subscribers can enter their answers online to earn instantaneous CME credits or MOC points. You can submit your answers using online answer sheets that are provided at mksap.acponline.org, where a record of your MKSAP 18 credits will be available. To earn CME credits or to apply for MOC points, you need to answer all of the questions in a test and earn a score of at least 50% correct (number of correct answers divided by the total number of questions). Please note that if you are applying for MOC points, you must also enter your birth date and ABIM candidate number.

Take either of the following approaches:

1. Use the printed answer sheet at the back of this book to record your answers. Go to mksap.acponline.org, access the appropriate online answer sheet, transcribe your answers, and submit your test for instantaneous CME credits or MOC points. There is no additional fee for this service.
2. Go to mksap.acponline.org, access the appropriate online answer sheet, directly enter your answers, and submit your test for instantaneous CME credits or MOC points. There is no additional fee for this service.

Earn CME Credits or MOC Points by Mail or Fax

Pay a $20 processing fee per answer sheet and submit the printed answer sheet at the back of this book by mail or fax, as instructed on the answer sheet. Make sure you calculate your score and enter your birth date and ABIM candidate number, and fax the answer sheet to 215-351-2799 or mail the answer sheet to Member and Customer Service, American College of Physicians, 190 N. Independence Mall West, Philadelphia, PA 19106-1572, using the courtesy envelope provided in your MKSAP 18 slipcase. You will need your 10-digit order number and 8-digit ACP ID number, which are printed on your packing slip. Please allow 4 to 6 weeks for your score report to be emailed back to you. Be sure to include your email address for a response.

If you do not have a 10-digit order number and 8-digit ACP ID number, or if you need help creating a username and password to access the MKSAP 18 online answer sheets, go to mksap.acponline.org or email custserv@acponline.org.

Disclosure Policy

It is the policy of the American College of Physicians (ACP) to ensure balance, independence, objectivity, and scientific rigor in all of its educational activities. To this end, and consistent with the policies of the ACP and the Accreditation Council for Continuing Medical Education (ACCME), contributors to all ACP continuing medical education activities are required to disclose all relevant financial relationships with any entity producing, marketing, re-selling, or distributing health care goods or services consumed by, or

used on, patients. Contributors are required to use generic names in the discussion of therapeutic options and are required to identify any unapproved, off-label, or investigative use of commercial products or devices. Where a trade name is used, all available trade names for the same product type are also included. If trade-name products manufactured by companies with whom contributors have relationships are discussed, contributors are asked to provide evidence-based citations in support of the discussion. The information is reviewed by the committee responsible for producing this text. If necessary, adjustments to topics or contributors' roles in content development are made to balance the discussion. Further, all readers of this text are asked to evaluate the content for evidence of commercial bias and send any relevant comments to mksap_editors@ acponline.org so that future decisions about content and contributors can be made in light of this information.

Resolution of Conflicts

To resolve all conflicts of interest and influences of vested interests, ACP's content planners used best evidence and updated clinical care guidelines in developing content, when such evidence and guidelines were available. All content underwent review by peer reviewers not on the committee to ensure that the material was balanced and unbiased. Contributors' disclosure information can be found with the list of contributors' names and those of ACP principal staff listed in the beginning of this book.

Hospital-Based Medicine

For the convenience of subscribers who provide care in hospital settings, content that is specific to the hospital setting has been highlighted in blue. Hospital icons (🏥) highlight where the hospital-only content begins, continues over more than one page, and ends.

High Value Care Key Points

Key Points in the text that relate to High Value Care concepts (that is, concepts that discuss balancing clinical benefit with costs and harms) are designated by the HVC icon [HVC].

Educational Disclaimer

The editors and publisher of MKSAP 18 recognize that the development of new material offers many opportunities for error. Despite our best efforts, some errors may persist in print. Drug dosage schedules are, we believe, accurate and in accordance with current standards. Readers are advised, however, to ensure that the recommended dosages in MKSAP 18 concur with the information provided in the product information material. This is especially important in cases of new, infrequently used, or highly toxic drugs. Application of the information in MKSAP 18 remains the professional responsibility of the practitioner.

The primary purpose of MKSAP 18 is educational. Information presented, as well as publications, technologies, products, and/or services discussed, is intended to inform subscribers about the knowledge, techniques, and experiences of the contributors. A diversity of professional opinion exists, and the views of the contributors are their own and not those of the ACP. Inclusion of any material in the program does not constitute endorsement or recommendation by the ACP. The ACP does not warrant the safety, reliability, accuracy, completeness, or usefulness of and disclaims any and all liability for damages and claims that may result from the use of information, publications, technologies, products, and/or services discussed in this program.

Publisher's Information

Copyright © 2018 American College of Physicians. All rights reserved.

This publication is protected by copyright. No part of this publication may be reproduced, stored in a retrieval system, or transmitted in any form or by any means, electronic or mechanical, including photocopy, without the express consent of the ACP. MKSAP 18 is for individual use only. Only one account per subscription will be permitted for the purpose of earning CME credits and MOC points and for other authorized uses of MKSAP 18.

Disclaimer Regarding Direct Purchases from Online Retailers

CME and/or MOC for MKSAP 18 is available only if you purchase the program directly from ACP. CME credits and MOC points cannot be awarded to those purchasers who have purchased the program from non-authorized sellers such as Amazon, eBay, or any other such online retailer.

Unauthorized Use of This Book Is Against the Law

Unauthorized reproduction of this publication is unlawful. The ACP prohibits reproduction of this publication or any of its parts in any form either for individual use or for distribution.

The ACP will consider granting an individual permission to reproduce only limited portions of this publication for his or her own exclusive use. Send requests in writing to MKSAP® Permissions, American College of Physicians, 190 N. Independence Mall West, Philadelphia, PA 19106-1572, or email your request to mksap_editors@acponline.org.

MKSAP 18 ISBN: 978-1-938245-47-3
(Gastroenterology and Hepatology)
ISBN: 978-1-938245-50-3

Printed in the United States of America.

For order information in the U.S. or Canada call 800-ACP-1915. All other countries call 215-351-2600, (Monday to Friday, 9 AM – 5 PM ET). Fax inquiries to 215-351-2799 or email to custserv@acponline.org.

Errata

Errata for MKSAP 18 will be available through the MKSAP Resource Site at mksap.acponline.org as new information becomes known to the editors.

Table of Contents

Colorectal Neoplasia

Disorders of the Liver

Disorders of the Gallbladder and Bile Ducts

Gastroenterology and Hepatology High Value Care Recommendations

The American College of Physicians, in collaboration with multiple other organizations, is engaged in a worldwide initiative to promote the practice of High Value Care (HVC). The goals of the HVC initiative are to improve health care outcomes by providing care of proven benefit and reducing costs by avoiding unnecessary and even harmful interventions. The initiative comprises several programs that integrate the important concept of health care value (balancing clinical benefit with costs and harms) for a given intervention into a broad range of educational materials to address the needs of trainees, practicing physicians, and patients.

HVC content has been integrated into MKSAP 18 in several important ways. MKSAP 18 includes HVC-identified key points in the text, HVC-focused multiple choice questions, and, for subscribers to MKSAP Digital, an HVC custom quiz. From the text and questions, we have generated the following list of HVC recommendations that meet the definition below of high value care and bring us closer to our goal of improving patient outcomes while conserving finite resources.

High Value Care Recommendation: A recommendation to choose diagnostic and management strategies for patients in specific clinical situations that balance clinical benefit with cost and harms with the goal of improving patient outcomes.

Below are the High Value Care Recommendations for the Gastroenterology and Hepatology section of MKSAP 18.

- In patients with gastroesophageal reflux symptoms without alarm features, empiric proton pump inhibitor therapy is the first therapeutic and diagnostic step.
- Attempts to stop or reduce long-term proton pump inhibitor therapy for uncomplicated gastroesophageal reflux disease should be considered at least annually (see Item 59).
- Women with gastroesophageal reflux disease do not require screening for Barrett esophagus.

- Patients 60 years and older with dyspepsia should undergo upper endoscopy.
- Patients younger than age 60 years with dyspepsia should be tested and treated for Helicobacter pylori infection.
- Enteral nutrition is preferred in patients with acute pancreatitis (see Item 26).
- Same-admission cholecystectomy reduces rates of gallstone-related complications for patients with mild gallstone pancreatitis (see Item 20).
- Asymptomatic patients with walled-off necrosis of the pancreas require no intervention (see Item 95).
- Biopsy and endoscopic retrograde cholangiopancreatography are not indicated in the diagnosis of chronic pancreatitis.
- Evaluation with imaging, endoscopy, and other testing is not indicated for irritable bowel syndrome or functional diarrhea.
- Irritable bowel syndrome can often be managed with reassurance, lifestyle modifications, and dietary modifications.
- The evaluation for centrally mediated pain syndrome does not require extensive laboratory testing or imaging.
- Acute diverticulitis usually does not require abdominal imaging.
- Patients with small hyperplastic polyps should undergo repeat colonoscopy no sooner than 10 years (see Item 11).
- Patients with uncomplicated diverticulitis should be treated with oral antibiotics (see Item 74).
- Ultrasonography is the most effective means of diagnosing ascites.
- Asymptomatic hepatic cysts require no follow-up.
- Focal nodular hyperplasia does not require follow-up.
- Incidentally diagnosed gallstones do not require cholecystectomy.
- The diagnosis of acute cholecystitis can be made by ultrasonography.
- In patients with upper gastrointestinal bleeding, a transfusion threshold of less than 7 g/dL (70 g/L) with a target hemoglobin level of 7-9 g/dL (70-90 g/L) is associated with decreased mortality and length of hospital stay (see Item 83).

Gastroenterology and Hepatology

Disorders of the Esophagus

Symptoms of Esophageal Disease

Dysphagia

Dysphagia represents a disruption in the swallowing mechanism, resulting in food not passing from the mouth to the stomach. Common descriptions of the sensations of dysphagia include food "hanging up" or feeling "lodged" or "stuck" during a meal. Determining whether the underlying cause is oropharyngeal or esophageal is important in developing a differential diagnosis and management plan. **Table 1** highlights the common causes of dysphagia.

Oropharyngeal Dysphagia

Oropharyngeal dysphagia, also known as transfer dysphagia, occurs when the patient is unable to transfer the food bolus

TABLE 1. Causes of Dysphagia	
Condition	**Diagnostic Clues**
Oropharyngeal Dysphagia	
Structural disorders	
Cervical osteophytes	High dysphagia, degenerative joint disease
Cricoid webs	High dysphagia, iron deficiency
Pharyngoesophageal (Zenker) diverticulum	Aspiration, neck mass, and regurgitation of foul-smelling food
Goiter	Neck mass
Neurologic/myogenic disorders	
Amyotrophic lateral sclerosis	Upper and lower motoneuron signs, fasciculations
Central nervous system tumor	Headache, vision changes, nausea, seizures, balance problem
Stroke	Focal neurologic deficits
Muscular dystrophy	Slow progression of muscular weakness over years
Myasthenia gravis	Weakness with repetitive activity
Multiple sclerosis	Episodes of neurologic dysfunction with variable degrees of recovery
Parkinson disease	Bradykinesia, rigidity, tremor
Dementia	Altered cognition
Sjögren syndrome	Dry mouth, dry eyes
Esophageal Dysphagia	
Structural disorders	
Dysphagia lusoria (vascular dysphagia)	Vascular extrinsic compression on the esophagus on imaging
Epiphrenic/traction diverticulum	Outpouching of the esophagus at any level on imaging
Esophageal strictures	Intermittent dysphagia, especially for solid food; history of reflux
Eosinophilic esophagitis	Food impactions, atopic history, rings or strictures on endoscopy
Esophageal webs or rings	Upper esophageal webs may be associated with iron deficiency anemia
Neoplasms	Rapidly progressive dysphagia for solids, then liquids; anorexia; weight loss
Motility disorders	
Achalasia	Concomitant liquid and solid dysphagia
Diffuse esophageal spasm	Chest pain
Systemic sclerosis	Tight skin, telangiectasias, sclerodactyly, gastroesophageal reflux disease, Raynaud phenomenon

from the mouth into the upper esophagus by swallowing. Symptoms commonly reported include choking, coughing, and nasal regurgitation of food. Patients are at risk for aspiration pneumonia. Other presenting symptoms include hoarseness (resulting from laryngeal nerve damage) and dysarthria (from weakness of the soft palate or pharyngeal constrictors), both representing an underlying neurologic disorder. A pharyngoesophageal (Zenker) diverticulum should be considered when undigested food is brought up several hours after a meal or if a patient reports hearing a gurgling noise in the chest.

The initial study for suspected oropharyngeal dysphagia is a modified barium swallow, with both a liquid and a solid phase to help identify the underlying cause. Management strategies include dietary changes and a swallowing exercise program implemented with a speech pathologist.

Esophageal Dysphagia

Patients with esophageal dysphagia are able to initiate the swallowing process, but often feel discomfort in the mid to lower sternum as the food bolus passes through the esophagus. Esophageal dysphagia is the result of one of two underlying causes: a mechanical obstruction or a motility disorder. Dysphagia occurring with solids alone suggests a mechanical obstruction, whereas dysphagia with either liquids alone or the combination of liquids and solids favors a motility disorder. Dysphagia that progresses from occurring with solids only to occurring with both solids and liquids suggests malignancy.

Achalasia often presents with nonacidic regurgitation of undigested food. Chest pain while taking liquids that are very hot or very cold may indicate esophageal spasm. Mechanical esophageal obstruction may be benign or malignant and may be caused by strictures, masses, esophageal ring (for example, a Schatzki ring [**Figure 1**]), or webs. Upper endoscopy allows for diagnostic (biopsy and inspection) and therapeutic intervention (dilation). Clinical management is based on the underlying cause.

Reflux and Chest Pain

The development of chest pain from an esophageal cause can mimic chest pain from cardiac disease. Reports of heartburn with history of Raynaud phenomenon could signify a systemic condition, such as scleroderma.

Once a cardiac cause is ruled out, the most common cause of chest pain is gastroesophageal reflux disease (GERD). Starting a course of an acid-reducing agent, such as an H$_2$ blocker or proton pump inhibitor (PPI), can be both diagnostic and therapeutic. Patients whose symptoms do not respond require further evaluation, including upper endoscopy and possibly ambulatory pH testing with or without esophageal manometry.

See Gastroesophageal Reflux Disease for information about diagnosis and management.

Odynophagia

A presentation of pain while swallowing defines odynophagia, which suggests active mucosal inflammation and

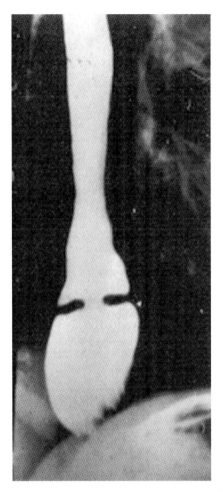

FIGURE 1. Barium esophagram showing a Schatzki ring, a subtype of esophageal ring located at the squamocolumnar junction and a common cause of dysphagia.

ulceration in the esophagus. Odynophagia is commonly associated with pill-induced damage, infection, or caustic ingestion, and is less commonly caused by GERD or esophageal cancer. Upper endoscopy with biopsies is the most appropriate diagnostic test to determine the degree of inflammation and underlying cause.

Globus Sensation

Patients commonly report globus sensation as a "lump in the throat" or "throat tightness," usually not linked to meals. Causes of globus include GERD (with or without heartburn), stress, and psychiatric conditions (anxiety, panic disorders, somatization). A diagnosis of globus should not be made if the patient reports other esophageal symptoms, such as dysphagia or odynophagia. Evaluation to determine the underlying cause should include evaluation for thyroid goiter and an underlying pharyngeal lesion, which can be diagnosed by transnasal endoscopy or barium swallow.

Treatment with acid suppression or cognitive behavioral therapy should be initiated once a structural cause has been ruled out.

KEY POINTS

- Oropharyngeal dysphagia occurs when the patient is unable to transfer the food bolus from the mouth into the upper esophagus by swallowing and should be evaluated with a modified barium swallow.

- Esophageal dysphagia occurring with solids alone suggests a mechanical obstruction, whereas dysphagia with either liquids alone or the combination of liquids and solids favors a motility disorder.

- Upper endoscopy is diagnostic and may be therapeutic for esophageal dysphagia.

- Chest pain is common in patients with gastroesophageal reflux disease, but a cardiac cause of chest pain must be ruled out first.

Nonmalignant Disorders of the Esophagus

Gastroesophageal Reflux Disease

GERD is characterized by food and acid refluxing from the stomach into the esophagus and throat. Its prevalence is 10% to 20% in the Western world, and there is a strong relationship between GERD and obesity. The most common symptoms reported are heartburn, regurgitation, and chest pain, for which a cardiac cause must be excluded. Reflux can be triggered by a number of factors (**Table 2**). Protective mechanisms to minimize the esophagus' exposure to acid consist of peristalsis, a competent lower esophageal sphincter (LES), and gastric emptying; reflux occurs when these physiologic protectors become ineffective. Uncontrolled GERD can negatively affect quality of life due to poor sleep, low productivity, and work absences. Longstanding GERD can lead to complications, including erosive esophagitis, stricture, Barrett esophagus, and

TABLE 2.	Factors Associated with Reflux
Category	**Factor**
Lifestyle	Cigarette smoking
	Obesity
Eating habits	Eating large meals
	Eating late at night
	Lying supine shortly after eating
Foods and beverages	Alcohol
	Chocolate
	Citrus fruits and juices
	Coffee
	Fatty and fried foods
	Onions
	Peppermint
Medications	Anticholinergic agents
	Aspirin and NSAIDs
	Calcium channel blockers
	Nitrates
	Progesterone
	Opioids (due to delayed gastric emptying)
Body position	Bending over, exercising (both result in increased intra-abdominal pressure)
Other	Pregnancy
	Tight-fitting clothing
	Hiatal hernia

esophageal cancer (**Figure 2**). Pregnant women may experience GERD during any trimester of pregnancy, but symptoms may worsen as the pregnancy progresses. Heartburn symptoms resolve after delivery.

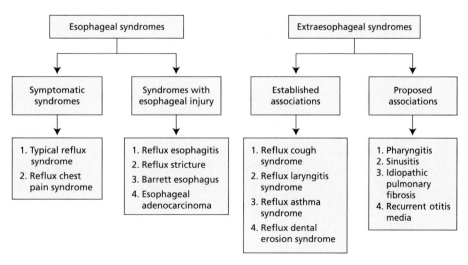

FIGURE 2. Classification of gastroesophageal reflux disease and its subsets.

Reprinted with permission from Vakil N, van Zanten SV, Kahrilas P, Dent J, Jones R; Global Consensus Group. The Montreal definition and classification of gastroesophageal reflux disease: a global evidence-based consensus. Am J Gastroenterol. 2006;101:1900-20; quiz 1943. [PMID: 16928254]. Copyright 2006, Springer Nature.

Diagnosis

Strategies for diagnosing GERD include use of clinical history, response to medical therapy, and testing, including endoscopy and ambulatory pH monitoring; there is no single gold-standard diagnostic test. Clinical symptoms of heartburn and regurgitation strongly suggest GERD. Patients with GERD symptoms, but without alarm features (such as dysphagia, unintentional weight loss, hematemesis, or melena) may undergo an empiric trial of a PPI. Symptom relief from medical therapy can confirm the diagnosis.

Upper endoscopy is warranted in patients reporting dysphagia to rule out an underlying ring, web, or malignancy, and in patients with suspected erosive esophagitis, stricture, or Barrett esophagus. Most patients with GERD have a normal upper endoscopy examination.

Ambulatory pH monitoring can assess the degree of acid exposure in the esophagus, especially in patients unresponsive to acid-reducing therapy. Impedance-pH testing can help differentiate between acid and nonacid reflux. Testing to detect active acid reflux can be done with a 24-hour transnasal catheter or a 48-hour wireless capsule, which patients generally tolerate better. Esophageal manometry has limited value in diagnosing GERD, but should be considered as part of the evaluation for antireflux surgery to rule out motility disorders such as achalasia.

Treatment

An algorithm outlining the management of GERD is presented in **Figure 3**.

Lifestyle Changes

Patients with recent weight gain or who are overweight should develop a weight-loss plan. Patients with nocturnal GERD should eat at least 2 to 3 hours before going to sleep and should consider raising the head of the bed.

Dietary modification should focus on eliminating foods that trigger an individual patient's GERD symptoms, rather than globally eliminating all common trigger foods (caffeine, chocolate, spicy foods, acidic foods such as citrus fruits, and fatty foods). Cessation of alcohol and tobacco use is universally supported.

Medical Therapy

Pharmacologic therapy includes antacids, H_2 blockers, and PPI therapy. A PPI once daily for 8 weeks is the therapy of choice for symptom relief, as well as for treatment of erosive esophagitis. PPI therapy is superior to H_2 blocker therapy for GERD with or without erosive esophagitis. The PPI should be taken once daily, 30 to 60 minutes before the first meal of the day. Patients with partial response to PPI therapy should increase the dosage to twice daily. Patients requiring long-term maintenance therapy should be placed on the lowest effective PPI dose, including on-demand or intermittent usage, and for patients with uncomplicated GERD, an attempt to stop or reduce chronic PPI therapy should be made once a year. Adverse effects of PPIs are shown in **Table 3**. Switching to a different PPI may be warranted for adverse reactions or for unresponsive symptoms. Initial studies suggested an interaction with clopidogrel; however, subsequent data suggest that

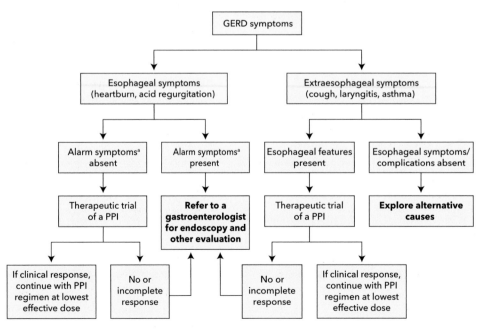

FIGURE 3. Management of gastroesophageal reflux disease.

GERD = gastroesophageal reflux disease; PPI = proton pump inhibitor.

^aAlarm symptoms include dysphagia, unintentional weight loss, hematemesis, and melena.

TABLE 3. Adverse Effects of Proton Pump Inhibitors

Common	Unusual	Proposed Associations
Headache	Vitamin B$_{12}$ deficiency	Kidney injury
Diarrhea	Hypomagnesemia	Dementia
Dyspepsia	Community-acquired pneumonia	
	Clostridium difficile infection	
	Hip fracture	

concurrent use does not increase risk for a cardiac event. PPIs are safe in pregnant patients.

Sucralfate has no role in the treatment of GERD. Prokinetic agents such as metoclopramide should not be used to treat GERD unless gastroparesis is present.

Antireflux Surgery
Surgical treatments for GERD are laparoscopic fundoplication or bariatric surgery for obese patients, as well as magnetic sphincter augmentation, a newer technique in which a magnetic ring is placed around the LES without surgical alteration of the stomach. Surgery is infrequently required; indications include failure of optimal therapy, wanting to stop medication, and intolerable medication side effects. Patients should undergo objective testing, such as impedance-pH monitoring, to confirm true acid reflux and correlation with symptoms before surgery. Surgery is most effective in patients with typical symptoms of heartburn and regurgitation that are responsive to therapy. However, about one third of patients require resumption of a PPI 5 to 10 years after surgery. Postoperative complications include dysphagia, diarrhea, and inability to belch from a tight fundoplication.

Endoscopic Therapy
Endoscopy-based therapies for GERD include thermal radiofrequency to augment the LES, silicone injection to the LES, and suturing of the LES. Early relief of reflux symptoms has been seen with these therapies, but long-term benefits have not been proven. None of these therapies has been associated with normalized esophageal pH levels. Newer approaches include transoral incisionless fundoplication, which is a full-thickness suture to create an endoscopic fundoplication, but there are no long-term data on its efficacy.

Extraesophageal Manifestations
Asthma, chronic cough, and laryngitis have been linked to GERD (see Figure 3). It is important to eliminate other non-GERD causes when these symptoms are present. Laryngoscopy often shows edema and erythema as signs of reflux-induced laryngitis. However, more than 80% of healthy persons also have these findings; therefore, laryngoscopy should not be used to diagnose GERD-related laryngitis. A PPI trial is recommended in patients who also have typical GERD symptoms. If a patient has atypical symptoms only, ambulatory esophageal pH monitoring should be considered before a PPI trial. Surgery is less effective in this group and should be considered only in patients whose symptoms respond to PPI therapy.

Refractory GERD
The first step in addressing refractory GERD is to optimize PPI therapy by emphasizing the importance of taking medication 30 to 60 minutes before eating, increasing the dosage to twice daily, or switching to another PPI. If symptoms are still unresponsive, alternative causes must be considered. For typical symptoms, use endoscopy to rule out eosinophilic esophagitis or erosive esophagitis. Esophageal impedance-pH testing may also be useful and should be performed while the patient is receiving optimized PPI therapy. For atypical symptoms, refer the patient to otorhinolaryngology, pulmonary, or allergy specialists to identify and treat the underlying cause. In these patients, medical therapy should be stopped before impedance-pH testing. A negative impedance-pH test likely means that the patient does not have GERD and PPI therapy should be discontinued. For patients with both types of symptoms, if further evaluation is unremarkable, impedance-pH testing should be performed.

Eosinophilic Esophagitis
Eosinophilic esophagitis (EE) is a condition commonly associated with dysphagia and food bolus obstruction. Most patients are diagnosed between the second and fifth decades of life, and EE is more commonly seen in men. Patients often have other atopic conditions such as asthma, rhinitis, dermatitis, and seasonal or food allergies. The reported prevalence is as high as 40 to 90 per 100,000 in the United States. The diagnostic criteria for EE are esophageal symptoms (dysphagia), esophageal biopsies showing 15 eosinophils/hpf or greater, persistent mucosal eosinophilia despite a trial of PPI therapy, and exclusion of other causes of eosinophilia. EE is a diagnosis made in the absence of peripheral eosinophilia.

Endoscopic findings include rings, longitudinal furrows, luminal narrowing, and white exudates and plaques. Patients with GERD may have elevated numbers of eosinophils in mucosal biopsies. Therefore, patients with prominent esophageal mucosal eosinophils should first undergo an 8-week trial of a PPI to rule out GERD. If there is no clinical improvement, repeat endoscopy with biopsy is recommended. If biopsies continue to show 15 eosinophils/hpf or greater, EE can be diagnosed and appropriate therapy initiated, with swallowed aerosolized topical glucocorticoids (fluticasone or budesonide). Diet modification has been suggested as a treatment option to prevent EE flares. An empiric elimination diet—removing the foods most commonly associated with food allergies, such as egg, soy, wheat, peanuts, cow's milk, and fish/shellfish—has been used. Endoscopic dilation should be considered in patients with continued dysphagia caused by esophageal stricture not responding to medical therapy.

Infectious Esophagitis

Infectious esophagitis can be caused by fungal, viral, bacterial (uncommon), and parasitic pathogens. Patients most commonly present with odynophagia or dysphagia. *Candida* esophagitis most commonly causes dysphagia, while viral esophagitis produces odynophagia. Other organisms associated with esophagitis include *Lactobacillus*, B-hemolytic streptococci, *Cryptosporidium*, *Pneumocystis jirovecii*, *Mycobacterium avium* complex, and *Mycobacterium tuberculosis*.

Candida infection can occur in immunocompetent or immunocompromised hosts. Diagnosis is usually made clinically based on the presence of compatible symptoms and oral candidiasis. Endoscopy and biopsy can be considered for patients who do not respond to empiric therapy or have atypical symptoms. Endoscopy shows small, white, raised plaques, and esophageal brushings confirm the diagnosis (**Figure 4**). The most common species is *Candida albicans*, treated with oral fluconazole.

Herpes simplex virus and cytomegalovirus are seen in immunodeficient or immunosuppressed individuals, but rarely in immunocompetent patients. Endoscopy with biopsy is needed to confirm the diagnosis. Herpes simplex virus infection is treated with acyclovir, and cytomegalovirus infection with ganciclovir.

Pill-Induced Esophagitis

Medications can cause esophageal injury resulting in esophagitis. Risk factors associated with pill-induced esophagitis include decreased salivary output, esophageal dysmotility, large pills, medications that increase the LES tone (opioids), and ingestion of medications in the supine position. Patients commonly report chest pain, dysphagia, and odynophagia occurring several hours to days after taking medication. Pill-induced esophagitis has been observed with alendronate, quinidine, tetracycline, doxycycline, potassium chloride, ferrous sulfate, and mexiletine. Medications associated with stricture formation include alendronate, ferrous sulfate, NSAIDs, and potassium chloride. Preventive strategies include drinking sufficient water with medication and remaining in an upright position for 30 minutes after pill ingestion.

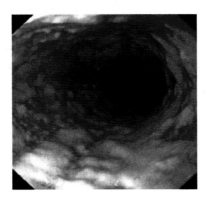

FIGURE 4. Upper endoscopy showing white adherent plaques suggestive of *Candida* esophagitis.

Esophageal Motility Disorders

The esophagus is a muscle that passes a food bolus from the hypopharynx to the stomach through peristalsis. The upper third of the esophagus is composed of skeletal muscle innervated by axons of lower motoneurons. The lower two thirds is smooth muscle innervated by the vagus nerve. The upper and lower esophageal sphincters relax during swallowing.

Additional peristaltic activity occurs when the esophagus is distended. High-resolution esophageal manometry is used to evaluate suspected esophageal motility disorders.

GERD is the most common cause of noncardiac chest pain. However, hypercontractile disorders of the esophagus should also be considered in patients with noncardiac chest pain. Esophageal manometry is used to differentiate these disorders.

Hypertonic Motility Disorders

Hypertonic motility disorders are characterized by dysphagia with both liquids and solids. Other symptoms can include regurgitation of undigested food, in particular when in a recumbent position. Treatment of hypertonic disorders of the esophagus is aimed at relieving symptoms.

Achalasia and Pseudoachalasia

Achalasia is a hypertonic motility condition defined by inadequate relaxation of the LES and aperistalsis. Achalasia can be idiopathic or associated with viral, autoimmune, and neurodegenerative disorders and infection (Chagas disease). Damage to the ganglion cells and myenteric plexus in the esophageal body and LES leads to uncontested cholinergic nerve activation, which prevents LES relaxation. Achalasia affects men and women equally, with an annual incidence of 1 in 100,000 individuals. It commonly occurs between 30 and 60 years of age. Patients present with dysphagia occurring with both solids and liquids along with nonacidic regurgitation of undigested food. Additional symptoms include heartburn, weight loss, and chest pain unresponsive to acid-reducing agents. Extrinsic compression from surgical procedures, such as fundoplication or bariatric surgery (gastric band), can also cause secondary achalasia. Barium esophagography is the initial diagnostic test, which shows dilation of the esophagus with narrowing at the gastroesophageal junction (GEJ), known as a "bird's beak" (**Figure 5**). Upper endoscopy reveals retained food and saliva, no signs of mechanical obstruction or mass, and "tightness" at the GEJ while advancing the scope into the stomach. Esophageal manometry showing incomplete LES relaxation and aperistalsis confirms the diagnosis of achalasia.

Pseudoachalasia is a result of malignant tumor infiltration or other secondary causes, and can present similarly to achalasia causing myenteric plexus damage. Unlike achalasia, this condition has been associated with sudden weight loss later in life, usually after age 50 years. Suspected pseudoachalasia should be evaluated with CT or endoscopic ultrasound.

Approaches to treatment of achalasia include endoscopic or surgical intervention with the goal of lowering LES

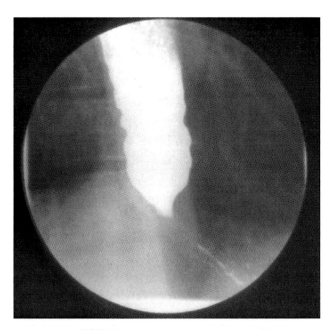

FIGURE 5. Barium esophagram showing the typical appearance of a dilated esophagus and "bird's beak" narrowing at the gastroesophageal junction in a patient with achalasia.

pressure, which relieves symptoms. Medical therapy is uncommonly used.

Endoscopic therapy involves injection of botulinum toxin, pneumatic dilation, or peroral endoscopic myotomy. Botulinum toxin injection into the LES inhibits acetylcholine release, causing LES relaxation. However, after 1 year, only 40% of patients have continued relief of symptoms. Botulinum toxin injection can be repeated, but successive treatments are often less effective for symptom management. Pneumatic dilation is an effective nonsurgical therapy. Dilators ranging from 30 mm to 40 mm in size are used to disrupt the circular muscle. Clinical symptom improvement ranges from 50% to 90%, and the most common complication is perforation. Peroral endoscopic myotomy is a newer endoscopic procedure in which the physician creates an esophageal submucosal tunnel extending to the level of the LES and then performs a myotomy. Studies have shown resolution of symptoms in over 80% of patients. Surgical treatment consists of laparoscopic myotomy of the circular muscle fibers. Fundoplication is also recommended to avoid reflux symptoms after myotomy. Determining whether a patient should receive endoscopic or surgical therapy often depends on local expertise.

Medical therapy is reserved for patients who are poor candidates for endoscopic or surgical therapy. LES pressure can be reduced with medical therapy, including calcium channel blockers (nifedipine) or long-acting nitrates.

Patients with achalasia for more than 10 years have increased risk for squamous cell carcinoma and may benefit from surveillance endoscopy, but there are no established guidelines for frequency of surveillance.

Diffuse Esophageal Spasm and Nutcracker Esophagus

Diffuse esophageal spasm is a hypercontractile state presenting with chest pain or dysphagia. Symptoms often respond to nitroglycerin, suggesting a flaw in esophageal nitric-oxide production. The esophagus has a "corkscrew" (**Figure 6**) or "rosary bead" appearance on esophagography. Esophageal manometry shows simultaneous high-amplitude (>30 mm Hg) esophageal contractions with intermittent aperistaltic contractions. Medical therapy with antidepressants (trazadone and imipramine) or a phosphodiesterase inhibitor (sildenafil) can relieve chest pain. Dysphagia may respond to calcium channel blockers. Botulinum toxin injection has been reported to alleviate dysphagia symptoms.

"Nutcracker" or "jackhammer" esophagus is found in patients with high-amplitude peristaltic contractions of greater than 220 mm Hg.

Hypotonic Motility Disorders

Hypotonic disorders of the esophagus are marked by lack of contractility and incomplete peristalsis. Patients may report symptoms of GERD, which result from decreased LES pressure or dysphagia from incomplete peristalsis. In most cases, the cause of hypotonic esophageal disease is unknown. However, secondary causes include smooth-muscle relaxants, anticholinergic agents, estrogen, progesterone, connective tissue disorders (scleroderma), and pregnancy. Esophageal manometry shows hypotonic, weak nonperistaltic contractions in the distal esophagus. Findings can mimic achalasia.

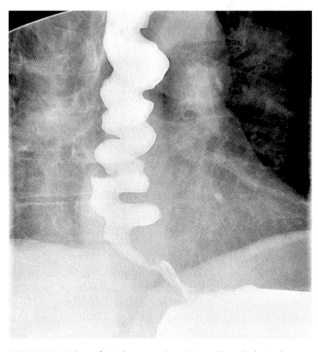

FIGURE 6. Findings of a "corkscrew esophagus" (caused by multiple simultaneous contractions) on esophagography are typical of diffuse esophageal spasm.

Treatment includes lifestyle changes, such as eating upright and eating liquid or semisolid rather than solid food. Medical therapy includes acid-reducing agents for GERD and low-dose antidepressants to reduce chest discomfort. Prokinetic agents, such as metoclopramide, are not recommended for treatment.

KEY POINTS

HVC
- In patients with symptoms of gastroesophageal reflux disease but without alarm features, an empiric trial of a proton pump inhibitor can relieve symptoms and confirm the diagnosis.

- Most patients with gastroesophageal reflux disease do not require surgery; indications include failure of optimal proton pump inhibitor therapy, wanting to stop medication, and intolerable medication side effects.

- The diagnostic criteria for eosinophilic esophagitis are esophageal symptoms (most commonly dysphagia), esophageal biopsies showing persistent counts of 15 eosinophils/hpf or greater despite a trial of proton pump inhibitor therapy, and exclusion of other causes of eosinophilia.

- Odynophagia and dysphagia are the most common presenting symptoms of infectious esophagitis.

- To prevent pill-induced esophagitis, patients should drink water with medication and remain upright for at least 30 minutes after ingestion.

Metaplastic and Neoplastic Disorders of the Esophagus

Barrett Esophagus

Epidemiology and Screening

Barrett esophagus is defined as the extension of the metaplastic columnar epithelium above the GEJ into the esophagus. Barrett esophagus is a consequence of GERD, even in patients who experience no clinical symptoms, and is classified as a premalignant condition because it has the potential to progress to esophageal cancer. Risk factors associated with Barrett esophagus include chronic GERD (for more than 5 years), age older than 50 years, male sex, white race, tobacco use, and obesity. Drinking alcohol is not associated with increased risk for Barrett esophagus, and wine consumption might be protective.

Risk factors associated with Barrett esophagus progression to dysplasia or esophageal cancer include older age, long Barrett esophagus length, obesity, and tobacco use. Some studies have suggested that the use of PPIs, NSAIDs, and statins may be protective; however, this has not been established, and the use of these agents for prevention of progression to dysplasia is not recommended. The annual cancer risk associated with Barrett esophagus without dysplasia is 0.2% to 0.5% per year. For Barrett esophagus with low-grade dysplasia, annual risk for cancer is 0.7% per year, and for Barrett esophagus with high-grade dysplasia, 7% per year.

About 10% of patients with GERD are found to have Barrett esophagus on endoscopy. Studies have suggested individuals with multiple risk factors for esophageal carcinoma and chronic GERD might benefit from screening. Men older than age 50 years with GERD symptoms for more than 5 years and additional risk factors (nocturnal reflux symptoms, hiatal hernia, elevated BMI, intra-abdominal distribution of body fat, tobacco use) may benefit from screening endoscopy. Women do not require routine endoscopic screening for Barrett esophagus. Evidence does not support routine screening for Barrett esophagus based on GERD symptoms for the general population.

Diagnosis and Management

The diagnosis of Barrett esophagus is established based on endoscopic findings (**Figure 7**) with biopsy, which are then confirmed by pathology showing specialized intestinal metaplasia with acid-mucin-containing goblet cells. Endoscopy measurements have categorized Barrett esophagus into short-segment (≤3 cm) or long-segment (>3 cm). The Prague classification more accurately assesses a segment of Barrett esophagus using the degree of circumferential disease (C followed by a number indicating the length in cm) along with maximal Barrett esophagus segment length (M followed by a number indicating the length in cm). For example, a patient with Barrett esophagus extending circumferentially for 2 cm above the squamocolumnar junction but with tongues of Barrett

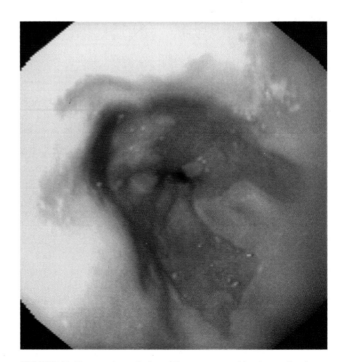

FIGURE 7. Upper endoscopic view of Barrett mucosa, with salmon-colored mucosa representing Barrett mucosa compared with the normal pearl-colored squamous mucosa.

esophagus extending 5 cm above the squamocolumnar junction would have a Prague classification of C2M5.

Barrett esophagus progresses along a pathway from intestinal metaplasia, to indefinite for dysplasia, to low-grade dysplasia, to high-grade dysplasia, to invasive adenocarcinoma. Surveillance and treatment recommendations are based on grade of Barrett esophagus and the presence of dysplasia (Table 4).

Chemoprevention is recommended in the form of PPI therapy, but dosing should be based on symptom control and healing of erosive esophagitis. Initial dosing is once daily. There is no strong evidence that antireflux surgery can prevent the progression of Barrett esophagus to adenocarcinoma when compared to medical therapy with PPIs. NSAIDs and aspirin should not be prescribed as an antineoplastic strategy.

Patients with a diagnosis of Barrett esophagus indefinite for dysplasia should start or optimize PPI therapy, followed by repeat upper endoscopy. Treatment to remove Barrett esophagus is recommended for patients with high-grade dysplasia and confirmed low-grade dysplasia. Endoscopy-based therapies include radiofrequency ablation and endoscopic mucosal resection, possibly used in combination. Endoscopic therapies have had similar outcomes to surgery (esophagectomy) in patients with high-grade dysplasia, but local expertise and patient preference will determine the best course of therapy. The Prague classification is useful to more accurately assess response to endoscopic therapy.

Esophageal Carcinoma

Epidemiology

The incidence of esophageal cancer varies widely between regions of the world; high-prevalence areas include Asia and southern and eastern Africa. Worldwide, squamous cell carcinoma comprises about 90% of all esophageal cancers, but incidence has been decreasing in Western countries as the incidence of adenocarcinoma is rising. Esophageal cancer occurs in the fifth to seventh decade of life and is three to four times more common in men. In the United States, about 16,000 new cases are reported annually, with 15,000 deaths occurring within the same year. The overall 5-year survival rate ranges from 15% to 25%, depending on the stage of the cancer at the time of initial presentation. The rate has remained relatively unchanged since 2000.

Risk Factors

Risk factors for the development of adenocarcinoma include GERD, Barrett esophagus, obesity, tobacco use, past thoracic radiation, a diet low in fruits and vegetables, older age, male sex, and the use of medications that relax the LES. Risk factors for squamous cell carcinoma include tobacco and alcohol use, caustic injury, achalasia, past thoracic radiation, nutritional deficiencies (zinc, selenium), poor socioeconomic status, poor oral hygiene, nonepidermolytic palmoplantar keratoderma (an autosomal dominant disorder associated with yellow, wax-like hyperkeratosis on the palms and soles, also known as tylosis), human papillomavirus infection, and nitrosamine exposure.

Diagnosis and Staging

The most common initial presentation of esophageal carcinoma is dysphagia with solid foods, but asymptomatic individuals have been diagnosed based on surveillance endoscopy. Other symptoms include weight loss, anorexia, anemia (secondary to gastrointestinal bleeding), and chest pain. Upper endoscopy with biopsy is the preferred diagnostic test.

Squamous cell carcinoma is most commonly located in the proximal esophagus, and adenocarcinoma is usually found in the distal esophagus.

TNM staging is often done with endoscopic ultrasound for locoregional disease and with CT and PET to identify metastatic disease. For treatment of esophageal carcinoma, see MKSAP 18 Hematology and Oncology.

> **KEY POINTS**
> - Barrett esophagus is a premalignant condition caused by longstanding gastroesophageal reflux disease.
> - Women with gastroesophageal reflux disease do not require routine screening for Barrett esophagus.
> - Patients with Barrett esophagus should receive proton pump inhibitor therapy with dosing based on symptom relief and healing of erosive esophagitis.
> - Dysphagia with solid foods is the most common presenting symptom of esophageal cancer.

HVC

TABLE 4. Practice Guidelines for Endoscopic Surveillance of Barrett Esophagus

Dysplasia Grade	Recommendation
None	If no dysplasia is present, repeat upper endoscopy every 3 to 5 years
Indefinite	Start or adjust proton pump inhibitor therapy, then repeat endoscopy in 3 to 6 months
	If still present, then repeat endoscopy in 1 year
Low-grade	Confirmation by expert pathologist, then proceed to endoscopic eradication therapy (surveillance endoscopy in 12 months is an alternative)
High-grade	Confirmation by expert pathologist
	Endoscopic eradication therapy is preferred

Adapted with permission from Shaheen NJ, Falk GW, Iyer PG, Gerson LB; American College of Gastroenterology. ACG clinical guideline: diagnosis and management of Barrett's esophagus. Am J Gastroenterol. 2016;111:30-50; quiz 51. [PMID: 26526079] doi:10.1038/ajg.2015.322.

Disorders of the Stomach and Duodenum

Dyspepsia

Clinical Features

Dyspepsia is a term used to describe epigastric pain. Associated symptoms can include early satiety, epigastric burning, nausea, and postprandial symptoms, including pain, bloating, or belching. Coexistent heartburn may be present, but it is not a primary symptom of dyspepsia. Recurrent or bothersome vomiting should raise concern for other conditions.

The list of possible organic causes of dyspepsia is extensive (**Table 5**); the most common conditions are peptic ulcer disease and gastroesophageal reflux disease (20% of patients with erosive esophagitis present with dyspepsia). If no organic cause of dyspepsia symptoms is identified after testing, the term *functional dyspepsia* applies.

Functional dyspepsia represents a heterogeneous group of functional gastrointestinal disorders predominated by one or more upper gastrointestinal symptoms. Diagnostic criteria from the fourth Rome working group for functional gastrointestinal disorders are shown in **Table 6**. Functional dyspepsia can be further categorized into postprandial distress syndrome if the patient's predominant symptoms are meal-induced (**Table 7**), or epigastric pain syndrome if the predominant symptoms of epigastric pain or burning are unrelated to meals (**Table 8**).

Evaluation and Management

The approach to testing for dyspepsia should be based on patient age, severity of symptoms, and risk for gastric cancer. Upper endoscopy is commonly ordered to exclude upper gastrointestinal neoplasia; however, it is invasive and costly. Given the low incidence of malignancy and consideration for cost effectiveness in the evaluation of dyspepsia in younger adults, the American College of Gastroenterology (ACG) and the Canadian Association of Gastroenterology (CAG) have jointly recommended routine use of upper endoscopy only in patients aged 60 years and older to exclude malignancy. The ACG/CAG guidelines recommend against the routine use of upper endoscopy in patients younger than age 60 years, even in the presence of alarm features including weight loss, anemia, dysphagia,

TABLE 5.	Organic Causes of Dyspepsia
Gastroesophageal	Gastroesophageal reflux disease, peptic ulcer disease, *Helicobacter pylori* gastritis, gastric cancer/lymphoma, gastric amyloidosis, Ménétrier disease, gastroparesis
Small bowel	Celiac disease, Crohn disease
Pancreatic	Pancreatitis, pancreatic cancer
Infectious	*Giardia lamblia, Strongyloides stercoralis*, tuberculosis, syphilis
Common medications	NSAIDs, aspirin, iron, antibiotics (erythromycin, ampicillin), narcotics, estrogens and oral contraceptives, theophylline, levodopa, digitalis
Other systemic conditions	Coronary artery disease, kidney disease, thyroid dysfunction, adrenal insufficiency, hyperparathyroidism, pregnancy

TABLE 6.	Rome 4 Diagnostic Criteria for Functional Dyspepsia

One or more of the following:[a]

    Bothersome postprandial fullness

    Bothersome early satiation

    Bothersome epigastric pain

    Bothersome epigastric burning

No evidence of structural disease (including upper endoscopy) that is likely to explain the symptoms

[a]Criteria fulfilled for the last 3 months with symptom onset at least 6 months before diagnosis.

Reprinted with permission from Stanghellini V, Chan FK, Hasler WL, Malagelada JR, Suzuki H, Tack J, et al. Gastroduodenal disorders. Gastroenterology. 2016;150:1380-92. [PMID: 27147122] doi:10.1053/j.gastro.2016.02.011. Copyright 2016, The AGA Institute.

TABLE 7.	Rome 4 Diagnostic Criteria for Postprandial Distress Syndrome	
Criteria[a]	**Supportive Remarks**	
Must include one or both of the following at least 3 days per week:	Postprandial epigastric pain or burning, epigastric bloating, excessive belching, and nausea can also be present	
Bothersome postprandial fullness (i.e., severe enough to affect usual activities)	Vomiting warrants consideration of another disorder	
Bothersome early satiation (i.e., severe enough to prevent finishing a regular-sized meal)	Heartburn is not a dyspeptic symptom but may often coexist	
	Symptoms that are relieved by evacuation of feces or gas should generally not be considered as part of dyspepsia	
No evidence of organic, systemic, or metabolic disease that is likely to explain the symptoms on routine investigations (including upper endoscopy)	Other individual digestive symptoms or groups of symptoms, such as from gastroesophageal reflux disease and irritable bowel syndrome, may coexist	

[a]Criteria fulfilled for the last 3 months with symptom onset at least 6 months before diagnosis.

Reprinted with permission from Stanghellini V, Chan FK, Hasler WL, Malagelada JR, Suzuki H, Tack J, et al. Gastroduodenal disorders. Gastroenterology. 2016;150:1380-92. [PMID: 27147122] doi:10.1053/j.gastro.2016.02.011. Copyright 2016, The AGA Institute.

TABLE 8.	Rome 4 Diagnostic Criteria for Epigastric Pain Syndrome
Criteria[a]	**Supportive Remarks**
Must include the following symptoms at least 1 day per week:	Pain may be induced by ingestion of a meal, relieved by ingestion of a meal, or may occur while fasting
Bothersome epigastric pain and/or burning (i.e., severe enough to affect usual activities)	Postprandial epigastric bloating, belching, and nausea can also be present
	Persistent vomiting suggests another disorder
No evidence of organic, systemic, or metabolic disease that is likely to explain the symptoms on routine investigations (including upper endoscopy)	Heartburn is not a dyspeptic symptom but may often coexist
	The pain does not fulfill biliary pain criteria
	Symptoms that are relieved by evacuation of feces or gas should generally not be considered as part of dyspepsia
	Other individual digestive symptoms or groups of symptoms, such as from gastroesophageal reflux disease and irritable bowel syndrome, may coexist

[a]Criteria fulfilled for the last 3 months with symptom onset at least 6 months before diagnosis.

Reprinted with permission from Stanghellini V, Chan FK, Hasler WL, Malagelada JR, Suzuki H, Tack J, et al. Gastroduodenal disorders. Gastroenterology. 2016;150:1380-92. [PMID: 27147122] doi:10.1053/j.gastro.2016.02.011. Copyright 2016, The AGA Institute.

persistent vomiting, a family history of gastric cancer, immigration from a region with increased risk for gastric cancer (Asia, Russia, and South America), and severe symptoms, because these features are poor predictors of organic pathology, such as malignancy, peptic ulcer disease, or esophagitis. The ACG/CAG guidelines also state that upper endoscopy can be considered regardless of age in patients with a combination of alarm features.

For patients younger than age 60 years with dyspepsia symptoms, the ACG/CAG guidelines recommend noninvasive testing for *Helicobacter pylori*. Other testing, such as routine laboratory testing, screening for celiac disease, abdominal imaging, or gastric emptying, should be considered on an individual basis.

Management of dyspepsia is directed at treatment of the underlying cause. Patients who test positive for *H. pylori* should receive eradication therapy. If *H. pylori* testing is negative or *H. pylori* eradication fails to relieve the dyspepsia, an empiric trial of a proton pump inhibitor (PPI) should be pursued for 4 weeks. Patients whose symptoms are not alleviated with PPI therapy should undergo further evaluation with an upper endoscopy. Patients diagnosed with functional dyspepsia after the exclusion of organic disease can be treated with a variety of interventions (**Figure 8**).

KEY POINTS

HVC • For patients with dyspepsia, routine upper endoscopy to exclude malignancy is reserved for patients older than age 60 years.

• Upper endoscopy should be considered for patients with alarm features such as a family history of gastric cancer, immigration from a region with increased risk for gastric cancer, or severe symptoms, regardless of age.

HVC • Patients younger than age 60 years with dyspepsia symptoms should be tested and treated for *Helicobacter pylori* infection.

Peptic Ulcer Disease

Clinical Features, Diagnosis, and Complications

The most frequently reported symptom of peptic ulcer disease (PUD) is epigastric pain, frequently described as worse during fasting and improved with eating or use of antacid or antisecretory therapy. Pain may be accompanied by other dyspeptic symptoms, such as early satiety, abdominal bloating, nausea, belching, or heartburn (from coexistent esophagitis). Epigastric pain may be minimal or absent in the elderly, immunosuppressed patients, and chronic NSAID users.

NSAIDs and *H. pylori* infection are the two most common causes of PUD, although idiopathic (NSAID-negative, *H. pylori*-negative) PUD is becoming more common in the United States. The causes of idiopathic PUD remain unclear; however, cocaine, methamphetamine, bisphosphonates, selective serotonin reuptake inhibitors, smoking, excessive alcohol consumption, and stress have been implicated. Rare causes of PUD include gastrinoma (Zollinger-Ellison syndrome), systemic mastocytosis, α_1-antitrypsin deficiency, COPD, chronic kidney disease, gastric cancer, gastric lymphoma, Crohn disease, eosinophilic gastroenteritis, or cytomegalovirus (in immunocompromised patients).

The diagnosis of PUD is most often made by upper endoscopy. Abdominal CT is the diagnostic study of choice for suspected perforating PUD, with a sensitivity of 98%.

Complications of PUD include bleeding, perforation, and obstruction. PUD is the most common cause of upper gastrointestinal bleeding. Overt bleeding presents with melena, hematemesis, and/or hematochezia, whereas obscure bleeding presents with iron deficiency anemia and/or stool positive for occult blood. Perforation is likely to present with sudden, severe epigastric pain that can become more generalized, along with peritoneal findings. Symptoms associated with obstruction may include vomiting, early satiety, abdominal distension, and weight loss.

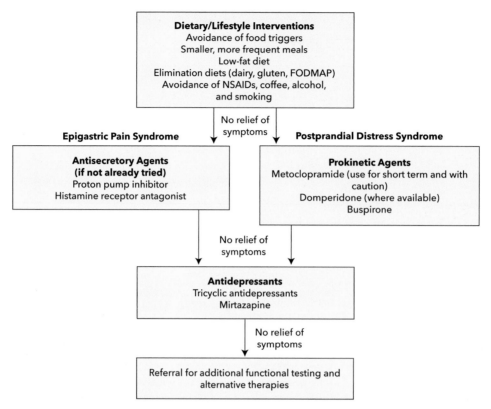

FIGURE 8. Treatment of functional dyspepsia.

FODMAP = Fermentable Oligosaccharides, Disaccharides, Monosaccharides, And Polyols.

Management

Following confirmation of uncomplicated PUD by upper endoscopy, *H. pylori* infection should be treated if identified and eradication confirmed after treatment. If *H. pylori* testing is negative, a once-daily PPI should be initiated and any agent causing PUD (such as an NSAID) should be discontinued.

In patients with bleeding PUD, risk factors that increase the risk for recurrent bleeding and death include tachycardia, hypotension, age older than 60 years, hemoglobin level less than 7 g/dL (70 g/L) (8 g/dL [80 g/L] in patients with cardiovascular disease), and comorbid illness. Interventions to address the modifiable risks should be pursued before upper endoscopy.

Upper endoscopy should be performed within 24 hours. The use of PPIs before upper endoscopy reduces the need for endoscopic therapy only in patients with high-risk ulcer findings. An intravenous dose of erythromycin 30 minutes before upper endoscopy reduces the need for repeat endoscopy by improving gastroduodenal visualization. Nasogastric tube placement is not required before upper endoscopy.

In patients with bleeding PUD related to low-dose aspirin use for secondary cardiovascular prevention, aspirin should be restarted 1 to 7 days after cessation of bleeding. PPI therapy can be discontinued after confirmation of *H. pylori* eradication in patients with *H. pylori*–associated bleeding PUD. NSAIDs should be discontinued in patients with NSAID-induced bleeding PUD. If there is no effective alternative to NSAIDs, a selective cyclooxygenase-2 inhibitor plus a once-daily PPI should be used. Patients with idiopathic ulcers that have bled should receive once-daily PPI therapy indefinitely because of the significant risk for rebleeding.

Repeat upper endoscopy is not performed routinely. Reasons for a follow-up upper endoscopy may include persistent symptoms after 8 to 12 weeks of therapy, ulcers of unknown cause, and if gastric ulcer biopsy was not performed during the initial upper endoscopy.

Perforated PUD is a surgical emergency with a mortality rate of up to 30%; older age, comorbidity, and delayed surgery confer increased risk. Prompt identification, urgent surgical intervention, and proper pre- and postoperative management of sepsis are essential. Postoperative upper endoscopy to rule out gastric cancer should be considered for patients with perforating gastric ulcers.

Gastric outlet obstruction resulting from inflammation or scarring at the pylorus or proximal duodenum should be biopsied at the time of diagnosis to exclude malignancy. For mild symptoms, PPI therapy, treatment of *H. pylori* infection if identified, and/or cessation of NSAIDs may be effective. For severe or persistent symptoms, endoscopic dilation should be pursued, reserving surgery for obstruction that persists after more than two attempts at endoscopic dilation.

KEY POINTS

- NSAIDs and *Helicobacter pylori* infection are the two most common causes of peptic ulcer disease.

- Upper endoscopy is the diagnostic test of choice for peptic ulcer disease.

- Repeat upper endoscopy is reserved for patients with persistent symptoms after 8 to 12 weeks of therapy, ulcers of unknown cause, or if gastric ulcer biopsy was not performed during the initial upper endoscopy.

Helicobacter pylori Infection

Indications for *Helicobacter pylori* Testing

Indications for *H. pylori* testing include active PUD, history of PUD without documented cure of *H. pylori* infection, gastric mucosa-associated lymphoid tissue lymphoma, or history of endoscopic resection of early gastric cancer. Other conditions in which *H. pylori* testing should be considered include dyspepsia in patients younger than age 60 years without alarm features warranting early upper endoscopy, before long-term low-dose aspirin or NSAID use, unexplained iron deficiency anemia, and idiopathic thrombocytopenic purpura in adult patients with gastrointestinal symptoms. Routine testing for *H. pylori* is not indicated in patients with typical gastroesophageal reflux disease symptoms, lymphocytic gastritis, hyperplastic gastric polyps, or hyperemesis gravidarum, or in asymptomatic individuals with a family history of gastric cancer.

Diagnosis

The diagnosis of *H. pylori* infection can be made with gastric biopsies during upper endoscopy, or noninvasively using ^{13}C-urea breath, stool antigen, or serologic testing. The ^{13}C-urea breath and the monoclonal stool antigen are the preferred noninvasive tests because both have sensitivity and specificity greater than 95% for evidence of active infection. Serologic testing for IgG antibodies against *H. pylori* is the cheapest and most convenient method; however, it has the significant disadvantage of being unable to distinguish between active and previous infection. Although the negative predictive value of serologic testing is reasonably high, a positive serologic result in a population with low prevalence of *H. pylori* infection, such as in the United States, requires confirmation with the ^{13}C-urea breath test, stool antigen test, or gastric biopsy. Also, conditions that lower the *H. pylori* density, such as PPI use, recent antibiotic use, atrophic gastritis, intestinal metaplasia, or mucosa-associated lymphoid tissue lymphoma, can result in false-negative results for any of the noninvasive studies. Serologic testing is most useful as an adjunct test in patients with bleeding PUD because of the decreased sensitivity of biopsy in the setting of acute bleeding. Any upper endoscopy for the evaluation of dyspepsia, or with the finding of gastric erosions or ulcers, should include gastric biopsies for *H. pylori* testing by histology or a rapid urea test.

Treatment

Any patient with a test result that is positive for active infection requires treatment with the goal of *H. pylori* eradication. The first course of treatment offers the best chance of eradication and should be carefully chosen. Several first-line treatments are available, with the choice based on resistance patterns of *H. pylori*, previous antibiotic use by the patient, and antibiotic allergies (**Table 9**). In most cases, duration of therapy is 14 days. Second-line therapy in the event of treatment failure should be for a minimum of 14 days, ideally using antibiotics different from those used for initial treatment (**Table 10**).

Eradication Testing

Testing for eradication of *H. pylori* should be done after completion of eradication therapy, using a ^{13}C-urea breath test, fecal antigen test, or biopsies obtained during upper endoscopy at least 4 weeks after completion of eradication therapy. Serologic testing is not used to confirm *H. pylori* eradication because it can remain positive in the absence of active infection.

KEY POINTS

- Patients with active peptic ulcer disease, history of peptic ulcer disease without documented cure of *Helicobacter pylori* infection, gastric mucosa-associated lymphoid tissue lymphoma, or history of endoscopic resection of early gastric cancer must be tested for *H. pylori* and treated if positive.

- Gastric biopsies during upper endoscopy or noninvasive testing methods, including ^{13}C-urea breath and stool antigen testing, can confirm the presence of *H. pylori* infection; negative serologic testing can exclude infection, but a positive serologic result requires confirmation.

- Treatment regimens for *H. pylori* consist of a minimum of three agents, including two antimicrobial agents and one antisecretory agent; treatment duration is 14 days in most cases.

- Testing for eradication of *H. pylori* is performed using a ^{13}C-urea breath test, fecal antigen test, or biopsies obtained during upper endoscopy at least 4 weeks after completion of eradication therapy.

Miscellaneous Gastropathy

Atrophic Gastritis

Chronic atrophic gastritis can present as either an environmental metaplastic atrophic gastritis (EMAG), also called multifocal atrophic gastritis, or an autoimmune atrophic gastritis (AMAG). EMAG is the result of *H. pylori* infection, and typically improves after *H. pylori* eradication. AMAG is caused by autoantibody formation to parietal cell antigens, and is

TABLE 9. First-Line Treatment Options for *Helicobacter pylori* Infection

Treatment Regimen	Duration of Therapy	Clinical Indicators
PPI, standard[a] or double dose twice daily (esomeprazole, once daily only) Clarithromycin, 500 mg twice daily Amoxicillin, 1 g twice daily	14 days	*H. pylori* clarithromycin resistance is known to be <15% No previous history of macrolide exposure for any reason
PPI, standard or double dose twice daily Clarithromycin, 500 mg twice daily Metronidazole, 500 mg three times daily	14 days	*H. pylori* clarithromycin resistance is known to be <15% No previous history of macrolide exposure for any reason Penicillin allergy
PPI, standard dose twice daily Bismuth subcitrate, 120-300 mg or subsalicylate, 300 mg four times daily Tetracycline, 500 mg three times daily Metronidazole, 250 mg four times daily or 500 mg three times daily	10-14 days	Previous macrolide exposure Penicillin allergy
PPI, standard dose twice daily Clarithromycin, 500 mg twice daily Amoxicillin, 1 g twice daily Nitroimidazole, 500 mg twice daily	10-14 days	May be an alternative to standard clarithromycin triple therapy Not validated in North America
PPI, standard dose twice daily Levofloxacin, 500 mg twice daily Amoxicillin, 1 g twice daily	10-14 days	May be an alternative to standard clarithromycin triple therapy Not validated in North America

PPI = proton pump inhibitor.

[a]Standard dose PPIs: esomeprazole, 40 mg; lansoprazole, 30 mg; omeprazole, 20 mg; pantoprazole, 40 mg; rabeprazole, 20 mg.

Adapted with permission from Chey WD, Leontiadis GI, Howden CW, Moss SF. ACG clinical guideline: treatment of *Helicobacter pylori* infection. Am J Gastroenterol. 2017;112:212-239. [PMID: 28071659] doi:10.1038/ajg.2016.563.

TABLE 10. Second-Line Treatment for *Helicobacter pylori* Infection after Failure of Initial Treatment

Treatment Regimen	Duration of Therapy	Clinical Indicators
PPI, standard dose twice daily Bismuth subcitrate, 120-300 mg, or subsalicylate, 300 mg four times daily Tetracycline, 500 mg three times daily Metronidazole, 250 mg four times daily, or 500 mg three times daily	14 days	Failure of clarithromycin-based or levofloxacin-based therapy
PPI, standard dose twice daily Levofloxacin, 500 mg twice daily Amoxicillin, 1 g twice daily	14 days	Failure of bismuth-based or clarithromycin-based therapy
PPI, standard or double dose twice daily Clarithromycin, 500 mg twice daily Amoxicillin, 1 g twice daily	14 days	Failure of bismuth-based therapy
PPI, standard or double dose twice daily Clarithromycin, 500 mg twice daily Metronidazole, 500 mg three times daily	14 days	Failure of bismuth-based therapy Penicillin allergy

PPI = proton pump inhibitor.

Adapted with permission from Chey WD, Leontiadis GI, Howden CW, Moss SF. ACG clinical guideline: treatment of *Helicobacter pylori* infection. Am J Gastroenterol. 2017;112:212-239. [PMID: 28071659] doi:10.1038/ajg.2016.563.

commonly associated with pernicious anemia. The achlorhydria from chronic atrophic gastritis can lead to iron deficiency, small intestinal bacterial overgrowth, and enteric infections. The hypergastrinemia associated with AMAG can promote the development of gastric carcinoid. Goals of therapy for patients with AMAG include the prevention of pernicious anemia and iron deficiency with vitamin B_{12} supplementation and iron replacement, and surveillance for gastric neoplasm. There are no universally accepted surveillance protocols for gastric neoplasm in the United States. A screening upper endoscopy with gastric biopsy is recommended in the setting of pernicious anemia.

Intestinal Metaplasia

Gastric intestinal metaplasia is a preneoplastic gastropathy arising from chronic inflammation associated with *H. pylori* infection. Other causes of chronic inflammation, including other gastric infections, chemical agents, and autoimmune disease, may also promote progression to gastric intestinal metaplasia. There is no conclusive evidence that long-term PPI use promotes the development of intestinal metaplasia. Gastric intestinal metaplasia is believed to be an intermediary stage in the multistage progression from chronic atrophic gastritis to gastric adenocarcinoma. Given the rare occurrence of gastric adenocarcinoma in the United States, there are no universally accepted surveillance strategies. Surveillance programs do exist in other parts of the world, and endoscopic surveillance should be considered in patients at increased risk, such as those with a family history of gastric cancer or who have immigrated from East Asia, Russia, or South America.

Eosinophilic Gastritis

Eosinophilic gastritis is a rare gastropathy characterized by infiltration of eosinophils in the stomach. Secondary causes of eosinophilia should first be excluded, including parasitic and bacterial infections of the stomach, inflammatory bowel disease, hypereosinophilic syndrome, myeloproliferative disorders, polyarteritis, allergic vasculitis, scleroderma, drug injury, and drug hypersensitivity. The cause of primary eosinophilic gastritis is unknown, but believed to be an allergic process. Symptoms vary widely based on depth of eosinophilia and organ involvement, as the small bowel may also be involved. Treatment includes avoidance of food allergens and use of elemental diets and/or glucocorticoids.

Lymphocytic Gastritis

Lymphocytic gastritis is a rare gastropathy typically presenting with mild, nonspecific dyspeptic symptoms and a normal-appearing stomach on endoscopy. On occasion, the stomach may have thickened folds covered by small nodules and aphthous ulceration. Celiac disease is the most common cause of lymphocytic gastritis. Other causes include HIV infection, Crohn disease, common variable immunodeficiency, and, rarely, *H. pylori* infection.

KEY POINTS

- Autoimmune atrophic gastritis is associated with pernicious anemia, iron deficiency, small intestinal bacterial overgrowth, and gastric cancer.
- *Helicobacter pylori* is associated with upper gastrointestinal conditions other than peptic ulcer disease including environmental metaplastic atrophic gastritis, gastric intestinal metaplasia, and, rarely, lymphocytic gastritis.

Gastrointestinal Complications of NSAIDs

Epidemiology and Risk Factors

Upper gastrointestinal complications associated with NSAID use can occur with short- or long-term NSAID use and are dose dependent, with a linear increase in incidence over time with chronic NSAID use. Nearly 1% to 2% of chronic NSAIDs users suffer a clinically significant upper gastrointestinal event (such as a bleeding ulcer, perforation, or obstruction) annually. The rate of upper gastrointestinal adverse events rises to 14% for elderly NSAID users. The greatest risk factor for an NSAID-related upper gastrointestinal bleed is a history of gastrointestinal bleeding. Other risk factors are listed in **Table 11**.

The use of low-dose aspirin for cardioprophylaxis is associated with a two- to fourfold increase in risk for upper gastrointestinal complications including bleeding ulcer, perforation, and obstruction. Use of enteric-coated aspirin does not lower this risk, and an increase in aspirin dosage is associated with an increased risk for upper gastrointestinal complications.

Prevention of NSAID-Induced Injury

Treatment strategies for the prevention of NSAID-related upper gastrointestinal adverse events include the avoidance of NSAIDs, addressing modifiable risk factors, use of a selective cyclooxygenase (COX)-2 inhibitor, or coadministration of gastroprotective agents, such as PPIs, misoprostol, or H_2 blockers. PPIs are the preferred gastroprotective agent for the treatment and prophylaxis of NSAID-related (including aspirin-related) upper

TABLE 11. Risk Factors for NSAID-Related Upper Gastrointestinal Complications
History of upper gastrointestinal bleeding
History of peptic ulcer disease
Helicobacter pylori infection
Age older than 65 years
Hemodialysis or peritoneal dialysis
Use of high-dose or multiple NSAIDs
Concomitant use of aspirin (even low-dose), nonaspirin antiplatelet agents, anticoagulants, oral glucocorticoids, selective serotonin reuptake inhibitors

gastrointestinal complications, and are specifically superior to H_2 blockers in the prevention of PUD and bleeding related to low-dose aspirin use. Misoprostol may be used instead of PPIs in patients with intolerance or unwillingness to take PPIs. However, side effects of misoprostol, such as diarrhea, abdominal discomfort, and nausea, can be limiting, particularly at therapeutic doses, and it is contraindicated in pregnancy.

When coadministered with aspirin, a selective COX-2 inhibitor provides no advantage over an NSAID in the prevention of an upper gastrointestinal adverse event. Given the increased risk for PUD with the concomitant use of either an NSAID or selective COX-2 inhibitor with low-dose aspirin, at-risk individuals should receive gastroprotective therapy. Compared to an NSAID plus a PPI in patients at high risk, a selective COX-2 inhibitor plus a PPI offers a lower risk for perforation, obstruction, and bleeding, as well as for NSAID and COX-2 withdrawal due to gastrointestinal adverse events.

After an NSAID-induced bleeding peptic ulcer, the safest strategy is avoidance of future NSAID use. If an NSAID must be used, the combination of a selective COX-2 inhibitor plus a PPI provides the best gastrointestinal protection, as this combination is more likely to prevent a rebleed than a selective COX-2 inhibitor alone or an NSAID plus a PPI. A treatment approach based on risk for NSAID-related ulcer complications and the need for low-dose aspirin for cardioprophylaxis is provided in **Table 12**.

KEY POINTS

- Upper gastrointestinal complications, such as bleeding, are common with the use of NSAIDs (both short- and long-term) and low-dose aspirin.

- Proton pump inhibitors are the preferred agent for the prevention and treatment of NSAID-related (including aspirin-related) upper gastrointestinal complications.

- In high-risk individuals without cardiovascular disease, including those with previous NSAID-induced gastrointestinal bleeding, the combination of a selective cyclooxygenase-2 inhibitor plus a proton pump inhibitor provides the best gastrointestinal protection if avoidance of NSAIDs is not possible.

Gastroparesis

Presentation

Gastroparesis is a heterogeneous clinical syndrome with three components to the diagnosis: the presence of specific symptoms, absence of mechanical outlet obstruction, and objective evidence of delay in gastric emptying into the duodenum. The most commonly reported symptoms in order of prevalence are nausea (90%), vomiting (84%), upper abdominal pain (72%), and early satiety (60%). Other symptoms may include abdominal fullness and bloating. Symptoms may be chronic or persistent, or may occur intermittently. More severe cases may involve weight loss and evidence of malnutrition and/or dehydration. A viral prodrome, such as gastroenteritis or respiratory infection before symptom onset, may suggest postviral gastroparesis, a condition that frequently resolves over time. Gastroparesis can result from a variety of causes (**Table 13**).

Diagnostic Testing

The first study performed to evaluate suspected gastroparesis is an upper endoscopy to exclude a gastric outlet obstruction. Once a structural cause for symptoms has been excluded, an objective test to assess gastric emptying is performed. There are three testing modalities available to assess gastric emptying: gastric scintigraphy, wireless motility capsule, and the radiolabeled carbon breath test using ^{13}C-labeled *Spirulina platensis* (**Table 14**). Gastric scintigraphy is the most commonly used modality. Narcotic and anticholinergic agents must be stopped at least 72 hours before a gastric emptying study. Once delayed emptying is objectively confirmed, additional testing maybe required to determine the underlying cause of the gastroparesis.

Management

The severity of gastroparesis-related symptoms does not correlate with the severity of delayed gastric emptying, particularly with regard to the symptoms of abdominal bloating and epigastric pain. This suggests that gastroparesis is not simply

---

TABLE 12.	Strategies for Prevention of NSAID-Related Ulcer Complications		
	No GI Risk Factors[a]	**One to Two GI Risk Factors[a,b]**	**More than Two GI Risk Factors[a]**
No aspirin	NSAID	NSAID plus PPI	Ideally, avoidance of NSAIDs
			If no alternative to NSAIDs, then a selective COX-2 inhibitor plus a PPI
Low-dose aspirin (81 mg/d) for cardiovascular prophylaxis	Naproxen plus PPI	Naproxen plus PPI	Avoid selective COX-2 inhibitors and use alternative analgesic

COX-2 = cyclooxygenase-2; GI = gastrointestinal; NSAID = nonsteroidal anti-inflammatory drug; PPI = proton pump inhibitor.

[a]GI risk factors: history of GI bleeding; history of peptic ulcer disease; concurrent use of NSAIDs and aspirin (including low-dose aspirin), nonaspirin antiplatelets, anticoagulants, or glucocorticoids; age older than 65 years; any chronic, debilitating illness.

[b]With no prior NSAID-related upper GI bleeding.

Adapted with permission from Lanza FL, Chan FK, Quigley EM; Practice Parameters Committee of the American College of Gastroenterology. Guidelines for prevention of NSAID-related ulcer complications. Am J Gastroenterol. 2009;104:728-38. [PMID: 19240698] doi:10.1038/ajg.2009.115.

TABLE 13.	Causes of Gastroparesis
Common causes	Diabetes mellitus (40% in long-standing type 1 diabetes mellitus, 20% in type 2 diabetes mellitus)
	Postsurgical (e.g., Nissen fundoplication, bariatric surgery, pancreatic surgery)
	Idiopathic (e.g., postviral)
Infrequent causes	Connective tissue disease (e.g., systemic sclerosis)
	Neurologic disease (e.g., Parkinson disease)
	Eating disorders
	Hypothyroidism
	Amyloidosis
	Paraneoplastic syndromes (e.g., small cell lung cancer)
	Mesenteric ischemia
	Medications (e.g., opiates, anticholinergic agents)

a motility disorder but one of altered sensation as well. Because poor glycemic control (blood glucose level >200 mg/dL [11.1 mmol/L]) can worsen symptoms as well as gastric emptying, tight glycemic control is the most important element of treatment of diabetic gastroparesis. Initial management also includes correction of dehydration and electrolyte abnormalities, and nutritional support if needed. Initial dietary intervention should consist of small, frequent meals that are low in fat and soluble fiber. Referral to a dietician may be beneficial.

Pharmacologic therapy is used to improve gastric emptying and to treat symptoms. Metoclopramide is the only prokinetic approved in the United States for the treatment of gastroparesis. To minimize the significant risk for neurologic side effects, including dystonia, Parkinsonian movements, and tardive dyskinesia, the lowest effective dose should be used.

Therapy must be stopped immediately if neurologic side effects develop.

Erythromycin improves gastric emptying, but its use should be limited to the treatment of flares or short-term use (2 to 3 weeks) due to the risk for tachyphylaxis.

Antiemetics for treatment of nausea and vomiting as well as centrally acting modulators, including tricyclic antidepressants and mirtazapine, can also provide relief of symptoms but have no beneficial effect on gastric emptying.

Interventional therapy, such enteral feeding via jejunostomy, gastric stimulator placement, pyloroplasty, and subtotal or total gastrectomy, can be considered in patients who do not respond to dietary and pharmacologic therapy.

KEY POINTS

- Gastroparesis is a heterogeneous clinical syndrome with three components to the diagnosis: the presence of specific symptoms, absence of mechanical outlet obstruction, and objective evidence of delay in gastric emptying into the duodenum.

- Initial management of gastroparesis includes correction of dehydration and electrolyte abnormalities; nutritional support; small, frequent meals that are low in fat and soluble fiber; and improved glycemic control in patients with diabetes mellitus.

- Metoclopramide is a prokinetic drug that improves gastric emptying but is associated with dystonia, tardive dyskinesia, and Parkinsonism.

Gastric Polyps and Subepithelial Lesions

Gastric Polyps

Polyps in the stomach include fundic gland polyps, hyperplastic polyps, and adenomas. All gastric polyps should be biopsied to determine polyp histology. Fundic gland polyps and

TABLE 14.	Diagnostic Tests Assessing Gastric Emptying		
Test Modality	**Advantages**	**Disadvantages**	**Clinical Pearls**
Gastric scintigraphy	Considered the gold standard	Radiation exposure (technetium radiolabeled meal)	4-Hour study is most accurate
		Requires specially trained personnel	Assesses solid emptying (liquid emptying is less accurate)
		Cost	Blood sugar should be less than 275 mg/dL (15.3 mmol/L)
Wireless motility capsule	Can also assess small bowel, colon, and whole gut transit	Cost	Consider in a patient with suspected global motility problem
	No radiation	Can't be used with pacemaker or defibrillator	Stop antisecretory agents as study relies on measurement of pH
	Ambulatory study	Risk for capsule retention	
Gastric emptying breath test	Low cost	Only recently commercially available	—
		Efficacy and accuracy limited to clinical trials	

hyperplastic polyps account for 70% to 90% of stomach polyps. Fundic gland polyps have no potential for malignancy and are commonly seen in the setting of PPI use. Multiple fundic gland polyps are also found in patients with familial adenomatous polyposis.

Hyperplastic polyps of the stomach are thought to have malignant potential, with 5% to 19% harboring dysplasia or malignancy. Risk factors for malignant potential of hyperplastic polyps include size greater than 1 cm and pedunculated morphology. All hyperplastic polyps greater than 0.5 to 1.0 cm in size should be resected.

Adenomas found in the stomach can be sporadic or associated with hereditary syndromes, including familial adenomatous polyposis and Lynch syndrome. Adenomas in the stomach should be resected and endoscopic surveillance should be performed 1 year after resection and then every 3 to 5 years thereafter.

Gastric Subepithelial Lesions

Gastrointestinal Stromal Tumors

Gastrointestinal stromal tumors (GISTs) are the most common mesenchymal tumors of the stomach. GISTs may present with symptoms, such as bleeding or abdominal pain, but are also found incidentally. Endoscopic ultrasonography is the best diagnostic modality for evaluation of a GIST. High-risk features on endoscopic ultrasonography include size greater than 2 cm, lobulated or irregular borders, invasion into adjacent structures, and heterogeneity. Biopsies of a GIST can be done, but the high-risk endoscopic features are better predictors of malignant potential. Treatment consists of surgical excision if the GIST is symptomatic or high-risk features are present. For GISTs without high-risk features, yearly endoscopic surveillance is indicated. See MKSAP 18 Hematology and Oncology for staging and treatment of GISTs.

Carcinoid Tumors

A carcinoid tumor is a well-differentiated neuroendocrine tumor originating in the digestive tract, lungs, or, rarely, the kidneys or ovaries. Carcinoid tumors can be encountered throughout the gastrointestinal tract, including the stomach. They may present symptomatically or may be found incidentally. Carcinoid tumors are usually sporadic but can be seen in the setting of Zollinger-Ellison syndrome, atrophic gastritis, and rare syndromes, such as multiple endocrine neoplasia type 1 and neurofibromatosis type 1. Carcinoid tumors are classified by their size, number, and anatomic distribution. Management includes endoscopic surveillance for lesions smaller than 1 cm in size, especially when multiple lesions are present. Endoscopic or surgical excision is indicated for carcinoid tumors with high-risk features, such as solitary lesions not found in the setting of atrophic gastritis or Zollinger-Ellison syndrome. See MKSAP 18 Hematology and Oncology for treatment of gastric neuroendocrine tumors.

KEY POINTS

- Polyps in the stomach include fundic gland polyps, which have no malignant potential; hyperplastic polyps; and, less commonly, adenomas, which should be resected.
- Gastrointestinal stromal tumors should be evaluated with endoscopic ultrasonography and excised if symptoms or high-risk features are present.
- Carcinoid tumors are well-differentiated neuroendocrine tumors that can occur throughout the gastrointestinal tract, including the stomach.

Gastric Adenocarcinoma

Epidemiology and Risk Factors

Stomach adenocarcinoma has an incidence rate of 6.7 in 100,000 persons and a mortality rate of 3.4 per 100,000 persons in the United States. Rates have steadily decreased since the 1990s. There are two types of gastric cancer: intestinal-type, which is more common, and diffuse-type. _H. pylori_ is a recognized risk factor for both types of cancer. Other risk factors primarily associated with intestinal-type gastric adenocarcinoma include male sex; ethnicity (incidence is highest in persons of Asian and Pacific Island descent, and mortality is highest in non-Hispanic white persons); geography (the highest rates worldwide occur in Asia, Eastern Europe, and Central and South America); diet high in smoked, salted, and pickled foods as well as nitrates and nitrites; smoking; and obesity. Additional risk factors include previous stomach surgery, pernicious anemia, and hereditary syndromes such as hereditary diffuse gastric cancer (associated with the diffuse type), Lynch syndrome, and familial adenomatous polyposis. Gastric intestinal metaplasia and dysplasia are also risk factors for gastric adenocarcinoma.

Screening and Surveillance

There is no recommendation for population-based screening for gastric adenocarcinoma in countries with a low incidence of gastric cancer, such as the United States. If intestinal metaplasia with high-grade dysplasia is identified, it should be resected because 25% of cases progress to adenocarcinoma. Screening and surveillance is indicated for patients with familial adenomatous polyposis and Lynch syndrome.

Clinical Manifestations and Diagnosis

Symptoms of gastric adenocarcinoma may be vague. They include poor appetite, weight loss, abdominal pain, early satiety, nausea, and vomiting. Signs of gastric adenocarcinoma include iron deficiency anemia. Diagnosis is typically made by upper endoscopy with biopsies.

For treatment of gastric cancer, see MKSAP 18 Hematology and Oncology.

KEY POINTS

- In countries with a low incidence of gastric cancer, screening for gastric cancer should be reserved for patients with genetic cancer syndromes.
- The primary nongenetic risk factor for gastric cancer is *Helicobacter pylori* infection.
- Upper endoscopy with biopsy is the diagnostic test of choice for gastric cancer.

Gastric Surgery Complications

For complications of bariatric surgery, see MKSAP 18 General Internal Medicine.

Partial or complete gastric resections are performed for benign and malignant disease. The extent of resection, type of reconstruction, and nature of the disease affect postoperative morbidity and mortality. Partial gastric resection allows for preservation of some function of the stomach, but in the setting of malignancy, it requires lifelong surveillance of the remaining stomach for recurrence. Patients who undergo partial gastrectomy for benign disease have an increased risk for cancer in the gastric remnant 15 to 20 years after surgery, with reported frequency ranging from 0.8% to 8.9%.

Dumping syndrome, which results from rapid gastric emptying after gastric surgery, can cause significant postprandial gastrointestinal and vasomotor symptoms. Clinical features of early dumping syndrome occur within 30 minutes of eating due to gastrointestinal hormone hypersecretion, autonomic dysregulation, and bowel distention. Symptoms include palpitations, flushing or pallor, diaphoresis, lightheadedness, hypotension, and fatigue, followed by diarrhea, nausea, abdominal bloating, cramping, and borborygmus. Late symptoms occur 1 to 3 hours after meals because of reactive hypoglycemia and can include decreased concentration, faintness, and altered consciousness. In severe cases, protein-wasting malnutrition can occur. It is estimated that 25% to 50% of all patients who have undergone gastric surgery experience some symptoms of dumping syndrome, but severe, persistent symptoms occur in only about 10%. Oral glucose challenge testing is useful to make the diagnosis, with a sensitivity as high as 100% and a specificity of 94%.

First-line treatment for dumping syndrome is dietary, with smaller, more frequent meals and ingestion of liquids after meals. Decreasing carbohydrate intake, especially simple carbohydrates, and increasing protein and fiber intake may also alleviate symptoms.

Acarbose, an α-glycosidase hydrolase inhibitor that interferes with the digestion of polysaccharides to monosaccharides, can be used for late symptoms of dumping syndrome. Other pharmacologic therapies include anticholinergics to slow gastric emptying, and antispasmodics. Severe cases of dumping rarely require octreotide. If a trial of subcutaneous injections is effective, monthly intramuscular injections of long-acting octreotide can be used.

KEY POINTS

- Patients who undergo partial gastrectomy for malignancy require lifelong surveillance for recurrence of cancer.
- Dumping syndrome results from rapid gastric emptying after gastric surgery; first-line treatment is smaller, more frequent meals with liquids taken following meals.

Disorders of the Pancreas

Acute Pancreatitis

Acute pancreatitis is an inflammatory process involving the pancreas and extrapancreatic organs. It is the most common gastrointestinal cause of hospitalization in the United States. Passage of gallstones, sludge, or biliary crystals (microlithiasis) is the most common cause of acute pancreatitis (**Table 15**).

TABLE 15.	Causes of Acute Pancreatitis
Common	
Biliary disease	
Gallstones	
Microlithiasis (1- to 2-mm stones that are not detected by imaging studies)	
Alcohol use	
Post-endoscopic retrograde cholangiopancreatography	
Occasional	
Medications	
Furosemide	
Didanosine	
Asparaginase	
Mesalamine	
Hydrochlorothiazide	
6-Mercaptopurine/azathioprine	
Simvastatin	
Hypertriglyceridemia	
Hypercalcemia	
Choledochocele	
Rare	
Autoimmune	
Infectious	
Viral (mumps, coxsackie B virus, cytomegalovirus)	
Parasitic (*Toxoplasma* species, *Ascaris lumbricoides*)	
Ischemia	
Trauma	
Neoplasia	
Celiac disease	
Genetic (only if attacks are recurrent)	

Premature activation of digestive enzymes and release of cytokines cause "autodigestion" of the pancreas and inflammation, which may involve surrounding tissues and distant organs.

Acute pancreatitis is classified as mild, moderately severe, or severe. Mild acute pancreatitis does not involve organ failure or local or systemic complications, usually resolves within 1 week, and has a low mortality rate. Twenty percent of patients with acute pancreatitis develop moderately severe or severe disease. Moderately severe acute pancreatitis involves local or systemic complications such as necrosis or transient organ failure (for less than 48 hours). Severe acute pancreatitis involves systemic inflammatory response syndrome (SIRS), persistent organ failure (usually kidney or respiratory failure), duration longer than 48 hours, and one or more local complications; it has a mortality rate as high as 50%.

Clinical Presentation and Diagnosis

The diagnosis of acute pancreatitis requires two of the following three criteria: (1) acute-onset abdominal pain characteristic of pancreatitis (severe, persistent for hours to days, and epigastric in location, often radiating to the back); (2) serum lipase or amylase levels elevated to three to five times the upper limit of normal; and (3) characteristic radiographic findings on contrast-enhanced CT (**Figure 9**), MRI, or transabdominal ultrasonography. The presence of high fever and leukocytosis is part of the cytokine cascade and does not necessarily indicate infection.

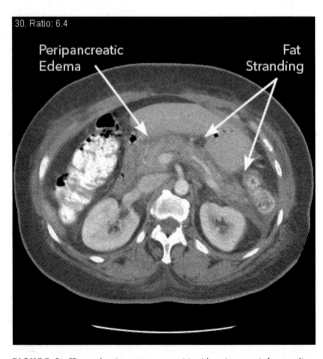

FIGURE 9. CT scan showing acute pancreatitis with peripancreatic fat stranding and inflammation. The hazy appearance of the mesenteric fat surrounding the pancreas in this image is called fat stranding, and the blurring of the margins of the pancreas is consistent with peripancreatic edema, features seen with inflammatory changes of acute pancreatitis.

Because acute pancreatitis is most commonly caused by biliary disorders, patients with acute pancreatitis should undergo transabdominal ultrasonography. Transabdominal ultrasonography is preferred over CT because it has a higher sensitivity for detection of gallstones, avoids the risks associated with intravenous contrast, and is more cost effective. However, abdominal air can limit the visualization of the pancreas in patients with acute pancreatitis. Magnetic resonance cholangiopancreatography (MRCP) may be considered in patients who do not have abnormal findings on ultrasonography. CT may be indicated if the diagnosis is in question or if clinical symptoms are not alleviated within the first 48 hours.

Acute liver-enzyme elevation at presentation suggests biliary obstruction. Serum amylase and lipase levels may be elevated in conditions other than acute pancreatitis, such as kidney disease, acute appendicitis, cholecystitis, intestinal obstruction or ischemia, peptic ulcer, or gynecologic disorders. Enzyme levels may be falsely low or normal in patients with hypertriglyceride-induced pancreatitis because of lipemic-serum interference with laboratory assays. Triglyceride levels should be measured in patients without a biliary cause of acute pancreatitis, and if the triglyceride level is greater than 1000 mg/dL (11.3 mmol/L), it can be considered the cause of the acute pancreatitis.

Prognostic Criteria

Risk factors for severe disease include age older than 55 years, medical comorbidities, BMI greater than 30, the presence of SIRS, signs of hypovolemia on presentation (for example, a serum blood urea nitrogen level greater than 20 mg/dL [7.1 mmol/L] and rising, a hematocrit greater than 44%, or an elevated serum creatinine), the presence of pleural effusions and/or infiltrates, and altered mental status. A systematic review of 18 multiple-factor scoring systems, including the Ranson criteria and the Acute Physiologic Assessment and Chronic Health Evaluation (APACHE) II score, for predicting outcome in acute pancreatitis found these systems to have limited clinical value and accuracy. Scoring systems only identify severe disease as it develops, without enough lead time for intervention, and they are too cumbersome for routine use. Data suggest serum hematocrit, elevated blood urea nitrogen levels, and the presence of SIRS to be as accurate as complex scoring systems in predicting outcome, and they are easier to use.

Management

Mainstays of management include fluid resuscitation, pain management, and antinausea medication.

Aggressive hydration (250-500 mL/h of intravenous lactated Ringer solution) should be given to patients with acute pancreatitis on presentation and is most beneficial in the first 12 to 24 hours. More rapid fluid resuscitation (boluses) may be needed in patients with severe volume depletion. Patients with organ failure or SIRS should be admitted to an ICU or

CONT.

intermediary care setting, with reassessment of fluid requirements every 6 hours for the first 24 to 48 hours.

Routine use of antibiotics is not warranted in acute pancreatitis, unless there is evidence of extrapancreatic infection, such as ascending cholangitis, bacteremia, urinary tract infection, or pneumonia. Use of prophylactic antibiotics in patients with sterile pancreatic necrosis to prevent infected necrosis is not recommended.

In mild acute pancreatitis, oral feedings can be started as soon as nausea and vomiting are controlled and clinical symptoms begin to subside. Enteral feeding should begin within 72 hours if oral feeding is not tolerated; it is usually required in patients with moderately severe or severe acute pancreatitis. Feeding with a nasojejunal tube has traditionally been preferred, but data suggest that nasogastric feedings are likely equally effective and easier to administer. Enteral feeding promotes a healthy gut-mucosal barrier to prevent translocation of bacteria into inflamed tissues.

If a biliary cause of acute pancreatitis is suspected, serial liver chemistry tests and clinical symptoms can show whether the biliary obstruction is ongoing or resolving. Endoscopic retrograde cholangiopancreatography (ERCP) is not indicated in patients with gallstone pancreatitis unless there is persistent elevation of liver chemistries or if choledocholithiasis is seen on imaging studies. Patients with cholangitis should undergo ERCP within 24 hours of admission. Patients with uncomplicated gallstone pancreatitis should be considered for cholecystectomy before discharge.

There is no value in rechecking serum amylase and lipase levels after the diagnosis is established.

Complications

There are two overlapping phases of acute pancreatitis with two peaks in mortality. The early phase is the first week of the disease, when the body is responding to local pancreatic injury and the cytokine cascade, and SIRS and organ failure are possible. The late phase occurs after the first week and may persist for weeks to months in patients with moderately severe or severe acute pancreatitis. Significant risk for infection in peripancreatic fluid collections and necrosis occurs in the late phase.

Proper classification of fluid collections in acute pancreatitis is important to guide management. An international consensus group updated the Atlanta classification and definitions of acute pancreatitis and its complications in 2012 to try to promote consistency in diagnosis and management. Four types of fluid collections were defined:

1. Acute peripancreatic fluid collections are collections that occur in edematous interstitial pancreatitis (no necrosis) within the first 4 weeks, are thought to occur because of rupture of main or side branch ducts as a result of inflammation, are sterile, and usually resolve spontaneously.

2. Pancreatic pseudocysts are acute peripancreatic fluid collections that have persisted for longer than 4 weeks,

developed a well-defined wall, and contain no solid debris (necrosis).

3. Acute necrotic collections (**Figure 10**) are areas of necrosis in the pancreatic parenchyma and/or peripancreatic tissues within the first 4 weeks of acute pancreatitis.

4. Walled-off necrosis (**Figure 11**) occurs after 4 weeks, when the body liquifies the necrosis and contains it within a well-defined wall.

Contrast-enhanced CT may not be able to distinguish solid from liquid content in fluid collections; therefore, necrotic collections are frequently misdiagnosed as pancreatic pseudocysts. Pancreatic pseudocysts do not require drainage

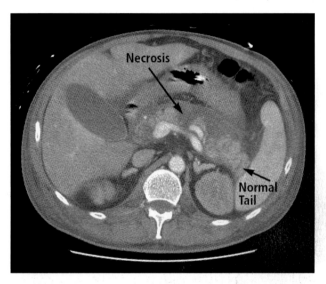

FIGURE 10. CT scan showing acute pancreatitis with hypoperfusion of the body of the pancreas as indicated by lack of enhancement following intravenous contrast infusion (necrosis) and normal perfusion of the pancreatic tail.

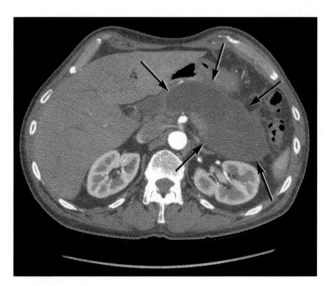

FIGURE 11. CT scan showing maturation and liquefaction of pancreas necrosis of nearly the entire pancreas over 4 weeks in duration with a well-defined rim or wall (*arrows*), known as walled-off necrosis.

CONT.

unless they cause significant symptoms, regardless of size. Because they contain only fluid, pseudocysts are easily drained under endoscopic or radiographic guidance. Walled-off necrosis is not as amenable to percutaneous or endoscopic drainage due to solid necrotic debris within the cavity and may require endoscopic, radiologic, or surgical debridement.

The management of suspected infected necrosis includes initiation of antibiotics (for example, imipenem-cilastatin, meropenem, or ciprofloxacin plus metronidazole) with consideration of fine-needle aspiration with Gram stain and culture under CT guidance. Drainage procedures or debridement should be delayed for at least 4 weeks if possible to allow encapsulation of the necrosis with a fibrous wall. H

KEY POINTS

- Biliary disease, such as gallstone or microlithiasis, is the most common cause of acute pancreatitis.
- Diagnosis of acute pancreatitis requires two of three criteria: (1) acute-onset upper abdominal pain, (2) serum lipase or amylase levels elevated at least three times greater than the upper limit of normal, and (3) characteristic findings on imaging.
- Patients with acute pancreatitis should undergo transabdominal ultrasonography to evaluate for biliary disease.
- Patients with acute pancreatitis should be hospitalized for fluid administration and close monitoring of cardiovascular, respiratory, and kidney status.

Chronic Pancreatitis

Chronic pancreatitis is thought to develop when the inflammatory response to acute pancreatitis persists and ongoing inflammation activates stellate cells, resulting in a fibroinflammatory response. This causes distorted tissue architecture, loss of normal parenchyma, activation of pancreatic nociceptors, and loss of acinar and islet cell function. Genetic variants affecting inflammatory response, enzyme activation, and tissue repair are thought to play important roles in the pathogenesis of chronic pancreatitis. Many genes have been identified as disease modifiers in chronic pancreatitis, but the gene-environment interaction is not fully understood.

Alcohol use has long been described as a risk factor for chronic pancreatitis, but less than 3% of heavy alcohol users develop pancreatic disease. Patients who drink more than five drinks per day (or 35 drinks per week) seem to be more susceptible to chronic pancreatitis. In the largest study of patients with chronic pancreatitis in North America, only 46% had a history of significant alcohol use. The higher prevalence of alcohol-associated pancreatitis among men could be partially explained by an X chromosome–linked genetic variant, the *CLDN2* gene. Tobacco is considered an independent risk factor. **Table 16** lists common causes of chronic pancreatitis.

Clinical Presentation and Diagnosis

Abdominal pain is the most common presenting symptom of chronic pancreatitis (seen in 85% of patients), but some patients have no pain. Pain patterns can vary from constant, daily pain to intermittent attacks of severe pain. Pancreatic enzyme levels may not increase during attacks of pain because of fibrosis and atrophy of acinar cells and decreased enzyme production. Constant daily pain in chronic pancreatitis causes significant reduction in quality of life, with increased use of health care resources, disability benefits, and time away from employment. Exocrine or endocrine insufficiency occurs in some patients as a result of significant tissue destruction.

Diagnosis of chronic pancreatitis remains challenging because hallmark anatomic features, such as pancreatic calcifications (**Figure 12**), only occur in 25% of patients, and other features of atrophy or duct dilation can occur normally with aging or other disease processes. If pancreatic calcifications are not present on CT imaging of the abdomen, diagnosis usually requires a combined approach in patients with symptoms,

TABLE 16.	Causes of Chronic Pancreatitis
Toxic or metabolic	
Alcohol, tobacco, hypercalcemia, hypertriglyceridemia, chronic kidney disease	
Genetic	
Mutations or polymorphisms of the *CFTR, PRSSI, SPINKI, CTRC, CASR, CLDN2* genes	
Recurrent and severe acute pancreatitis	
Vascular disease/ischemia	
Obstructive	
Pancreatic tumor, intraductal papillary mucinous neoplasm	
Posttraumatic (pancreatic duct stricture)	
Autoimmune (type 1 and type 2)	
Idiopathic	

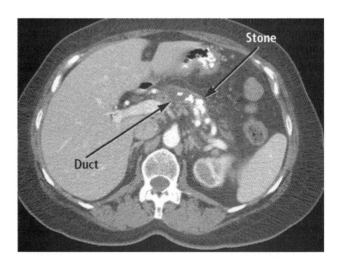

FIGURE 12. CT scan showing chronic calcific pancreatitis with multiple stones in the main duct and side branches of the pancreas.

with advanced imaging using MRI, MRCP, or endoscopic ultra-sonography and evidence of pancreatic dysfunction. Pancreatic biopsy is not indicated. ERCP is no longer used as a diagnostic tool for chronic pancreatitis. MRI and MRCP are safer and more readily available; however, sensitivity and specificity are variable. Endoscopic ultrasonography for the diagnosis of chronic pancreatitis has relatively high sensitivity but low specificity, and is not reliable as a single diagnostic test.

Management

The management of chronic pancreatitis focuses on treating symptoms. No effective treatment exists to reverse or halt disease progression. Patients should be counseled to avoid alcohol and tobacco, as this may lessen attacks of inflammation and pain. Intermittent attacks of severe acute pain are treated as in acute pancreatitis. Complications of chronic pancreatitis, including pseudocyst, pancreatic duct stones causing upstream obstruction, and malignancy, should be evaluated with imaging when a patient's symptom pattern changes. Constant, daily pain is more challenging to manage and frequently involves the use of medications such as tramadol, gabapentinoids, and possibly narcotics, although long-term use of narcotics should be avoided due to hyperesthesia and development of tolerance or addiction. Pancreatic enzymes are used to treat steatorrhea but have not been shown to effectively treat pain or prevent attacks of pancreatitis. Two large randomized trials using antioxidants to treat chronic pancreatitis pain showed conflicting results, and guidelines do not support their use. Nerve blocks and neurolysis procedures are not recommended because the response rate is low, and pain relief, if achieved, only lasts a few weeks.

Surgery offers the best long-term results for chronic, refractory pain management and, depending on anatomy and cause, may include lateral pancreaticojejunostomy, duodenal-preserving pancreatic head resection, pancreaticoduodenectomy, distal pancreatectomy, or even total pancreatectomy with or without auto–islet cell transplantation. These procedures have been shown to improve outcomes in patients at high-volume pancreas referral centers. Pancreatic endocrine insufficiency may require specialty referral for labile diabetes management and nutritional consultation.

> **KEY POINTS**
>
> - Abdominal pain, which may occur as intermittent attacks or as ongoing, daily pain, is the most common symptom of chronic pancreatitis.
>
> **HVC** - Pancreatic biopsy and endoscopic retrograde cholangio-pancreatography are not indicated in the diagnosis of chronic pancreatitis.
>
> - Symptomatic management is the cornerstone of treatment for chronic pancreatitis, including patients with refractory pain.
>
> - Patients with chronic pancreatitis should be counseled to avoid alcohol and tobacco use.

Autoimmune Pancreatitis and IgG4 Disease

Autoimmune pancreatitis (AIP) is a frequent manifestation of IgG4-related disease. Other organs that can be affected include the lacrimal and salivary glands, central nervous system, kidneys, thyroid gland, lungs, biliary tract and liver, prostate gland, retroperitoneum, and lymph nodes. Storiform fibrosis and obliterative phlebitis are characteristics seen in the pancreas and biliary tract. The most common pancreatic manifestation of IgG4-related disease is type 1 AIP, with abundant infiltration of IgG4-positive plasma cells and lymphocytes. Type 2 AIP has no or few IgG4-positive cells but is characterized by idiopathic duct-centric neutrophil infiltration, known as a granulocytic epithelial lesion. Type 2 AIP is a pancreas-specific disease with occasional association with ulcerative colitis. The 2011 International Consensus of Diagnostic Criteria for Autoimmune Pancreatitis endorsed the concept of type 1 and type 2 disease, but there is some debate over whether type 2 should be considered an IgG4-related disease.

For more information on IgG4-related disease, see MKSAP 18 Rheumatology.

Clinical Presentation and Diagnosis

Diagnostic criteria for AIP require image findings of a narrowed main pancreatic duct and parenchymal swelling (the "sausage-shaped" pancreas [**Figure 13**]) and response to glucocorticoids. Patients with type 1 AIP have elevated levels of IgG4-positive cells in pancreatic tissue (>10 IgG4-positive cells/hpf), and 60% to 80% of patients have associated sclerosing cholangitis, sclerosing sialoadenitis, or retroperitoneal fibrosis. A significant elevation of serum IgG4 level is helpful in diagnosing type 1 AIP. Patients with type 2 AIP will have no elevation of IgG4-positive cells in pancreatic tissue. Patients with both types may present with abdominal pain or

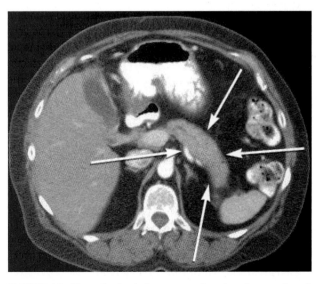

FIGURE 13. CT scan showing the homogeneous, hypodense "sausage-shaped" swelling (*arrows*) seen in autoimmune pancreatitis.

obstructive jaundice with or without a mass. In patients presenting with obstructive jaundice or with a mass, pancreatic malignancy must be considered. Many patients with malignancy have a dilated upstream main pancreatic duct, whereas patients with AIP may have a narrow main duct. Endoscopic ultrasonography and biopsy may be required to differentiate AIP and pancreas neoplasm. Ten percent of patients with type 1 AIP may develop chronic pancreatitis or pancreatic stone formation.

Treatment

Glucocorticoids are effective treatment for types 1 and 2 AIP, starting with oral prednisolone, 0.6 to 1.0 mg/kg/d, and tapered over 2 to 3 months. Response is determined by symptom relief and imaging features. Failure of clinical symptoms to respond to glucocorticoids suggests an incorrect diagnosis, and other causes should be investigated. Up to 60% of patients may relapse. Readministration of glucocorticoids or immunomodulators, such as 6-mercaptopurine, azathioprine, mycophenolate, or rituximab, may be used to treat recurrent AIP.

KEY POINTS

- Diagnosis of autoimmune pancreatitis requires the presence of a narrowed main pancreatic duct and parenchymal swelling ("sausage-shaped" pancreas) on imaging and disease response to glucocorticoids.

- Type 1 autoimmune pancreatitis is characterized by elevated numbers of IgG4-positive cells in pancreatic tissue; most patients also have a significant elevation of IgG4 in serum.

- Patients with type 2 autoimmune pancreatitis have normal IgG4-positive cell counts.

- Types 1 and 2 autoimmune pancreatitis are treated with glucocorticoids, with a relapse rate of up to 60%.

Pancreatic Adenocarcinoma

Pancreatic ductal adenocarcinoma has a poor prognosis and increasing incidence. In 2015, there were approximately 49,000 cases diagnosed in the United States and 41,000 deaths. It is predicted to become the second leading cause of cancer-related death in the United States over the next decade, with an overall 5-year survival rate of less than 6%.

Epidemiology and Risk Factors

Risk factors for pancreatic cancer include age older than 50 years, smoking history, obesity, chronic pancreatitis, and mucinous cystic lesions of the pancreas. Inherited conditions associated with pancreatic cancer include Peutz-Jeghers syndrome, *BRCA2* germline mutations, hereditary pancreatitis, familial atypical multiple mole melanoma, Lynch syndrome, and familial pancreatic cancer with at least two affected first-degree relatives.

There are no standard guidelines for screening high-risk or average-risk patients because no means of accurately detecting tumors at a curable stage has been identified.

Clinical Presentation

Symptoms in patients with pancreatic adenocarcinoma include abdominal pain, back pain, weight loss, and jaundice if the lesion is located in the head of the pancreas obstructing the common bile duct. Pancreatic cancer is highly associated with diabetes mellitus, and two thirds of patients develop new-onset diabetes mellitus in the 36 months surrounding the diagnosis. Venous thromboembolic events and depression have been observed to occur at higher rates in patients with pancreatic adenocarcinoma than in patients with other malignancies.

Diagnosis

Pancreas protocol CT uses multiphasic arterial and venous phases with thin cuts (3 mm) through the abdomen to view the primary tumor's relationship to mesenteric vasculature and to detect metastatic lesions. Some studies suggest that pancreas protocol MRI may be superior to CT for pancreatic disease. Histopathologic confirmation of pancreatic adenocarcinoma is increasingly recommended before initiation of therapy. Endoscopic ultrasound-guided biopsy is preferable to CT-guided biopsy in patients with potentially resectable disease because of ultrasonography's higher diagnostic yield, safety, and lower risk for peritoneal seeding. Patients are considered for primary surgical resection if they have no involvement of mesenteric vasculature or metastatic disease and are healthy enough for major intra-abdominal surgery. Preoperative chemotherapy and/or radiotherapy may be recommended for patients with locally advanced disease.

For staging and treatment of pancreatic adenocarcinoma, see MKSAP 18 Hematology and Oncology.

KEY POINTS

- Diagnosis of pancreatic cancer is suggested by weight loss, abdominal pain, jaundice, and new-onset diabetes mellitus; pancreas protocol CT or MRI help support the diagnosis and delineate the extent of disease.

- Endoscopic ultrasound-guided fine-needle aspiration of the pancreas is recommended to provide histological confirmation of cancer.

Ampullary Adenocarcinoma

Adenocarcinoma of the ampulla of Vater accounts for 0.2% of gastrointestinal malignancies and usually presents early because of obstruction of the biliary system. Endoscopic ultrasonography with biopsy is the preferred method for staging and tissue diagnosis, with 90% accuracy. At least 50% of patients with familial adenomatous polyposis syndrome develop adenomatous changes of the periampullary region; upper endoscopy screening in patients with this syndrome should begin at age 25 to 30 years. See Colorectal Neoplasia for more information on adenomatous polyposis syndromes.

Cystic Lesions of the Pancreas

Pancreatic cysts are found incidentally in 15% of patients undergoing abdominal imaging. The detection of a cystic lesion in the pancreas causes anxiety in patients and clinicians and is a growing driver of health care use in the United States.

Cystic neoplasms of the pancreas are subcategorized as mucin-producing and non–mucin-producing cysts. Mucin-producing cysts are thought to have malignant potential, but most never become malignant. Intraductal papillary mucinous neoplasms (IPMNs) are the most commonly found cystic lesions of the pancreas. Most IPMNs arise from a branched duct and have a very low rate of malignant transformation. In contrast, the rate of malignant transformation is greater than 65% in IPMNs involving the main pancreatic duct (**Figure 14**). Other high-risk features are the presence of symptoms, cyst size greater than 3 cm, and a solid component to the cyst.

Mucinous cystic neoplasms are mucin-producing cysts seen almost exclusively in women (more than 98%) and found in the pancreas body or tail in 90% of cases. They have a thick fibrous capsule with epithelioid cells similar to ovarian stroma surrounding the tumor. Differentiating mucinous cysts from serous cysts, pseudocysts, and cystic neuroendocrine tumors of the pancreas can be challenging, as there is no definitive test with high sensitivity and specificity. Endoscopic ultrasonography with fine-needle aspiration is used for cyst fluid analysis in worrisome lesions; carcinoembryonic antigen levels are frequently elevated in patients with mucinous cysts, whereas serum amylase levels are often elevated in patients with pseudocysts. Cytology of cyst fluid has a low sensitivity (<60%) and is an unreliable predictor of malignant transformation.

Surgical resection of high-risk cysts is currently the only option for treatment. In 2018, the American Gastroenterological Association published guidelines based on expert opinion for the management of asymptomatic cystic neoplasms of the pancreas. Worrisome features include symptoms related to the cyst (jaundice, pancreatitis), size of 3 cm or greater, dilated main pancreatic duct, and a solid component. MRI is preferred for surveillance. Surveillance can be discontinued if no worrisome features develop over 5 years or if the patient is no longer a surgical candidate.

KEY POINTS

- Most pancreatic cysts never become malignant, with the exception of intraductal papillary mucinous neoplasms involving the main pancreatic duct.
- Cystic lesions are managed with surveillance and surgical resection of high-risk cysts.

Pancreatic Neuroendocrine Tumors

Pancreatic neuroendocrine tumors are rare, representing 3% of primary pancreatic neoplasms. Ten to twenty-five percent of pancreatic neuroendocrine tumors are functional and hypersecrete hormones. Tumors may be sporadic or part of an inherited disorder. Initial evaluation includes blood and urine tests for chromogranin A, 5-hydroxyindoleacetic acid, gastrin, glucagon, insulin and proinsulin (if clinically indicated; requires fasting with concurrent glucose), pancreatic polypeptide, and vasoactive intestinal polypeptide to determine functional status. Most functional pancreatic neuroendocrine tumors secrete gastrin (gastrinoma) or insulin (insulinoma). Genetic testing for multiple endocrine neoplasia type 1 is recommended in all young patients with gastrinomas or insulinomas, and in any patient with a family or personal history of other endocrinopathies or multiple pancreatic neuroendocrine tumors. Genetic testing for other associated inherited disorders, such as von Hippel-Lindau syndrome, tuberous sclerosis, or neurofibromatosis-1, should be considered based on clinical and family history.

Imaging is recommended with multiphasic CT or MRI of the abdomen. Endoscopic ultrasonography (90% sensitive) or octreotide scintigraphy may be needed to detect small lesions. For functional pancreatic neuroendocrine tumors, surgery is recommended if more than 90% of the tumor can be resected. For nonfunctional tumors associated with multiple endocrine neoplasia type 1 and von Hippel-Lindau syndrome, surgery is usually recommended if the tumors are greater than 2 to 3 cm in size. Medical management of gastrinomas includes oral proton pump inhibitors two or three times daily or somatostatin analogs. High-volume or progressive disease is best managed in conjunction with a gastroenterologist.

KEY POINTS

- Ten to twenty-five percent of pancreatic neuroendocrine tumors are functional and hypersecrete hormones, most commonly gastrin or insulin.
- Genetic testing for inherited tumor syndromes should be considered based on patient age and history.

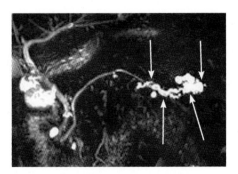

FIGURE 14. Magnetic resonance cholangiopancreatogram of a main-duct intraductal papillary mucinous neoplasm of the tail of the pancreas. Cystic dilation of the main pancreatic duct in the tail is seen (*arrows*).

Disorders of the Small and Large Bowel

Diarrhea

Classification

Diarrhea is a condition marked by passage of a greater number of less-formed stools than normal. The classification of diarrhea as acute or chronic is determined by duration of symptoms: acute diarrhea is defined by duration of less than 2 weeks, whereas chronic diarrhea is defined by duration of at least 4 weeks. Acute diarrhea is usually caused by infectious agents; chronic diarrhea is most commonly noninfectious.

Acute Diarrhea

Causes

Causes of acute diarrhea are primarily infectious, including bacteria, viruses, and parasites. These can be divided into noninvasive and invasive causes. Noninvasive causes lead to watery diarrhea; they include *Clostridium difficile*, viruses (such as norovirus and rotavirus), *Escherichia coli*, cholera, cryptosporidia, and *Giardia lamblia*. Invasive causes lead to dysentery or bloody diarrhea and include *Campylobacter*, hemorrhagic *E. coli*, *Entamoeba histolytica*, *Shigella*, and *Salmonella*. Persistent diarrhea (lasting between 14 and 30 days) is usually caused by a parasitic infection. For example, *Giardia lamblia* can begin as an acute infection but then become persistent or even chronic. See MKSAP 18 Infectious Disease for further discussion of infectious diarrhea.

Evaluation

Acute diarrhea may be accompanied by abdominal cramping, tenesmus, flatulence, fever, nausea, and vomiting. For all patients with acute diarrhea, evaluation of hydration status is important. Stool testing for infectious causes depends on many factors, including suspicion of disease outbreak, severity of symptoms, duration of symptoms (>7 days), and whether an individual is considered at increased risk for infectious diarrhea (such as a worker in day care, health care, or food preparation). For example, individuals with *Giardia* present with watery diarrhea that can be explosive and is associated with bloating due to malabsorption. A stool enzyme–linked immunosorbent assay is the best diagnostic test for *Giardia* infection.

Management

Fluid therapy is the mainstay of treatment for acute diarrhea. In patients with severe diarrhea or travelers with cholera-like diarrhea, balanced electrolyte rehydration solutions should be used. Confirmed infection with *C. difficile* should be treated with metronidazole, vancomycin, or other agents, depending on patient comorbidities and clinical severity (see MKSAP 18 Infectious Disease for discussion of *C. difficile* infection). Treatment of diarrhea in travelers includes bismuth and loperamide to relieve symptoms and consideration of empiric antibiotics if symptoms are moderate or severe.

Chronic Diarrhea

Causes

Chronic diarrhea can be grouped into six categories according to type of cause: (1) osmotic, (2) secretory, (3) steatorrhea, (4) inflammatory, (5) motility, and (6) miscellaneous (**Table 17**). These categories may overlap because some diseases have multiple mechanisms that cause diarrhea. The most common

TABLE 17.	Types of Chronic Diarrhea
Diarrhea Type	**Causes (examples)**
Osmotic	Medications (laxatives)
	Undigested sugars (lactose, fructose, sorbitol, mannitol)
Secretory	Medications (nonosmotic laxatives, antibiotics)
	Endocrine (carcinoid, gastrinoma, VIPoma, adrenal insufficiency, hyperthyroidism)
	Bile salt malabsorption (ileal resection, cholecystectomy)
	Noninvasive infections (giardiasis, cryptosporidiosis)
	Small intestinal bacterial overgrowth
Steatorrhea	Maldigestion (decreased bile salts, pancreatic dysfunction)
	Malabsorption (celiac disease, tropical sprue, giardiasis, Whipple disease, chronic mesenteric ischemia, short bowel syndrome, bacterial overgrowth, lymphatic obstruction)
Inflammatory	Inflammatory bowel disease (ulcerative colitis, Crohn disease, microscopic colitis)
	Malignancy (colorectal cancer, lymphoma)
	Invasive infections (*Clostridium difficile*, cytomegalovirus, *Entamoeba histolytica*, tuberculosis)
	Ischemia
	Radiation colitis/enteritis
Motility	Postsurgical (vagotomy, dumping)
	Endocrine (diabetes mellitus, hyperthyroidism)
	Scleroderma
Miscellaneous	Irritable bowel syndrome
	Functional diarrhea[a]
	Factitious
	Overflow
	Fecal incontinence

[a]Frequent or loose or watery stools without abdominal discomfort in the absence of other identifiable causes.

Adapted with permission from Schiller LR, Pardi DS, Spiller R, Semrad CE, Surawicz CM, Giannella RA, et al. Gastro 2013 APDW/WCOG Shanghai working party report: chronic diarrhea: definition, classification, diagnosis. J Gastroenterol Hepatol. 2014;29:6-25. [PMID: 24117999] doi:10.1111/jgh.12392

causes of chronic diarrhea are irritable bowel syndrome with predominant diarrhea (IBS-D) and functional causes. Medications are also an important cause of chronic diarrhea (**Table 18**).

Evaluation

The evaluation of chronic diarrhea includes a careful history and physical examination. Because IBS-D and functional causes are the most common causes, further diagnostic studies should be reserved for patients whose symptoms suggest another cause.

History and Physical Examination

The pattern of diarrhea can help determine the most likely diagnosis. Steatorrhea is often described as malodorous, greasy, or oily stools that float. The relation of symptoms to eating can also provide clues to the cause of diarrhea. Osmotic diarrhea occurs with eating and subsides with fasting, whereas secretory diarrhea does not subside with fasting. Information about specific dietary factors that commonly cause osmotic diarrhea, such as lactose, fructose, or artificial sweeteners (sorbitol) should be obtained. The patient should be asked about new medications (both prescription and nonprescription) and the timing of the initiation of medication in relation to the onset of diarrhea. Nocturnal symptoms are often related to inflammatory conditions, such as inflammatory bowel disease (IBD). Abdominal pain accompanying diarrhea suggests IBS-D, especially when a bowel movement relieves the pain. In

TABLE 18. Medications that Cause Diarrhea
Common
Antacids, proton pump inhibitors
Chemotherapy
Antibiotics
Colchicine
Metformin
NSAIDs, mesalamine
Cholesterol-lowering drugs
Rarer
ACE inhibitors
Angiotensin receptor blockers
β-adrenergic receptor antagonists
Carbamazepine
Lipase inhibitors
Lithium
Prostaglandin
Vitamin/mineral supplements

Adapted with permission from Schiller LR, Pardi DS, Spiller R, Semrad CE, Surawicz CM, Giannella RA, et al. Gastro 2013 APDW/WCOG Shanghai working party report: chronic diarrhea: definition, classification, diagnosis. J Gastroenterol Hepatol. 2014;29:6-25. [PMID: 24117999] doi:10.1111/jgh.12392.

evaluating chronic diarrhea, special attention should be given to features suggestive of malignancy, including rectal bleeding, weight loss, and age older than 50 years. Conditions such as IBS and microscopic colitis are more common in women than in men. IBS is most common in the third and fourth decades of life, whereas microscopic colitis is most common in the seventh and eighth decades.

Physical examination should assess for hydration and nutrition status, perineal disease suggestive of Crohn disease, and sphincter defects suggestive of fecal incontinence.

Additional Testing

The decision to do additional testing, including serologies, stool studies, imaging, and endoscopy, depends on the clinical scenario and likelihood of disease.

Evaluation of the small intestine may include imaging with small-bowel radiography, CT enterography, or MR enterography to identify conditions that could lead to bacterial overgrowth, such as small intestinal diverticular disease, inflammation, or strictures. Upper endoscopy is indicated when small-bowel mucosal disease (such as celiac disease or chronic infection) is suspected. Capsule endoscopy can be used to visualize the small intestine but does not allow for sampling. Device-assisted enteroscopy (balloon or spiral overtubes) can be used in selected patients who require sampling of small-intestinal tissue based on abnormalities found on imaging or capsule endoscopy. The diagnostic yields for capsule endoscopy and device-assisted enteroscopy are low in patients with chronic diarrhea and normal laboratory or imaging studies.

Colonoscopy is the primary diagnostic tool for evaluating causes of diarrhea related to the colon, such as IBD, microscopic colitis, chronic colonic infections, and malignancy. By definition, colon biopsies are required to exclude microscopic colitis. Colonoscopy is especially important in patients with rectal bleeding and/or age older than 50 years.

In cases of chronic diarrhea without an underlying diagnosis, stool studies can help clarify the cause. Analysis of stool includes fecal weight, stool electrolytes, fecal pH, fat content, fecal calprotectin, and presence of blood and leukocytes. In watery stools, fecal electrolytes can be used to calculate the fecal osmotic gap:

$$290 - (2 \times [\text{stool sodium} + \text{stool potassium}])$$

An osmotic gap of less than 50 mOsm/kg (50 mmol/kg) suggests secretory diarrhea, and a gap greater than 100 mOsm/kg (100 mmol/kg) suggests osmotic diarrhea.

The presence of blood or leukocytes in the stool suggests an inflammatory cause. A positive 72-hour stool collection for fecal fat confirms steatorrhea; a random fecal fat assessment may be helpful if a timed collection is not possible. When laxative abuse is suspected, a stool or urine laxative screen can aid in the diagnosis.

Additional testing may be warranted in immunocompromised patients, patients with secretory diarrhea, and those in whom celiac disease is suspected. Patients found to have a small-bowel tumor in the setting of diarrhea should be considered for additional testing including radioimmunoassays for peptides and/or 24-hour urine 5-hydroxyindoleacetic acid measurement for carcinoid tumors. Testing for carcinoid tumors should be limited to patients with chronic diarrhea and flushing.

Management

The management of chronic diarrhea is determined by its underlying cause. IBS-D and chronic diarrhea with a functional cause are treated with various medications aimed at slowing motility (loperamide), binding bile acids (cholestyramine), altering the gut microbiome (rifaximin), decreasing bowel contractions (eluxadoline), and modulating neurotransmitters (antidepressants).

Treatment of osmotic diarrhea requires avoiding offending agents, such as following a low-Fermentable Oligosaccharides, Disaccharides, Monosaccharides, And Polyols (FODMAP) (**Table 19**) and lactose-free diet.

Treatment of secretory diarrhea is aimed at identification of the underlying cause as well as careful management of hydration. Repletion of fat-soluble vitamins is important in cases of fat malabsorption. Probiotics are not recommended for treatment of diarrhea.

Diarrhea induced by medications necessitates changing medications unless the benefits exceed the potential harms and the diarrhea is manageable from the standpoint of the patient.

KEY POINTS

- Acute diarrhea (of less than 2 weeks' duration) is usually caused by infectious agents; chronic diarrhea (of more than 4 weeks' duration) is most commonly noninfectious.
- Maintaining hydration is the primary goal of treatment for acute diarrhea.
- The primary causes of chronic diarrhea are irritable bowel syndrome with predominant diarrhea, functional causes, and medications.
- Evaluation with imaging, endoscopy, and additional testing should be reserved for patients whose symptoms do not suggest irritable bowel syndrome or a functional cause of chronic diarrhea.

HVC

TABLE 19. Sources of FODMAP Carbohydrates
Fructose: honey, apples, pears, peaches, mangos, fruit juice, dried fruit
Lactose: milk, custard, ice cream, yogurt, soft cheeses
Fructans: wheat, rye, onions, leeks, zucchini
Galactans: legumes
Sugar alcohols: xylitol, sorbitol, maltitol, mannitol

FODMAP = Fermentable Oligosaccharides, Disaccharides, Monosaccharides, And Polyols.

Celiac Disease and Nonceliac Gluten Sensitivity

Celiac disease is an immune-mediated disease that primarily affects the small intestine in response to dietary gluten. It is one of the most common causes of malabsorption, and only affects individuals who are genetically predisposed. The immune reaction leads to destruction of the small intestinal villi starting in the proximal duodenum. Although antibodies are produced as part of the immune reaction, they are not thought to be involved in the pathogenesis of celiac disease.

Testing

Testing should be pursued in patients with typical gastrointestinal symptoms or extraintestinal manifestations, and in those with increased risk (patients with type 1 diabetes mellitus, autoimmune thyroid disease, or a first-degree family member with celiac disease). Gastrointestinal symptoms of celiac disease typically include chronic diarrhea, bloating, and weight loss, but may also include atypical symptoms, such as constipation and dyspepsia. Other manifestations include iron deficiency anemia, bone loss, abnormal liver aminotransferase levels, neurologic symptoms, and dermatitis herpetiformis (**Figure 15**). Patients may also be asymptomatic.

Ideally, testing for celiac disease should be done while the patient is on a gluten-containing diet. The best initial step is to test for IgA tissue transglutaminase antibodies. Because IgA deficiency is more common in patients with celiac disease, total IgA levels may also need to be measured. Testing for anti-deamidated gliadin peptide IgG antibodies may also be used. Anti-endomysial antibodies are highly specific and can be

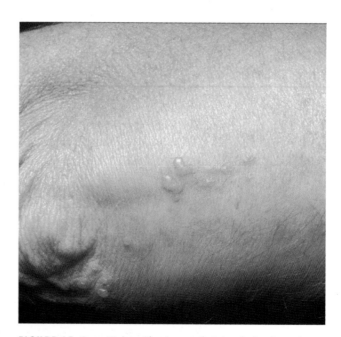

FIGURE 15. Dermatitis herpetiformis, a manifestation of celiac disease, is characterized by pruritic papules and transient, almost immediately excoriated blisters on the elbows, knees, and buttocks.

helpful in making the diagnosis of celiac disease, but measurement with immunofluorescent microscopy is not reliable. Testing for anti-gliadin antibodies (IgA and IgG) should not be used because of low sensitivity and specificity. If clinical suspicion is high and initial testing is negative, additional testing should be pursued. Antibody testing is less reliable if the patient is on a gluten-free diet. In such patients, genetic testing for *HLA-DQ2* or *HLA-DQ8* should be considered.

The vast majority of patients with celiac disease carry *HLA-DQ2* or *HLA-DQ8* genetic susceptibility; however, these genes can be found in up to 40% of the general population. Therefore, genetic testing can rule out disease but not confirm it.

Diagnosis

A positive serologic test for celiac disease requires upper endoscopy with biopsies from the duodenum for confirmation of the disease. There are specific recommendations for the biopsy procedure to minimize false-negative results. Celiac disease is confirmed by the presence of increased intraepithelial lymphocytosis and villous blunting or atrophy of the duodenal villi.

Management and Monitoring

Patients with a diagnosis of celiac disease should be educated about the gluten-free diet by a knowledgeable registered dietician. The treatment of celiac disease is lifelong avoidance of wheat, rye, and barley. Patients should be aware of gluten in medications and over-the-counter products. Dietary oats are generally safe in patients with celiac disease. Monitoring includes clinical assessment of symptoms and signs of celiac disease, assessment of dietary adherence, and confirmation of normalization of antibody levels. Repeat upper endoscopy with biopsies should be considered for individuals with ongoing symptoms while adhering to a gluten-free diet. Assessment of bone density at the time of diagnosis should be considered to ensure adequate bone health.

Nonresponsive Celiac Disease

The most common cause of refractory celiac disease symptoms is gluten exposure. When a patient's symptoms do not resolve completely with adherence to a gluten-free diet, the accuracy of the original diagnosis of celiac disease should be reassessed. Other conditions that may account for ongoing symptoms include IBS, lactose or fructose intolerance, bacterial overgrowth, microscopic colitis, or IBD. Additional evaluation to exclude these as causes is critical before considering the patient to have refractory celiac disease.

A very small number of patients develop refractory celiac disease, in which small-intestinal inflammation persists despite adherence to a strict gluten-free diet. Individuals with refractory sprue are typically older than age 65 years and present with diarrhea, weight loss, dehydration, and nutritional deficiencies. Possible medication-induced sprue should be managed by discontinuing the offending medication. Patients

with refractory celiac disease should be managed in a specialized celiac disease center.

Nonceliac Gluten Sensitivity

Nonceliac gluten sensitivity is defined by gastrointestinal and extraintestinal symptoms that occur with gluten ingestion and subside with avoidance of gluten. By definition, celiac disease must be excluded. Because gluten is a nonabsorbable carbohydrate, it can cause gastrointestinal symptoms due to osmotic mechanisms, as well as fermentation by colonic bacteria. Other than assessing symptom response after withdrawal of gluten, there is no diagnostic test for nonceliac gluten sensitivity.

KEY POINTS

- The best initial test for celiac disease is testing for IgA tissue transglutaminase antibodies.
- Up to 40% of the general population carries the *HLA-DQ2*   **HVC** or *HLA-DQ8* mutation, so genetic testing alone cannot be used to diagnose celiac disease.
- The treatment of celiac disease is lifelong avoidance of gluten.
- The most common cause of refractory celiac disease symptoms is gluten exposure.

Malabsorption

Small Intestinal Bacterial Overgrowth

Small intestinal bacterial overgrowth (SIBO) is caused by various conditions, including impaired motility, strictures (for example, in Crohn disease), or blind loops (for example, small-bowel diverticula). There is some evidence that SIBO could contribute to symptoms in IBS-D.

Classically, SIBO is defined by the presence of more than 10^5 colony-forming units per mL of jejunal aspirate. Based on its use in research studies, jejunal aspirate is considered the gold standard but is often not used in clinical practice due to the requirement for endoscopy to obtain cultures, the patchy nature of small intestinal overgrowth, and oropharyngeal contamination of the specimen. Glucose and lactulose breath tests have acceptable specificity (around 80%) but poor sensitivity (30%-40%) for diagnosing SIBO. Diagnosis requires typical symptoms and a confirmatory test, usually breath testing. Treatment consists of antibiotic therapy and often requires repeated courses if the underlying condition cannot be resolved.

Short Bowel Syndrome

Short bowel syndrome is defined by a small-intestine length of less than 200 cm, with loss of absorptive area leading to maldigestion, malabsorption, and malnutrition. Surgery for strangulated bowel, Crohn disease, ischemia, trauma, and weight loss can all lead to short bowel syndrome.

Treatment depends on whether the patient has an intact ileocecal valve and colon or an ostomy. Patients with short bowel syndrome and an ostomy usually require parenteral nutrition and hydration. Those with extensive ileal resection should be tested and treated for vitamin B_{12} deficiency. Adjunctive therapies include antimotility and antisecretory drugs. Glucagon-like peptide 2 and its analog, teduglutide, are new pharmacologic agents for treatment of short bowel syndrome. Both have been evaluated in randomized trials and found to increase intestinal wet weight absorption and decrease parenteral fluid support in patients with short bowel syndrome.

Carbohydrate Malabsorption

Carbohydrates can be classified as monosaccharides (glucose, fructose), disaccharides (lactose, sucrose), oligosaccharides (maltodextrose), or polyols (sorbitol, mannitol). These short-chain carbohydrates are osmotically active and can lead to increased luminal water retention and gas production through colonic fermentation. These two actions can cause gastrointestinal symptoms, including gas, bloating, and diarrhea.

Lactose malabsorption is commonly due to loss of the brush border lactase enzyme in adulthood. Fructose malabsorption can also lead to gastrointestinal symptoms such as bloating and diarrhea. Although both lactose and fructose breath tests are available, testing is often not required, as symptoms subside with exclusion of the sugar from the diet and recur with ingestion.

KEY POINTS

- Small intestinal bacterial overgrowth is caused by various conditions, including impaired motility, strictures, or blind loops, and is treated with antibiotic therapy.

- Short bowel syndrome is defined by a small-intestine length of less than 200 cm, resulting in maldigestion, malabsorption, and malnutrition.

- Lactose malabsorption is common, with symptoms occurring when lactose is ingested and subsiding with exclusion of lactose from the diet.

Inflammatory Bowel Disease

IBD is an idiopathic chronic inflammatory condition of the gut that includes ulcerative colitis and Crohn disease. In addition, microscopic colitis is considered a type of IBD with distinct clinical and pathologic features. The pathogenesis of IBD likely involves host genetic predisposition and abnormal immunologic responses to endogenous gut bacteria.

Risk Factors

The primary risk factor for development of IBD is family history, with a risk of approximately 10% for first-degree relatives of affected patients. Individuals of Ashkenazi Jewish descent have increased risk for IBD. Tobacco smoking increases the risk for Crohn disease and is protective for ulcerative colitis.

IBD has a bimodal age presentation, with an initial peak incidence in the second to fourth decades of life followed by a less prominent second peak in the seventh and eighth decades.

Clinical Manifestations

Ulcerative Colitis

The major symptoms of ulcerative colitis include diarrhea, abdominal discomfort, rectal bleeding, and tenesmus, with symptoms varying depending on the extent and severity of disease. Symptoms typically have a slow, insidious onset and often have been present for weeks or months by the time the patient seeks care, although ulcerative colitis may present acutely, mimicking infectious colitis.

Rectal inflammation (proctitis) causes frequent defecatory urges and passage of small liquid stools containing mucus and blood. Although bloody diarrhea is considered the hallmark presentation of ulcerative colitis, diarrhea is not always present. Patients with proctitis or proctosigmoiditis may have constipation. Abdominal pain is usually not a prominent symptom of ulcerative colitis; however, most patients with active disease experience vague lower-abdominal discomfort relieved with defecation. Physical examination in patients with mild or moderate ulcerative colitis is usually normal but may reveal mild lower-abdominal discomfort over the affected colonic segment. The presence of fever, nausea, vomiting, or severe abdominal pain indicates a severe attack or complication such as superimposed infection or toxic megacolon.

Crohn Disease

The clinical presentation of Crohn disease may be subtle and varies depending on the location and severity of inflammation along the gut axis as well as the presence of intestinal complications such as abscess, stricture, or fistula. Compared with ulcerative colitis, abdominal pain is a more common symptom of Crohn disease. The ileocecal area is the most common bowel segment affected by Crohn disease, and it often presents insidiously with mild diarrhea and abdominal cramping. Abdominal examination may reveal fullness or a tender mass in the right hypogastrium. Some patients present initially with a small-bowel obstruction caused by impaction of indigestible vegetables or fruit. Occasionally, the main presenting symptom is acute pain in the right lower quadrant, mimicking appendicitis. In patients with Crohn colitis, tenesmus is less common than in patients with ulcerative colitis because the rectum is often less inflamed than other colonic segments. Perianal disease is a common presentation of Crohn disease with anal fissures, ulcers, and stenosis.

Fistulae are a frequent manifestation of the transmural nature of Crohn disease and consist of abnormal connections between two epithelial surfaces (perianal, enteroenteric, enterocutaneous, rectovaginal, enterovesical). Drainage of fecal material from fistulae leads to symptoms such as passage of feces through the vagina (rectovaginal fistula). Intra-abdominal abscesses may form; the classic presentation is spiking fevers and focal abdominal tenderness, which may be masked by the use of glucocorticoids. Strictures represent long-standing inflammation and may occur in any segment of the gastrointestinal tract, although the terminal ileum is the most common site. Strictures may be secondary to fibrosis or severe inflammatory luminal narrowing. Patients with intestinal strictures often initially present with colicky postprandial abdominal pain and bloating that may progress to complete intestinal obstruction.

Table 20 summarizes the features of ulcerative colitis and Crohn disease.

Extraintestinal Manifestations

Inflammatory conditions involving extraintestinal structures, including the joints, eyes, liver, and skin, may occur in patients with IBD. These extraintestinal manifestations are categorized as either associated with active bowel disease or independent of bowel inflammation. Up to 30% of patients with IBD

experience an extraintestinal manifestation at some time during the course of their disease; peripheral arthritis is the most common. See MKSAP 18 Rheumatology for discussion of IBD-related arthritis.

The two most common dermatologic extraintestinal manifestations are erythema nodosum and pyoderma gangrenosum. Erythema nodosum most commonly presents as single or multiple tender nodules on extensor surfaces of the lower extremities (**Figure 16**). Pyoderma gangrenosum typically presents as a papule that rapidly develops into an ulcer with undermined and violaceous borders (**Figure 17**). Both manifestations usually correspond to underlying IBD activity. See MKSAP 18 Dermatology for discussion of cutaneous manifestations of IBD.

Ocular extraintestinal manifestations of IBD include episcleritis and uveitis. Episcleritis is more common and consists of injection of the sclera and conjunctiva. It does not affect visual acuity and occurs in association with active bowel disease. Uveitis presents with headache, blurred vision, and

TABLE 20. Features of Ulcerative Colitis and Crohn Disease		
Feature	**Ulcerative Colitis**	**Crohn Disease**
Depth of inflammation	Mucosal	Transmural
Pattern of disease	Contiguous and symmetric	Skips areas and asymmetric
Location	Colorectum	Mouth to anus
Rectal involvement	Nearly 100%	Less common
Ileal disease	Backwash ileitis (15%)	Common
Fistulas, abscess, and strictures	Rare	Common
Perianal disease	Rare	Common
Granulomas	Unlikely	In approximately 30%
Overt rectal bleeding	Common	Less common
Tobacco use	Protective	Exacerbates

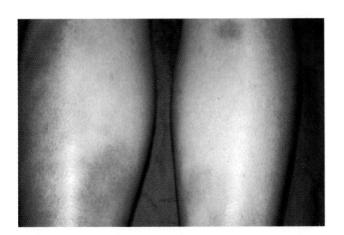

FIGURE 16. Erythema nodosum, a manifestation of inflammatory bowel disease, typically appears as ill-defined erythema overlying subcutaneous, tender nodules most commonly symmetrically located on the anterior shins.

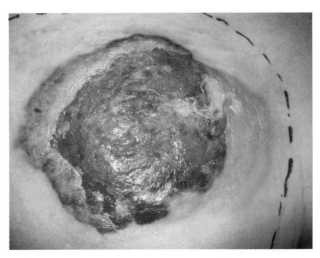

FIGURE 17. Pyoderma gangrenosum, a manifestation of inflammatory bowel disease, typically begins as a small pustule or red nodule that rapidly expands with an edematous, infiltrated, actively inflamed border and a painful, exudative wet ulcer. The border is characteristically violaceous with an edge that overhangs the ulcer.

photophobia. Uveitis is an ocular emergency requiring prompt referral to an ophthalmologist. See MKSAP 18 General Internal Medicine for discussion of episcleritis and uveitis.

Primary sclerosing cholangitis is a major liver manifestation of IBD, occurring in 5% of patients. Patients most often present with isolated elevations in the serum alkaline phosphatase level. The liver disease is typically progressive and independent of the outcome of the IBD. See Disorders of the Liver for discussion of primary sclerosing cholangitis.

Diagnosis

The diagnosis of IBD relies on the integration of the clinical presentation, exclusion of infectious enteropathogens, endoscopic appearance, histologic assessment of mucosal biopsies, and radiologic features. IBD should be considered in any patient with chronic or bloody diarrhea. It is paramount to exclude infection, particularly with *C. difficile* and Shiga toxin–producing *E. coli*, by stool tests, especially in patients with acute onset of symptoms. Fecal calprotectin should be considered to help differentiate IBD from irritable bowel syndrome. Laboratory testing helps to assess disease activity. Common findings include anemia and hypoalbuminemia. Many patients develop iron deficiency anemia from chronic blood loss. Hematologic changes, such as thrombocytosis and leukocytosis, reflect active inflammatory disease. Persistently abnormal serum alkaline phosphatase levels should prompt further investigation for primary sclerosing cholangitis.

Endoscopy (either sigmoidoscopy or colonoscopy) with biopsy is needed to help make the diagnosis of IBD. Colonoscopy is most commonly used to assess the extent and severity of disease. At presentation, 50% of patients with ulcerative colitis have disease limited to the rectum and sigmoid (proctosigmoiditis), 20% have left-sided disease (to the splenic flexure), and 30% present with pancolitis (to the cecum). Endoscopic findings range from decreased vascular pattern with erythema and edema in mild disease to large and deep ulcerations in severe disease. Histopathology characteristically shows features of chronic colitis with distorted and branching colonic crypts along with crypt abscesses.

Crohn disease has a different pattern of distribution from ulcerative colitis: 50% of patients have ileocolonic disease, 30% have isolated small bowel disease, and 20% have colonic disease. A minority of patients have isolated upper gastrointestinal tract or perianal disease in the absence of inflammation in the small bowel or colon. The earliest endoscopic findings of Crohn disease include aphthous ulcers, which can coalesce to form stellate ulcers, and a "cobblestone" mucosal appearance. A characteristic mucosal feature of Crohn disease is the so-called "skip lesion," consisting of affected areas separated by normal mucosa. Granulomatous inflammation is characteristic of Crohn disease but uncommonly found on mucosal biopsies. Histopathology in small-intestinal Crohn disease will show chronic jejunitis or ileitis, and Crohn colitis will have histology similar to that in ulcerative colitis, with exception of granulomas.

Radiographic studies establish the location, extent, and severity of IBD. Patients with a severe attack of IBD require a plain abdominal radiograph to assess for a dilated colon (indicative of evolving toxic megacolon) or small-bowel obstruction (**Figure 18**). CT or MR enterography provides information about the location and severity of small bowel disease and the presence of complicating fistula, abscess, or stricture. Video capsule endoscopy is a highly sensitive modality for detection of small inflammatory lesions of the intestine, although it is not commonly required.

Treatment

The goals of therapy for IBD are to induce and maintain remission, and to prevent disease- and treatment-related complications. Four categories of drugs are used to treat IBD: 5-aminosalicylates, glucocorticoids, immunomodulators, and biologics. Stratification based on clinical severity is important in guiding IBD management. Currently, there are no validated or consensus definitions of mild, moderate, or severe IBD. However, three domains are relevant to the evaluation of disease severity in IBD: impact of the disease on the patient (clinical symptoms, quality of life, and disability); inflammatory burden (extent, location, and severity of bowel involvement); and disease course, including structural

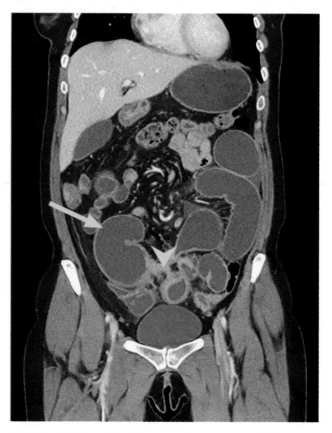

FIGURE 18. CT scan of the abdomen and pelvis in a patient with Crohn disease, showing small-bowel obstruction with dilated loops of small intestine (*arrow*) and matted loops of bowel (*arrowhead*) in the pelvis.

damage. Surgery is reserved for refractory symptoms and complications.

Patients with IBD are at markedly increased risk for venous thromboembolism. The cause of thromboembolism is multifactorial and related to severity of disease, immobilization, and hospitalization. It is important that all hospitalized patients with IBD be given venous thromboembolism prophylaxis with subcutaneous heparin. Only in cases of massive gastrointestinal bleeding with severe anemia, tachycardia, and hypotension should nonpharmacologic prophylaxis with intermittent pneumatic compression of the lower extremities be used.

Pharmacotherapy

5-Aminosalicylates

5-Aminosalicylates (5-ASAs) are believed to have an anti-inflammatory mechanism of action. Various formulations and controlled-release systems are available, with some preparations purported to deliver 5-ASAs to the small bowel.

5-ASAs are the mainstay of treatment of mild to moderate ulcerative colitis, with a dose-dependent response when used to induce disease remission. Three major factors need to be considered when choosing therapy for ulcerative colitis (**Figure 19**). Patients with proctitis or left-sided disease should receive topical therapy with 5-ASA suppositories and enemas. In mild to moderate ulcerative colitis, combined 5-ASA therapy (oral and topical) is superior for induction of remission compared with oral or topical therapies alone. Once remission is achieved, 5-ASAs are effective in maintaining it. Of the available agents, sulfasalazine has the most adverse effects, including fever, rash, nausea, vomiting, and headache. In addition, sulfasalazine may cause reversible sperm abnormalities and impair folate absorption.

Despite the availability of several formulations designed to deliver the drug to the small bowel, 5-ASAs have not proved to be efficacious in small-bowel Crohn disease.

Glucocorticoids

Oral and intravenous glucocorticoids are commonly used to treat moderate to severe flares of IBD and are effective in inducing remission. However, glucocorticoids are not effective for

maintenance therapy and have significant adverse effects. One formulation of oral budesonide is a controlled-release glucocorticoid with high first-pass metabolism in the liver and minimal systemic adverse effects. It is effective in inducing remission in mild to moderate ileocolonic Crohn disease. Another oral formulation is multimatrix (MMX) budesonide, designed to release the drug throughout the colon. It is effective in inducing remission in mild to moderate ulcerative colitis.

Immunomodulators

Thiopurines (azathioprine and mercaptopurine [6-MP]) are immunomodulators used as glucocorticoid-sparing agents. They have a slow onset of action (2-3 months) and patients require a tapering glucocorticoid regimen to bridge the time interval until the thiopurines take effect. Thiopurine methyltransferase, a key enzyme involved in the metabolism of azathioprine and 6-MP, exhibits a population polymorphism that greatly increases the risk for bone marrow toxicity with use of these agents. Therefore, before initiation of thiopurine therapy, testing for the *TPMT* genotype or phenotype (enzyme activity) is recommended to help prevent toxicity by identifying individuals with low or absent *TPMT* enzyme activity. However, regardless of *TPMT* status, all patients require monitoring with complete blood counts and liver chemistry testing because 70% of patients who develop leukopenia while using these agents do not have *TPMT* mutations. Azathioprine and 6-MP are reported to cause the rare hepatosplenic T-cell lymphoma. Azathioprine and 6-MP are effective in maintaining remission in patients with ulcerative colitis and should be considered in glucocorticoid-dependent patients. This includes patients who require two courses of glucocorticoids for induction of remission within 1 year, or patients who require intravenous glucocorticoids for acute disease flare.

Methotrexate is an immunomodulator that is beneficial in inducing and maintaining remission in Crohn disease but not in ulcerative colitis. Side effects of methotrexate include hepatotoxicity and interstitial pneumonitis, which can manifest with cough and dyspnea of insidious onset.

Biologic Agents

Tumor necrosis factor (TNF)-α is a proinflammatory cytokine that plays a critical role in the pathogenesis of both Crohn disease and ulcerative colitis. The anti-TNF agents infliximab, adalimumab, and certolizumab are used to treat moderate to severe Crohn disease. Infliximab is administered by intravenous infusion; adalimumab and certolizumab are given subcutaneously. Combination therapy with infliximab and azathioprine is more efficacious than monotherapy with either agent alone in achieving glucocorticoid-free remission and mucosal healing. There is increasing evidence for the use of biologic agents early in the course of disease. Before initiation of anti-TNF agents, patients should undergo testing for latent tuberculosis because of an increased risk for reactivation of tuberculosis during therapy. If latent tuberculosis is present,

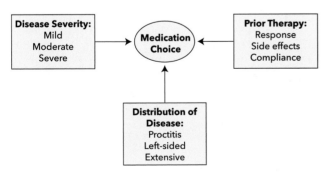

FIGURE 19. Factors to consider when choosing medical therapy for ulcerative colitis.

treatment with isoniazid should occur for at least 2 months before initiation of anti-TNF therapy. Patients should also be assessed for chronic hepatitis B viral infection before starting anti-TNF therapy and receive treatment if needed.

The anti-TNF agents infliximab, adalimumab, and golimumab are used to treat moderate to severe ulcerative colitis. Combination therapy with infliximab and azathioprine is more effective than monotherapy with either agent in achieving glucocorticoid-free remission and mucosal healing.

The anti-adhesion agents natalizumab and vedolizumab are effective in inducing and maintaining remission for moderate to severe Crohn disease. Ustekinumab, a monoclonal antibody that blocks the biologic activity of interleukin-12 and -23 by inhibiting receptors for these cytokines on T-cells, is efficacious in severe Crohn disease. These agents are typically used after anti-TNF therapies prove ineffective.

Surgery

Indications for surgery in patients with Crohn disease include medically refractory fistula, fibrotic stricture with obstructive symptoms, symptoms refractory to medical therapy, and cancer. The guiding principle of surgery in Crohn disease is the preservation of bowel length and function, as the rate of disease recurrence after segmental resection is high. Patients with Crohn disease who undergo surgery require aggressive pharmacologic treatment with anti-TNF agents and/or immunomodulators to decrease the rate of postoperative recurrence of Crohn disease.

In patients with ulcerative colitis, total proctocolectomy with end-ileostomy or ileal pouch-anal anastomosis is performed for medically refractory disease, toxic megacolon, or carcinoma.

Health Care Considerations

Patients with IBD are at increased risk for vaccine-preventable illnesses, and vaccines are underutilized in this patient population. Inactivated vaccines can be safely administered to all patients with IBD, regardless of immunosuppression. Patients with IBD should receive a seasonal influenza vaccine as well as the 13-valent pneumococcal conjugate vaccine and the 23-valent pneumococcal polysaccharide vaccine. Ideally, pneumococcal vaccination should occur before beginning immunosuppressive therapy. Live vaccines such as measles, mumps, rubella; varicella; and herpes zoster are contraindicated in immunosuppressed patients with IBD. See MKSAP 18 General Internal Medicine for discussion of vaccination strategies.

Women with IBD are at increased risk for developing cervical dysplasia; this risk is greater in women with Crohn disease than in those with ulcerative colitis, and is also greater in women using immunosuppressive therapy. Women with IBD should undergo Pap testing annually, and human papillomavirus vaccination is recommended.

All patients with IBD should be encouraged to stop smoking. Smoking increases Crohn disease activity and the risk for

extraintestinal manifestations. Patients with IBD are at increased risk for metabolic bone disease due to use of glucocorticoids and diminished vitamin D and calcium absorption. Patients with Crohn disease are at greater risk than those with ulcerative colitis. Screening for osteoporosis should be considered in patients at increased risk.

Patients with IBD are at increased risk for developing cancers of the colorectum, cervix, and skin. Longstanding inflammation of the colorectum increases the risk for cancer. In patients with IBD (ulcerative colitis with disease proximal to the sigmoid colon and Crohn disease with more than one third of the colon involved), surveillance colonoscopy should begin 8 years after diagnosis and recur every 1 to 2 years thereafter. Primary sclerosing cholangitis increases the risk for colorectal cancer, and surveillance colonoscopy should begin at the time of diagnosis and recur yearly thereafter.

Patients with IBD are at increased risk for both melanoma and nonmelanoma skin cancers. Most of the risk has been associated with specific treatments; however, there is some evidence that IBD is associated with an increased risk for melanoma, independent of treatment. All patients with IBD should be advised to use sunscreen, wear protective clothing, avoid tanning beds, and have a yearly skin examination.

Microscopic Colitis

Microscopic colitis is a distinct type of IBD characterized by macroscopically normal mucosa with inflammatory changes seen only on histopathology of colon biopsies. It is subclassified into lymphocytic colitis and collagenous colitis (**Figure 20**) based on predominating histologic features. It predominantly affects middle-aged women and is associated with other autoimmune conditions, particularly celiac disease. It presents with abrupt or gradual onset of watery diarrhea that has a relapsing and remitting course over months to years, sometimes accompanied by mild weight loss.

Several classes of medications, including NSAIDs, selective serotonin reuptake inhibitors, and proton pump inhibitors

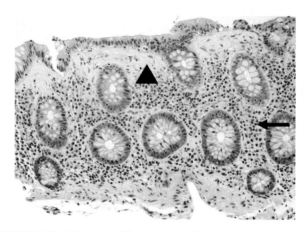

FIGURE 20. Collagenous colitis: colon mucosal biopsy showing a pink, abnormal subepithelial collagen band (*arrowhead*) and lamina propria expanded by inflammatory cells (*arrow*).

have been associated with development of microscopic colitis. The first step in management is to discontinue any potentially causative medication. First-line treatments include supportive treatment with antidiarrheal agents such loperamide or bismuth subsalicylate. The next step is oral budesonide, which is efficacious but has a high rate of recurrent symptoms when discontinued. Unlike Crohn disease and ulcerative colitis, there is no long-term increased risk for colorectal cancer in patients with microscopic colitis.

KEY POINTS

- The major symptoms of ulcerative colitis include diarrhea, abdominal discomfort, rectal bleeding, and tenesmus, with a slow onset of symptoms.
- Fistula, abscess, and stricture are characteristic complications of Crohn disease.
- Endoscopy with biopsy is needed to help make the diagnosis of inflammatory bowel disease.
- The goals of therapy are to induce and maintain remission of inflammatory bowel disease, and to prevent disease- and treatment-related complications.
- Unlike patients with Crohn disease or ulcerative colitis, patients with microscopic colitis are not at increased risk for colorectal cancer.

Constipation

Constipation is one of the most common gastrointestinal symptoms, affecting 20% of the general population. Constipation can present with symptoms including infrequent, difficult, or incomplete defecation. It can be acute or chronic, and either secondary or idiopathic in nature. Medications are the most common cause of secondary constipation; other causes include mechanical obstruction, systemic illnesses, altered physiologic states, and psychosocial conditions (**Table 21**).

Once secondary causes have been excluded, chronic constipation is considered to be functional (idiopathic). The definition of functional constipation has been refined by the fourth Rome working group for functional gastrointestinal disorders. Functional constipation is subtyped into categories of slow transit, normal transit, or dyssynergic defecation. Slow transit constipation is defined as the delayed passage of fecal contents through the colon based on objective transit testing (radiopaque marker study, scintigraphy, or the wireless motility capsule). Normal transit constipation is idiopathic constipation in which colonic transit times are adequate based on objective transit testing. Dyssynergic defecation (also termed pelvic floor dyssynergia, obstructed defecation, or outlet obstruction) refers to difficulty with or inability to expel stool as a result of some combination of abnormalities in contraction and/or relaxation of the muscles of the pelvic floor during defecation. In some cases, functional constipation can be the result of slow transit constipation and coexistent dyssynergic defecation.

TABLE 21. Secondary Causes of Constipation

Medications

Opioids

Antidiarrheals

Anticholinergics (antispasmodics, antiparkinsonian drugs, tricyclic antidepressants, antipsychotics)

Antihistamines

NSAIDs

Iron supplements

Calcium supplements

Bismuth

Antihypertensives (calcium channel blockers, diuretics, clonidine)

Serotonergic antagonists (ondansetron)

Mechanical Causes

Colorectal cancer

Rectocele

Rectal intussusception

Rectal prolapse

Sigmoidocele

Enterocele

Anastomotic stricture

Anal stenosis/stricture

Extrinsic compression from pelvic/abdominal process

Systemic Illnesses

Endocrinologic
- Diabetes mellitus
- Hypothyroidism
- Panhypopituitarism
- Pheochromocytoma
- Glucagonoma

Neuropathy/myopathy

Altered Physiologic State

Hypercalcemia

Hypokalemia

Pregnancy

Porphyria

Heavy-metal poisoning (arsenic, lead, mercury)

Psychosocial

Depression

Cognitive impairment

Immobility

Evaluation

A careful medical, surgical, and medication history identifies most causes of secondary constipation. The medication history should focus on the temporal relationship between medications and the development of constipation symptoms. The history should include an assessment for the presence of alarm features: hematochezia, acute constipation in elderly patients, unintentional weight loss, family history of colorectal cancer, unexplained anemia, and age older than 50 years with no previous colonoscopy. Anorectal examination, including a digital examination during Valsalva maneuver, is an important part of the physical examination because it may identify anatomic or functional causes of an evacuation disorder.

A flat plate radiograph of the abdomen is the most useful initial study because it can assess for the presence and distribution of excessive stool in the colon and/or rectum. Colonoscopy is used to assess blood in the stool, a sudden change in bowel habits, or unexplained anemia. It is also used for colon cancer screening in patients at average and increased risk due to family history of colorectal cancer. Additional imaging or laboratory studies should only be considered if clinically indicated. Physiologic testing, including colon transit testing, anorectal manometry, balloon expulsion testing, or defecography, is reserved for patients with constipation symptoms that do not respond to initial trials of laxative therapy.

Functional (idiopathic) constipation is diagnosed once secondary causes have been excluded.

Management

Various treatment strategies may benefit patients with constipation when lifestyle and dietary interventions have been ineffective. Treatment options include bulking agents, stimulant laxatives, osmotic laxatives, stool softeners, secretagogues, and/or biofeedback (**Table 22**). The evidence for treatment

TABLE 22. Treatments for Constipation

Intervention	Mechanism of Action	Considerations
Bulk Laxative Soluble fiber (psyllium, methylcellulose, calcium polycarbophil, wheat dextrin) Insoluble fiber (bran, rye, flax seed)	Increases ability of stool to retain water Bulks stool Speeds movement of stool through colon	Start with a low dose and increase slowly Soluble fiber works better than insoluble fiber Bloating, distension, flatulence, and cramping may be limiting
Stool Softener Docusate sodium, docusate calcium	A detergent that allows water to penetrate the stool	Minimal effectiveness in clinical trials Only role is in mild constipation symptoms Well tolerated Few side effects
Osmotic Laxative Polyethylene glycol 3350 Lactulose Magnesium hydroxide/magnesium citrate Sorbitol	Poorly absorbed compounds Creates an osmotic gradient Water moves into the bowel lumen	Polyethylene glycol 3350 and lactulose improve stool frequency and consistency; others have not been tested in clinical trials Bloating and gas can be limiting Caution with use of magnesium in renal insufficiency
Stimulant Laxative Anthraquinones (senna, cascara) Diphenylmethanes (bisacodyl, sodium picosulfate)	Irritates the colon wall, increasing contractions Stimulates sensory nerves lining the colon May inhibit water absorption in the colon	Quickest acting (works within 8-12 hours of ingestion) Senna can cause melanosis coli (benign pigmentation of the colon) Diarrhea, cramping, bloating, and nausea can be limiting
Secretagogue Lubiprostone Linaclotide Plecanatide	Lubiprostone activates type-2 chloride channels on enterocytes lining the gut lumen, causing chloride ions to move into the colonic lumen with sodium and water following the ionic gradient Linaclotide and plecanatide activate guanylate cyclase C receptors on enterocytes, leading to chloride channel activation through a series of processes within the cell	Lubiprostone improves stool form and frequency, straining, and abdominal pain; nausea is a common side effect Linaclotide and plecanatide improve stool form and frequency, straining, bloating, and abdominal pain; diarrhea is a common side effect
Serotonergic Agent Prucalopride	Increases intestinal contractions Increases intestinal secretion	Not available in the United States Available in Canada and Europe
Neuromuscular Reeducation (biofeedback)	Retrains the skeletal muscle involved in defecation (abdominal wall, pelvic floor, anorectal) Corrects altered rectal sensation	Effective for dyssynergic defecation Requires a specially trained physical therapist

efficacy is strongest for polyethylene glycol, lubiprostone, and linaclotide. Fiber supplements, polyethylene glycol, magnesium, senna, docusate, and bisacodyl have the advantage of being available without a prescription. For refractory cases of constipation, combination therapy should include agents with different mechanisms of action, such as an osmotic plus a stimulant laxative.

Although lubiprostone has an FDA indication for the treatment of opioid-induced constipation, initial treatment should be the same as for other forms of constipation. Three peripherally acting μ-opioid receptor antagonists (methylnaltrexone, naloxegol, and alvimopan) have also been approved for the treatment of opioid-induced constipation in selected patients.

KEY POINTS

- The most common cause of secondary constipation is medication.
- Treatment strategies include dietary and lifestyle modification, addressing causes of secondary constipation, and various pharmacologic agents.

Irritable Bowel Syndrome

IBS represents a heterogeneous group of functional bowel disorders defined by the presence of abdominal pain in association with defecation and/or a change in bowel habits. Abdominal pain may worsen or subside with defecation. The altered bowel habits may include constipation, diarrhea, or a mix of both types. Other commonly reported symptoms include abdominal bloating and abdominal distention. The exact cause of IBS remains unknown, and there are no all-encompassing pathophysiologic mechanisms to explain the symptoms. IBS is more common in women and adults younger than age 50 years, and is frequently seen in association with psychosocial disturbance. There are no specific anatomic or physiologic abnormalities, nor are there any reliable biomarkers to define IBS. The diagnosis of IBS requires symptoms of recurrent abdominal pain at least 1 day a week for a period of 3 months, along with at least two of the following three additional criteria: pain related to defecation, change in stool frequency, or change in stool consistency. IBS can then be further subtyped into IBS with predominant constipation (IBS-C), IBS with predominant diarrhea (IBS-D), IBS with mixed bowel habits, or IBS unclassified.

Evaluation

The diagnosis of IBS is no longer one of exclusion; instead, the diagnosis can reliably be made by clinical criteria in the absence of alarm features. Therefore, evaluation for IBS relies on a comprehensive history and physical examination.

Management

Management of IBS includes lifestyle and dietary modifications, and reassurance that the disease is benign. The focus is

control of symptoms. There is limited evidence to suggest that exercise, stress management, and correction of impaired sleep can alleviate the symptoms of IBS.

The most common dietary intervention is an increase in fiber, either through diet or use of fiber supplements. Water-soluble fiber supplements such as psyllium are more effective than insoluble dietary fiber such as bran. Dietary restrictions can include avoidance of trigger foods, gluten (in the absence of celiac disease), dairy products, and FODMAPs (see Table 19). Randomized trials have shown that a low-FODMAP diet alleviates symptoms in patients with IBS. When these initial measures fail to relieve symptoms, medications, typically directed at the primary symptoms of IBS such constipation, diarrhea, or abdominal pain, are employed. The evidence supporting the use of the various agents is variable, with few rigorous studies showing long-term effectiveness.

Therapy for Irritable Bowel Syndrome with Predominant Constipation

Several peripherally acting medications have demonstrated efficacy and safety in the treatment of IBS-C (see Table 22). The American Gastroenterological Association (AGA) has given a strong recommendation based on high-quality evidence for the use of linaclotide, followed by a conditional recommendation for the use of lubiprostone based on moderate-quality evidence and a conditional recommendation for the use of polyethylene glycol based on low-quality evidence in the treatment of IBS-C. Probiotics may offer benefit particularly for symptoms of pain, bloating, and flatulence, although specifics regarding the most beneficial species and strains is unknown.

Therapy for Irritable Bowel Syndrome with Predominant Diarrhea

Prescription medications with FDA approval for the treatment of IBS-D include rifaximin, eluxadoline, and alosetron. A 14-day course of rifaximin has shown superiority to placebo in relieving the global symptoms, bloating, abdominal pain, and loose stools associated with IBS-D for up to 10 weeks after treatment. A retreatment study of patients with recurring IBS-D symptoms after an initial course of rifaximin showed that a second 14-day treatment of rifaximin was superior to placebo in relieving abdominal pain and improving stool frequency for 4 weeks after treatment.

Eluxadoline (combination of a μ-opioid receptor agonist and a δ-opioid receptor antagonist) was superior to placebo in the treatment of men and women with IBS-D for up to 26 weeks based on a composite response of decreased abdominal pain and improved stool consistency in two randomized trials. Use of eluxadoline is contraindicated in patients without a gallbladder and in those with known or suspected biliary obstruction, Sphincter of Oddi disease or dysfunction, ingestion of three or more alcoholic beverages a day, history of pancreatitis or structural disease of the pancreas, severe hepatic impairment, or history of severe constipation.

Alosetron (a selective 5-HT$_3$ antagonist) has alleviated abdominal pain and the global symptoms of women with IBS-D in pooled data from several randomized trials. The AGA has given it a conditional recommendation for the treatment of women with IBS-D based on moderate-quality evidence. Due to the risk for severe constipation and ischemic colitis, prescribers must be enrolled in an FDA-mandated risk evaluation and mitigation strategy program in order to prescribe alosetron.

Other medications with clinical evidence for the treatment of IBS-D include loperamide, antispasmodics, and tricyclic antidepressants. The AGA has given a conditional recommendation for loperamide use in patients with IBS-D. Although loperamide has not demonstrated global relief of IBS-D symptoms, this recommendation is based on its ability to reduce stool frequency in other diarrheal conditions, as well as its low cost, favorable safety profile, and wide availability. Antispasmodics (for example, cimetropium-dicyclomine, peppermint oil, pinaverium, and trimebutine) decreased abdominal pain and global symptoms of IBS in a meta-analysis of 22 randomized trials. Although the overall quality of studies was low, the AGA gave a conditional recommendation for the use of antispasmodics in IBS-D. Based on data from several randomized trials, tricyclic antidepressants offer modest relief of the abdominal pain and global symptoms of IBS-D. The AGA has given a conditional recommendation based on low-quality evidence for the use of tricyclic antidepressants in the treatment of IBS-D.

KEY POINTS

- Irritable bowel syndrome is diagnosed based on clinical criteria and is no longer a diagnosis of exclusion.
- **HVC** Many cases of irritable bowel syndrome can be effectively managed with reassurance, lifestyle modifications, and dietary modifications.
- Pharmacotherapy should target predominant symptoms and be used if conservative treatment is not effective.

Management of Patients with Indeterminate Abdominal Pain

When abdominal pain is the primary symptom and is unrelated to food intake and defecation, centrally mediated abdominal pain syndrome (CAPS) should be considered. Abdominal pain is described as constant, nearly constant, or frequently recurring. The pain is not localized and may include extraintestinal symptoms such as musculoskeletal pain. It can be associated with impairment in activities of daily living and psychosocial issues. CAPS is a result of central sensitization with disinhibition of pain signals. Limited evaluation is needed in the setting of chronic pain meeting the diagnostic criteria for CAPS. Initial evaluation should include a detailed medical and psychosocial history, physical examination, and limited laboratory studies to exclude gastrointestinal bleeding and inflammation.

Successful treatment depends on the patient-physician relationship, and should focus on setting appropriate goals and expectations. A combination of pharmacologic and/or psychological therapies may be needed, including tricyclic antidepressants, selective serotonin reuptake inhibitors, or serotonin-norepinephrine reuptake inhibitors. Four classes of psychotherapy have shown benefits in CAPS when combined with medical therapy: cognitive-behavioral therapy, psychodynamic-interpersonal therapy, mindfulness- and acceptance-based therapy, and hypnotherapy.

Narcotic bowel syndrome, also known as opiate-induced gastrointestinal hyperalgesia, is characterized by the paradoxical increase in abdominal pain with increasing doses of narcotics despite clinical evidence showing improvement or stability of the underlying condition. Often these patients fear tapering off narcotics and believe the narcotics are "the only thing that helps." The only treatment is complete detoxification and cessation of narcotic use, which requires a trusting patient-physician relationship and understanding of the pathophysiology of the pain. Enrollment in a supervised detoxification program is recommended.

KEY POINTS

- The evaluation for centrally mediated pain syndrome in the setting of chronic abdominal pain requires a detailed medical and psychosocial history and physical examination with limited laboratory testing. **HVC**
- Narcotic bowel syndrome, also known as opiate-induced gastrointestinal hyperalgesia, is characterized by the paradoxical increase in abdominal pain with increasing doses of narcotics.

Diverticular Disease

A diverticulum is the herniation of the mucosa and submucosa through a weakness in the muscle wall. Diverticulosis (the presence of diverticula) is the most common finding identified during colonoscopy. Most patients with diverticulosis are asymptomatic, but 15% will develop complications. The causative mechanism is thought to be multifactorial, involving diet, microbiota, genetics, and colonic motility. The incidence of diverticulosis continues to rise in the Western world and increases with age, with a reported prevalence of 80% in persons aged 85 years and older. Diverticulosis may also cause bleeding, more commonly in the right colon, which often resolves spontaneously.

Diverticulitis is the consequence of a diverticulum becoming blocked, trapping bacteria, and subsequently developing inflammation. Diverticulitis can be classified as uncomplicated or complicated. In some patients, a focal area of colitis can develop in a segment of diverticulosis, called segmental colitis associated with diverticulosis.

The clinical presentation of uncomplicated diverticulitis is colicky abdominal pain that is relieved with flatus or a bowel movement. On physical examination, left-lower-quadrant abdominal tenderness is often present. Patients with complicated diverticulitis may present with dysuria, urinary frequency, pneumaturia, fecaluria, and recurrent urinary infection concerning for colovesical fistula. It is uncommon for patients with diverticulitis to present with rectal bleeding.

Acute diverticulitis is often a clinical diagnosis, usually not requiring imaging. However, a CT scan will help to differentiate uncomplicated from complicated diverticulitis.

The medical management of diverticulitis is based on the degree of the patient's symptoms and severity of diverticular disease. Uncomplicated diverticulitis is treated with oral antibiotics (ciprofloxacin or metronidazole) and a liquid diet. Intravenous antibiotics and hospitalization are required in patients unable to tolerate an oral diet; patients with severe comorbidities, advanced age, or immunosuppression; and patients for whom oral antibiotics have been ineffective.

Treatment of complicated diverticulitis depends on the severity of illness and CT findings. If the CT scan shows a large (>5 cm) abscess, CT-guided drainage may be needed. Surgery is indicated for patients presenting with, or who develop, peritonitis or persistent sepsis.

A high-fiber diet is recommended to prevent recurrence of diverticulitis. There is no evidence supporting restriction of foods such as nuts, berries, and seeds to prevent recurrent diverticulitis.

KEY POINTS

- Diverticulitis is the consequence of a diverticulum becoming blocked, trapping bacteria, and subsequently developing inflammation.

- The main presenting symptom of diverticulitis is colicky abdominal pain that is relieved with flatus or a bowel movement.

HVC
- Acute diverticulitis is often a clinical diagnosis, usually not requiring abdominal imaging.

Ischemic Bowel Disease

Ischemic bowel disease is a broad term describing a decrease in blood flow to the small or large intestine, which is insufficient to meet intestinal cellular metabolic function. It represents a spectrum of conditions that can be related to acute or chronic alterations of arterial or venous intestinal blood flow. Ischemic bowel disease can be broadly subcategorized into three major clinical syndromes: acute mesenteric ischemia, chronic mesenteric ischemia, and colonic ischemia.

Acute Mesenteric Ischemia

Clinical Features

Acute mesenteric ischemia (AMI) is a rare condition caused by an abrupt decrease in blood flow to the small intestine that can be obstructive or nonobstructive in nature. Obstructive causes of AMI include emboli from a cardiac source (such as atrial or ventricular thrombus) or thrombosis related to underlying atherosclerotic disease. Nonobstructive AMI is most commonly caused by vasoconstriction of the mesenteric vasculature in the setting of severe sepsis or marked reduction in effective circulating volume (low-flow states). Mesenteric vein thrombosis may cause AMI and often is associated with malignancy, hypercoagulable states, or intra-abdominal inflammatory conditions. If the reduction of blood flow is prolonged, bowel infarction occurs, which is the most important prognostic factor for adverse outcome.

AMI most commonly presents with abrupt onset of severe, periumbilical abdominal pain followed by the urge to defecate. The abdominal pain is constant and the patient may subsequently have loose, nonbloody stools. Hematochezia occurs in a minority of cases of AMI (15%) and its presence signifies concomitant right colon ischemia. In the early course of AMI, the abdominal examination may be falsely reassuring: despite the patient's reporting severe abdominal pain, the physical examination reveals a soft, nontender, nondistended abdomen without peritoneal signs. This is called "pain out of proportion to physical examination findings" and should immediately raise suspicion for early AMI. With delayed or late presentation, intestinal ischemia progresses to infarction and peritoneal signs develop. This represents late AMI, which carries a high mortality rate.

Diagnosis

Laboratory studies and abdominal imaging findings in the early course of AMI, before the development of intestinal infarction, are nonspecific. Most patients with AMI will have elevated leukocyte counts. A serum lactate concentration may be normal, and this should not exclude the diagnosis.

CT angiography is the recommended method of imaging for the diagnosis of AMI. CT angiography depicts the vessel origins and length of vessels, and characterizes the occlusion. While MR angiography avoids the risks of radiation and contrast exposure, it takes longer and is less sensitive for distal and nonocclusive disease. Duplex ultrasonography is an effective, low-cost method to assess the proximal mesenteric vessels, but an adequate ultrasound examination often cannot be performed in patients with AMI. The classic angiographic finding in obstructive AMI is either an embolus or thrombus in the superior mesenteric artery.

Treatment

After aggressive resuscitation and administration of broad-spectrum antibiotics, angiography with selective catheterization of the mesenteric vessels is indicated. Findings signifying mesenteric infarction, such as pneumatosis intestinalis (presence of gas within the wall of the intestine) or portal venous gas, require emergent surgery.

Chronic Mesenteric Ischemia

Clinical Features

Chronic mesenteric ischemia (CMI) is an uncommon condition that involves a gradual decrease in blood flow to the small intestine over months to years. It most commonly results from atherosclerotic narrowing of the mesenteric arteries. CMI occurs when two of the three adjacent mesenteric vessels (celiac, superior mesenteric, and inferior mesenteric) are severely narrowed.

The classic symptom triad of CMI is postprandial abdominal pain, sitophobia (fear of eating), and weight loss. However, this triad is seen in only 30% of patients with CMI, and CMI should be suspected in the setting of recurrent postprandial abdominal pain. The pain begins approximately 30 minutes after food ingestion and results from "shunting of blood" away from the small intestine to meet the increased functional demand of the stomach. Due to fixed narrowing of the mesenteric arteries, blood flow cannot increase sufficiently to meet the intestinal metabolic demand and ischemia results.

Diagnosis

The diagnosis of CMI requires symptoms (the CMI triad), exclusion of alternative causes of postprandial abdominal pain and weight loss, and compatible radiographic findings. Imaging modality should be chosen based on patient characteristics and availability. CT or MR angiogram findings suggestive of CMI include severe stenosis (>70%) of two of the three mesenteric arteries. If the patient has compatible symptoms and suggestive angiographic findings, and alternative explanations for postprandial abdominal pain have been excluded, then the diagnosis of CMI is secure.

Treatment

CMI is treated with percutaneous endovascular stenting or surgical revascularization. Choice of therapy depends on operative risk and occlusive lesion characteristics. Periprocedural morbidity and mortality are lower with endovascular stenting; however, it is less durable than surgical revascularization.

Colonic Ischemia

Colonic ischemia is the most common form of ischemic bowel disease. It most commonly results from a nonocclusive low-flow state in microvessels, which occurs in the setting of hypovolemia or hypotension. Risk factors include age (older than 60 years), female sex, vasoconstrictive medications, constipation, thrombophilia, and COPD.

Clinical Features

Colonic ischemia presents with the abrupt onset of lower abdominal discomfort that is mild to moderate and cramping, and is followed within 24 hours by hematochezia. The onset of bleeding often prompts the patient to seek medical attention.

Diagnosis

Physical examination most commonly reveals mild lower abdominal tenderness over the involved bowel segment without peritoneal signs. Laboratory studies may show a mild elevation in the leukocyte count and blood urea nitrogen level.

Abdominal CT is indicated to assess the severity, phase, and distribution of colonic ischemia. CT findings in colonic ischemia are nonspecific and include bowel-wall thickening (**Figure 21**) and pericolonic fat stranding (increase in density within the pericolonic fat secondary to inflammation). Infections that can mimic colonic ischemia, such as cytomegalovirus, *C. difficile*, and enterohemorrhagic *E. coli*, must be excluded. Colonoscopy with biopsy is the test of choice to confirm the diagnosis of colonic ischemia.

Because colonic ischemia is most commonly caused by a nonocclusive low-flow state, dedicated imaging of the mesenteric vasculature is of low yield and generally not indicated. The exception to this rule is right-sided colonic ischemia, which can be the harbinger of AMI caused by a focal thrombus or embolus of the superior mesenteric artery. Therefore, patients with right-sided colonic ischemia require noninvasive imaging of the mesenteric vasculature to exclude occlusive process of the superior mesenteric artery.

Treatment

Most cases of colonic ischemia are mild and transient with rapid spontaneous resolution. Patients with more severe

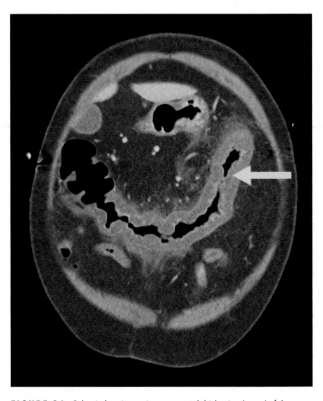

FIGURE 21. Colon ischemia causing segmental thickening (*arrow*) of the transverse colon wall on CT.

disease require hospitalization for supportive care with bowel rest, restoration of intravascular volume, antimicrobial therapy in select cases, and close observation. Only a small percentage of patients require operative intervention for necrotic bowel or irreversible complications such as stricture.

KEY POINTS

- Acute abdominal pain out of proportion to physical examination findings should immediately raise suspicion for early acute mesenteric ischemia.

- CT angiography is the recommended imaging method for the diagnosis of acute mesenteric ischemia.

- The classic symptom triad of chronic mesenteric ischemia is postprandial abdominal pain, sitophobia (fear of eating), and weight loss.

- Colonic ischemia is the most common form of ischemic bowel disease, and most cases resolve spontaneously and rapidly.

Anorectal Disorders

Perianal Disorders

Perianal disorders can range from relatively common and benign disorders, such as hemorrhoids, to potentially disabling conditions, such as anal fissure or fecal incontinence, to the life-threatening condition of anal cancer. Perianal symptoms, including bright red blood per rectum, anal pain, anal itching, or a reported anal mass, should prompt a detailed evaluation of the anus, anal canal, and rectum that includes visual inspection of the anus and digital rectal examination. Further evaluation with anoscopy or proctoscopy may be required to establish the diagnosis. Colonoscopy is indicated when additional alarm features are present; these include age older than 50 years, altered bowel habits, anemia, IBD, unexplained weight loss, and/or family history of colorectal cancer.

Hemorrhoids

Hemorrhoids are submucosal, arteriovenous sinusoids that are part of normal anorectal anatomy and are believed to play an important role in anal canal function. Risk factors for symptomatic hemorrhoids include ascites, pregnancy, excessive sitting or squatting, systemic rheumatic disorders, low dietary-fiber intake, obesity, and sedentary lifestyle. Recurrent straining and persistent bowel alterations (either constipation or diarrhea) can lead to engorgement of hemorrhoid plexuses, causing symptoms of bleeding, prolapse, and swelling. Age-related changes can cause the hemorrhoid beds to slide back and forth during defecation, resulting in mucoid anal discharge, as well as perianal wetness, soiling, irritation, and/or pruritus. Pain is not a common symptom of uncomplicated hemorrhoids and should raise suspicion for hemorrhoid complications, including thrombosis, ischemia, or incarceration from prolapse, or for an alternative diagnosis such as anal fissure, perirectal infection, or perianal abscess.

Other conditions to consider in the differential diagnosis are perianal dermatitis, lichen sclerosis, condyloma, solitary rectal ulcer syndrome, colorectal or anal polyps or cancer, and IBD. Hemorrhoids are categorized as internal if proximal to the dentate line, external if distal to the dentate line, or mixed if crossing the dentate line.

The evaluation of hemorrhoids should always include a careful perianal and digital rectal examination. Symptomatic hemorrhoids can be confused with rectal mucosal prolapse, full thickness rectal prolapse, or a prolapsed rectal polyp. The presence of prolapsed concentric folds indicates rectal prolapse as opposed to a prolapsed hemorrhoid or anal polyp (**Figure 22**). Further direct evaluation of the anorectum can be considered with anoscopy or flexible sigmoidoscopy.

First-line therapy for hemorrhoids includes increased fiber intake, adequate liquid intake, and avoidance of straining. Although various topical agents may reduce hemorrhoid symptoms, they are not necessary for curative therapy. Patients with internal hemorrhoids unresponsive to medical therapy should be considered for banding. Other options, including sclerotherapy and infrared coagulation, are less effective.

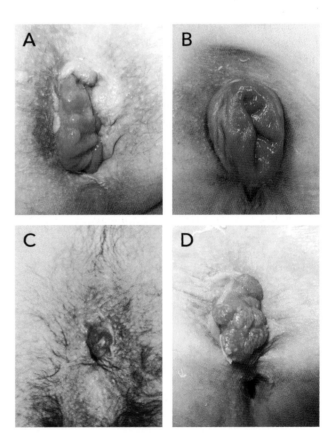

FIGURE 22. Hemorrhoids are vascular cushions that support the muscles of the anal sphincter by swelling up as needed to maintain stool continence. Prolapsed hemorrhoids (A) are internal hemorrhoids that protrude out of the rectum. The hallmark of rectal prolapse (B) is the identification of concentric rings of the rectum protruding through the anus. Prolapsed polyps (C, D) present as mucosa-covered globular masses protruding from the anus.

Images courtesy of Richard E. Burney, MD, Professor of Surgery, Michigan Medicine at the University of Michigan.

Thrombosed external hemorrhoids are best treated with surgical excision within 72 hours of symptom onset. Surgical hemorrhoidectomy should be reserved for refractory hemorrhoids, large external hemorrhoids, or combined internal and external hemorrhoids with rectal prolapse.

Anal Fissure

Anal fissures are longitudinal mucosal tears in the anal canal characterized by anorectal pain worsened by bowel movements and sitting (**Figure 23**). Rectal bleeding with bowel movements or wiping is frequently reported. Anal fissures are either idiopathic or the result of trauma due to the passage of hard stool, receptive anal intercourse, or the insertion of a foreign body such as an enema or endoscope. Anal fissures occurring laterally should raise concern for other entities including Crohn disease, ulcerative colitis, tuberculosis, syphilis, HIV, psoriasis, or anal cancer. Anal fissures lasting more than 8 to 12 weeks are considered chronic and may be characterized by edema and fibrosis as well as the presence of a sentinel pile (appearing as a skin tag) or hypertrophied anal papilla within the anal canal.

Acute anal fissures generally resolve within a few weeks with the use of sitz baths, psyllium, and bulking agents. Topical anesthetics and anti-inflammatory agents can be considered to address pain or bleeding, but their use is not required to promote fissure healing. Rectal spasm is the major reason for anal fissures becoming chronic and should be treated with either topical calcium channel blockers or nitrates. Patients with chronic fissures unresponsive to these measures should be referred for internal sphincter botulinum toxin injection or surgical sphincterotomy.

Fecal Incontinence

Fecal incontinence, also called accidental bowel leakage, is defined as the recurrent, uncontrolled passage of fecal material

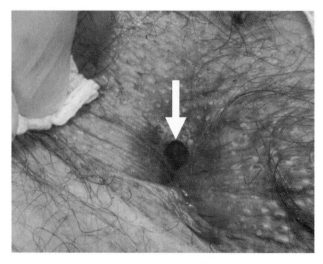

FIGURE 23. Anal fissures are painful longitudinal mucosal tears in the anal canal.

Image courtesy of Richard E. Burney, MD, Professor of Surgery, Michigan Medicine at the University of Michigan.

of at least 3 months' duration. Fecal incontinence does not include the passage of clear mucus or flatus incontinence. Fecal incontinence is grossly underreported due to associated embarrassment, and health care providers should inquire about it during clinic visits, particularly in patients at risk. Fecal incontinence is more common in multiparous women and in patients with advanced age, obesity, diarrhea or urinary incontinence, or history of obstetric complications, anorectal surgery or anorectal disease. Various factors can contribute to fecal incontinence, including loose stool, impairment of rectal storage capacity, altered rectal sensation, and reduced anal sphincter tone. Constipation with resultant fecal loading and overflow diarrhea can also cause fecal incontinence.

A digital rectal examination is essential in the evaluation. This can identify reduced anal sphincter tone, prolapse of hemorrhoids or rectum, or rectal stool impaction. Additional diagnostic testing is determined by the history and rectal examination. If fecal loading is suspected, an abdominal radiograph can be diagnostic. If diarrhea is present, stool testing and/or colonoscopy should be considered. If weak sphincter tone is appreciated or rectal urgency is reported, evaluation may include anorectal manometry to assess anal sphincter pressure and rectal sensation, anal endosonography for anal sphincter defects, or defecography for structural evaluation of the pelvic floor.

Initial treatment should be directed at the treatment of reversible factors such as diarrhea, constipation, offending medications, smoking, obesity, and physical inactivity. Effective dietary modifications include fiber supplementation and avoidance of trigger foods. If there is lack of response to conservative measures, the next step is pelvic floor muscle training with specially trained physical therapists. In the event of lack of response to biofeedback therapy, other treatment options include the use of anal plugs, anal wicking, various minimally invasive procedures (for example, the use of injectable bulking agents or sacral nerve stimulation), or surgery such as sphincteroplasty.

Anal Cancer

Anal cancer (**Figure 24**) is rare, with a yearly incidence of 8000 cases in the United States. Squamous cell cancer is the most common type, representing 80% of all anal cancers. The incidence has been rising by 2.2% each year for the last decade. Delayed diagnosis by up to 2 years in more than half of cases has resulted in increased need for aggressive surgical intervention.

Human papillomavirus infection and presence of intraepithelial neoplasia are strongly linked with anal cancer. Risk is increased in men who have sex with men, in patients with HIV infection, history of condylomata, and kidney or liver transplantation. Presenting symptoms of anal cancer may include bleeding, pain, or pruritus; however, 25% of cases present without any anorectal symptoms. Anal squamous cell cancer occurs in patients with IBD or ulcerative colitis at a rate of 1 in 100,000, and at a rate of 2 in 100,000 in patients with Crohn disease, largely in those with perianal disease, warranting

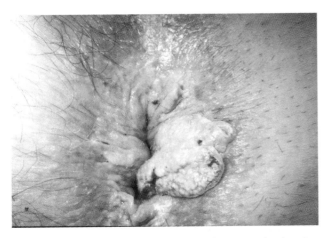

FIGURE 24. Anal cancer presenting as an ulcerated mass protruding from the anal canal. The presentation of anal cancer can vary from an obstructing anal mass to a nonprotruding polyp or flat growth in the anal canal.

Image courtesy of Richard E. Burney, MD, Professor of Surgery, Michigan Medicine at the University of Michigan.

heightened vigilance in patients with longstanding perianal disease. Cancer occurs at a young age in patients with Crohn disease (mean age of 42 years) with a typical presentation of anal pain. Anal cancer is aggressive in patients with Crohn disease; most patients require radical surgery, and cumulative overall and disease-free survival is 37% at 5 years.

Although no formal recommendations address screening for anal dysplasia in at-risk populations, screening modalities to consider include digital rectal examination, anal Pap test, human papillomavirus testing, and high-resolution anoscopy.

Biopsy is required to make the diagnosis of anal cancer. Unlike colorectal cancer, staging of anal cancer is based on tumor size and does not involve depth of invasion. Only anal cancers involving the vagina, urethra, or bladder are classified as T4 lesions, regardless of size. Invasion of the rectum, skin, or sphincter muscles does not classify lesions as T4. Lymph node metastasis is divided into perirectal, iliac, and/or inguinal lymph nodal involvement.

For treatment and follow-up of anal cancer, see MKSAP 18 Hematology and Oncology.

KEY POINTS

- First-line therapy for hemorrhoids includes increased fiber intake, adequate liquid intake, and avoidance of straining.

- Fecal incontinence is grossly underreported due to embarrassment, and health care providers should inquire about it during clinic visits, particularly in patients at risk.

- Presenting symptoms of anal cancer may include bleeding, pain, or pruritus; however, 25% of cases present without any anorectal symptoms.

- Patients with Crohn disease with longstanding perianal disease are particularly at risk for anal cancer.

Colorectal Neoplasia

Epidemiology

Colorectal cancer is the third most common cancer and second most common cause of cancer-related mortality among men and women in the United States. Its annual incidence rate among adults in the United States is 42 cases per 100,000, and its mortality rate is 15.5 deaths per 100,000. The incidence of colorectal cancer is approximately 25% higher in men than in women.

The incidence and mortality rates for colorectal cancer have decreased over the past 30 years, largely because of early detection through screening and changes in risk factors (such as decreased smoking). However, there has been a steady increase in the number of colorectal cancer cases in patients younger than age 50 years, for unknown reasons. Survival rates are greater than 90% when the disease is localized, underscoring the importance of early detection. Between 20% and 53% of adults older than age 50 years have premalignant adenomas of the colon detected on screening, and 3% to 8% of the adenomas have advanced histological features. Despite strong evidence supporting colorectal cancer screening, only about 59% of Americans older than age 50 years are up-to-date for recommended testing.

KEY POINT

- Colorectal cancer is the third most common cancer and second most common cause of cancer-related mortality among men and women in the United States.

Pathogenesis

Colorectal cancer develops through one of three mechanisms: chromosomal instability, microsatellite instability, and serrated neoplasia.

Chromosomal instability is the most common mechanism, accounting for approximately 85% of colorectal cancers. Chromosomal instability is characterized by cancer cells that gain or lose whole chromosomes or large fractions of chromosomes (aneuploidy) at an increased rate compared with normal cells. Stepwise accumulation of mutations leads to progression from normal colon to adenoma to cancer. The most commonly mutated gene in this pathway is the adenomatous polyposis coli (*APC*) gene, a multifunctional tumor suppressor gene. Deregulation caused by mutations in *APC* is implicated in the development and spread of colon cancer. Germline mutations in the *APC* gene lead to hereditary familial adenomatous polyposis.

Microsatellites are dozens to hundreds of repetitive nucleotide sequences seen throughout the human genome. The term *microsatellite instability* refers to the presence of mismatched bases at repeated DNA microsatellites. Microsatellite instability accounts for about 15% of colorectal cancers and is characterized by defective DNA mismatch repair, leading to multiple mutations, adenomas, and cancer. Defective mismatch repair can occur if there is a germline mutation in one of the mismatch repair genes in Lynch syndrome (including *MLH1*, *MSH2*, *MSH6*, *PMS2*) or in the epithelial cell adhesion molecule gene (*EPCAM*), or as a result of sporadic methylation of the *MLH1* promoter.

A more recently described mechanism involves hypermethylation of tumor suppressor genes and the development of serrated polyps and cancer. Serrated polyps are a heterogeneous group of lesions classified by their saw-toothed appearance on histology. Serrated polyps are often found in the proximal colon and may be flat and difficult to distinguish from normal mucosa (**Figure 25**). Hyperplastic polyps that are benign also develop through this mechanism. Interval colon cancers, which are defined as cancers that develop after a negative colonoscopy and before the next recommended screening colonoscopy, most commonly develop through the serrated neoplasia mechanism. A hereditary condition called serrated polyposis syndrome has been described, but its genetic basis has not been elucidated.

KEY POINT

- Chromosomal instability is the most common mechanism responsible for the development of colorectal cancer, accounting for 85% of cases.

Risk Factors

Several risk factors have been established for colorectal cancer. Nonmodifiable risk factors include age (50 years and older), male sex, black race, and a personal or family history of colon adenomas or colorectal cancer. The risk doubles with a family history of colorectal cancer in a first-degree relative.

Long-standing (≥8 years) colonic inflammatory bowel disease (both Crohn disease and ulcerative colitis) is associated with about a 2.7-fold increased risk and is dependent on the severity and extent of bowel involvement. Patients with ureterocolic anastomoses after extensive bladder surgeries and adult survivors of childhood malignancy who received abdominal radiation are also at increased risk for colorectal cancer.

Modifiable risk factors associated with increased risk include diets high in red and processed meat; low intake of fruits, vegetables, fiber, and dairy; use of alcohol and tobacco; type 2 diabetes mellitus; sedentary lifestyle; and obesity.

KEY POINTS

- Nonmodifiable risk factors for colorectal cancer include age (50 years and older), male sex, black race, and a personal or family history of colorectal cancer.

- Modifiable risk factors for colorectal cancer include diets high in red and processed meat; low intake of fruits, vegetables, fiber, and dairy; use of alcohol and tobacco; type 2 diabetes mellitus; sedentary lifestyle; and obesity.

- Longstanding inflammatory bowel disease (both ulcerative colitis and Crohn disease) is associated with increased risk for colorectal cancer.

Chemoprevention

Substantial epidemiological and experimental data show that aspirin use prevents colorectal cancer. The U.S. Preventive Services Task Force updated their guidelines in 2015 to include the use of low-dose aspirin (81 mg/d) for preventing colorectal cancer and cardiovascular disease in individuals aged 50 and 59 years who are at increased risk for cardiovascular disease. Aspirin use is associated with a 30% decreased risk for colorectal cancer based on cohort and case-control studies. However, randomized controlled trials have not shown a benefit of aspirin in prevention of colorectal cancer. Randomized controlled trials have shown that aspirin decreases the risk for recurrent adenomas.

Studies of other NSAIDs for prevention of colon cancer and adenomas have also yielded positive results; however, benefits of aspirin and other NSAIDs must be weighed against harms, most notably gastrointestinal bleeding.

Some evidence suggests that selective cyclooxygenase-2 inhibitors prevent recurrent adenomas and decrease the incidence of advanced lesions; however, the associated increased cardiovascular risk confounds a recommendation of their use for chemoprevention.

KEY POINT

- The U.S. Preventive Services Task Force recommends the use of low-dose aspirin for preventing colorectal cancer and cardiovascular disease in individuals aged 50 and 59 years who are at increased risk for cardiovascular disease.

Screening

Screening individuals at average risk is discussed in MKSAP 18 General Internal Medicine.

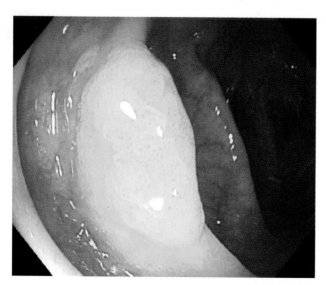

FIGURE 25. A serrated polyp in the ascending colon, showing flat morphology that can make these polyps difficult to identify on colonoscopy.

Screening strategies for individuals at increased risk for colorectal cancer are described in **Table 23**.

Key quality indicators for screening colonoscopy are adequate bowel preparation, preparation sufficient to identify polyps 6 mm in size or larger, visualization of the entire colon to the cecum, and longer duration of colonoscopy.

Because adenomas are an intermediary step in the progression from normal colonic mucosa to colon cancer, the identification and management of polyps is critical. Adenomas can be found throughout the colon. They are classified based on morphology, histology, and degree of dysplasia (**Table 24**). Adenomas with any degree of villous histology or high-grade dysplasia have greater malignant potential. Risk is also substantially increased in polyps larger than 1 cm in size. The progression of adenoma to carcinoma takes approximately 8 to 10 years.

KEY POINTS

- Screening for colon cancer should be individualized in patients at increased risk.
- The risk for colon cancer depends on the size of the adenoma, degree of villous histology, and presence of dysplasia.

Clinical Presentation

Colorectal cancer may be asymptomatic, or it may present with iron deficiency anemia, gastrointestinal bleeding, altered bowel habits, abdominal pain, colonic obstruction, and weight loss in more advanced cases.

Diagnosis and Staging

The diagnosis of colorectal cancer is usually made by colonoscopy with biopsy. Staging is based on tumor size and extent of invasion into local tissues, lymph node involvement, and evidence of metastasis (TNM system). Cross-sectional imaging of the chest, abdomen, and pelvis is used for staging in the initial evaluation after diagnosis. Management of colon cancer depends on stage, evidence of microsatellite instability, and presence of specific mutations, including *KRAS/NRAS* and *BRAF*.

For treatment of colorectal cancer, see MKSAP 18 Hematology and Oncology.

Favorable characteristics include stage 1 to 2, lack of angiolymphatic involvement, and negative margins after polyp removal. Endoscopic resection of polyps is curative in some cases. Malignant sessile or flat polyps are associated with higher risk for recurrence and local or distant spread.

KEY POINTS

- The diagnosis of colorectal cancer is usually made by colonoscopy with biopsy.
- Staging of colon cancer is based on tumor size and extent of invasion into local tissues, lymph node involvement, and evidence of metastasis.

TABLE 23.	Screening for Colorectal Cancer in Individuals at Increased Risk	
Risk Category	**Criteria**	**Screening Recommendations (age; modality; interval)**
Increased	Family history of CRC:	
	CRC diagnosed in FDR <60 years old or two or more FDRs at any age	Begin at age 40 years or 10 years earlier than age of youngest FDR at diagnosis, whichever comes first; colonoscopy; repeat every 5 years[a]
	CRC diagnosed in FDR >60 years old	Begin at age 50 years; any modality; repeat every 10 years[a]
	Personal history of CRC	Perform at time of diagnosis; colonoscopy; repeat at 1 year, 3 years, and, if normal, every 5 years thereafter until the benefit of continued screening is outweighed by risks
High	Familial adenomatous polyposis	Begin at age 10-12 years; flexible sigmoidoscopy or colonoscopy; repeat every 1-2 years until colectomy
	Lynch syndrome	Begin at age 20-25 years or 10 years earlier than youngest cancer in family; colonoscopy; repeat every 1-2 years
	Inflammatory bowel disease (Crohn disease or ulcerative colitis)	Begin after 8 years of chronic colitis; colonoscopy with biopsies; repeat every 1-2 years

CRC = colorectal cancer; FDR = first-degree relative (parent, sibling, or child).

[a]If baseline examination is normal.

Data from Rex DK, Johnson DA, Anderson JC, Schoenfeld PS, Burke CA, Inadomi JM; American College of Gastroenterology. American College of Gastroenterology guidelines for colorectal cancer screening 2009 [corrected]. Am J Gastroenterol. 2009;104:739-50. [PMID: 19240699] doi:10.1038/ajg.2009.104; Rubenstein JH, Enns R, Heidelbaugh J, Barkun A; Clinical Guidelines Committee. American Gastroenterological Association Institute Guideline on the Diagnosis and Management of Lynch Syndrome. Gastroenterology. 2015;149:777-82; quiz e16-7. [PMID: 26226577] doi:10.1053/j.gastro.2015.07.036; Syngal S, Brand RE, Church JM, Giardiello FM, Hampel HL, Burt RW; American College of Gastroenterology. ACG clinical guideline: Genetic testing and management of hereditary gastrointestinal cancer syndromes. Am J Gastroenterol. 2015;110:223-62; quiz 263. [PMID: 25645574] doi:10.1038/ajg.2014.435.

TABLE 24. Classification of Colorectal Polyps
Adenomatous Polyps[a]
Tubular adenoma
Tubulovillous adenoma
Villous adenoma
Serrated Polyps
Hyperplastic polyp
Sessile serrated polyp with or without cytologic dysplasia
Traditional serrated adenoma
Other
Hamartomatous polyp
Inflammatory polyp
[a]With or without high-grade dysplasia.

Surveillance

Surveillance for colorectal cancer after screening or polypectomy is based on findings on the baseline examination (**Table 25**).

Hereditary Colorectal Cancer Syndromes

Lynch Syndrome

Lynch syndrome is characterized by germline mutations in the mismatch repair genes (*MLH1*, *MSH2*, *MSH6*, *PMS2*) or the epithelial cell adhesion molecule gene (*EPCAM*), leading to an increased risk for neoplasia of the colon and other organs. Another name for this syndrome, hereditary nonpolyposis colorectal cancer, is no longer used because the syndrome is associated with colorectal polyps as well as extracolonic cancers. The syndrome follows an autosomal dominant inheritance pattern and new mutations are rare.

Individuals with Lynch syndrome are at increased risk for colorectal and endometrial cancers (most common), as well as other cancers, including tumors of the stomach, ovary, hepatobiliary and urinary tracts, small bowel, brain, and pancreas, and sebaceous skin adenoma or cancer.

In persons with Lynch syndrome, the lifetime risk for colorectal cancer depends on the location of the gene mutation, and the risk can be as high as 50% to 80%. Colorectal cancer in Lynch syndrome is more likely to occur in the proximal colon and can display characteristic pathological features, such as tumor-infiltrating lymphocytes and medullary growth pattern. Colorectal tumors in Lynch syndrome result from microsatellite instability that can be assessed using polymerase chain reaction or immunohistochemistry (see Pathogenesis). All colorectal cancers should be screened for Lynch-syndrome genetic mutations or microsatellite instability.

Clinical criteria to evaluate for Lynch syndrome include the Amsterdam and Bethesda criteria, as well as newer models such as the PREdiction Model for gene Mutations 5 (PREMM$_5$). The Amsterdam II criteria follow the "3-2-1-1-0 rule," which states that a diagnosis is warranted if all of the following criteria are met:

- Three family members are affected with a Lynch syndrome–associated cancer
- Two successive generations are affected
- One affected family member is a first-degree relative of the other two affected family members
- One of the cancers was diagnosed before age 50 years
- A familial polyposis syndrome has been ruled out
- Tumors have been verified histologically

These criteria are specific but not sensitive for the diagnosis of Lynch syndrome. The Bethesda criteria have good sensitivity but poor specificity. Genetic counseling and testing should be offered to patients with a personal and/or family history consistent with Lynch syndrome, as well as patients whose tumor shows evidence of microsatellite instability or loss of mismatch repair protein expression. When a mutation is identified in a family, testing of first-degree relatives should be performed and surveillance instituted.

Screening for colorectal cancer in patients with Lynch syndrome should begin at age 20 to 25 years (or 2-5 years

TABLE 25. Surveillance for Colorectal Cancer After Screening or Polypectomy	
Adenomatous Polyps	**Interval to Next Colonoscopy**
1-2 tubular adenomas <10 mm in size	5-10 years
3-10 adenomas ≥10 mm in size, villous histology, or high-grade dysplasia	3 years
≥10 adenomas on single examination	<3 years; a genetic cause of disease should be investigated
Serrated Polyps	**Interval to Next Colonoscopy**
Rectosigmoid hyperplastic polyps <10 mm in size	10 years
SSP <10 mm in size	5 years
SSP ≥10 mm in size or SSP with dysplasia or TSA	3 years
Serrated polyposis syndrome	1 year
SSP = sessile serrated polyps; TSA = traditional serrated adenomas.	

before the age of diagnosis of the earliest cancer in the family). Screening should be done by colonoscopy and repeated every 1 to 2 years. Risk-reducing total hysterectomy and bilateral salpingo-oophorectomy should be considered starting at age 40 to 45 years after childbearing is completed in women who carry Lynch syndrome mutations.

Screening with upper endoscopy for stomach and small-bowel cancers can be considered starting at age 30 to 35 years and repeated every 2 to 5 years. Testing for *Helicobacter pylori* is also recommended in patients at risk for or with Lynch syndrome.

Adenomatous Polyposis Syndromes

Syndromes that predispose to multiple adenomatous polyps in the colon include familial adenomatous polyposis (FAP), *MutYH*-associated polyposis (MAP), and polymerase proof-reading-associated polyposis (PPAP).

Familial Adenomatous Polyposis

FAP is an inherited disorder characterized by multiple (usually more than 100) adenomatous colon polyps. FAP is caused by germline mutations in the *APC* gene that are inherited in an autosomal dominant pattern, although *de novo* mutations occur in about 25% of cases. Adenomas in classic FAP are more numerous in the distal colon than in the proximal colon. Adenoma and cancer develop in 100% of classic FAP cases if surgery is not performed. The average age of colorectal cancer onset is 39 years, with a risk of 93% by age 50 years. An attenuated form of FAP (AFAP) causes fewer polyps (<100 synchronous polyps) with more proximal colonic distribution. The risk for colon cancer in patients with AFAP is about 70% by age 80 years, with an average age of onset of 58 years.

Both FAP and AFAP are associated with extracolonic intestinal manifestations (**Figure 26**). Duodenal adenomas

require surveillance because the lifetime risk for duodenal adenocarcinoma is estimated at 4%. Fundic gland polyps of the stomach do not have malignant potential but can mask gastric adenomas and cancer. Risk for gastric cancer is estimated at less than 1%. Risk for desmoid tumors is increased, especially after surgery to remove the colon. Risk for papillary thyroid cancer is also increased, especially in women. Nonmalignant findings include extra teeth, cysts, osteomas, and congenital hypertrophy of the retinal pigmented epithelium.

Screening in classic FAP mutation carriers should begin at age 10 to 12 years with sigmoidoscopy or colonoscopy and repeated every 1 to 2 years. Screening in patients with AFAP can be delayed until age 20 to 25 years and should be performed with colonoscopy. For individuals with FAP and AFAP, screening with upper endoscopy should begin at age 25 to 30 years and include visualization of the papilla with a duodenoscope. Fundic gland polyps in the stomach should be randomly sampled. Surveillance of the upper gastrointestinal tract is determined by findings in the duodenum. Annual thyroid ultrasound is also recommended.

Colectomy is the treatment of choice for classic FAP and may be pursued in patients with AFAP. Absolute indications for surgery include cancer and significant symptoms such as rectal bleeding. Relative indications include multiple adenomas greater than 6 mm size, increase in number of polyps, an adenoma with high-grade dysplasia, and multiple diminutive polyps, which can prevent identification of adenomas. The type of surgery depends on the polyp burden in the rectum; total colectomy with ileorectal anastomosis is indicated for patients with a small rectal polyp burden, and total procto-colectomy with ileo-pouch anastomosis is indicated for patients with a large rectal polyp burden. Postsurgical surveillance is yearly sigmoidoscopy for those with an intact rectum and ileoscopy every 2 years for patients with an ileostomy.

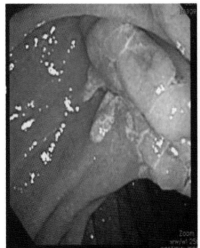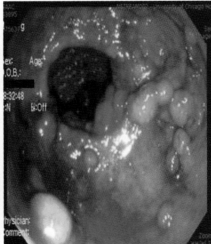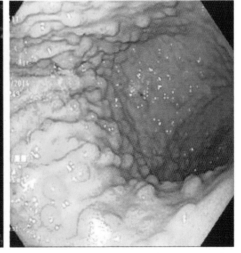

FIGURE 26. Intestinal features of familial adenomatous polyposis (FAP). Patients with FAP can develop polyps throughout the gastrointestinal tract. Adenomatous polyps always develop in the colon. Duodenal adenomas can also develop in patients with FAP, especially involving the ampulla of Vater. Regular upper endoscopic surveillance is indicated to remove polyps larger than 10 mm (*left*). If a patient with FAP has had surgery and has an ileorectal anastomosis, that patient must continue to be surveyed regularly because rectal polyps can develop in the remaining rectum (*center*). Numerous fundic gland polyps of the stomach can develop in FAP (*right*).

MutYH-Associated Polyposis

MAP is an inherited syndrome characterized by fewer adenomas than classic FAP. MAP is caused by mutations in the *MutYH* gene, a component of base excision repair. MAP is a recessive condition in which an affected patient has inherited two mutated copies from their parents. Most patients have between 20 and 99 adenomatous colon polyps. Some individuals can develop cancer with only a few or no synchronous adenomas. Mean age of cancer onset is about 52 years. In addition, other polyp types can be encountered in patients with MAP, including serrated and hyperplastic polyps. Duodenal cancer risk in MAP is estimated at 4% and surveillance with upper endoscopy is similar to that indicated in patients with FAP. Surgical management of the colon is similar to that of FAP.

Polymerase Proofreading-Associated Polyposis

This more recently described syndrome is inherited in an autosomal dominant manner. PPAP appears to have features of both FAP and Lynch syndrome and is caused by mutations in polymerase proofreading genes *POLE* and *POLD1*. Endometrial cancer has been described in this syndrome, and tumor testing has been reported to show microsatellite instability. Management guidelines have not been established for PPAP, but management of colonic polyps follows similar principles as for other adenomatous polyp syndromes.

Hamartomatous Polyposis Syndromes

Hamartomas refer to polyps caused by overgrowth of normal tissue. There are three primary syndromes associated with hamartomas in the gastrointestinal tract: juvenile polyposis syndrome (JPS), Peutz-Jeghers syndrome (PJS), and *PTEN* hamartoma syndrome, also known as Cowden syndrome.

Juvenile Polyposis Syndrome

JPS is caused by mutations in the *BMPR1A* and *SMAD4* genes. It has an incidence of approximately 1 in 130,000 live births. Multiple juvenile polyps (>5 polyps) are found in the colon (98%), stomach (14%), and small bowel (14%) of patients with JPS (**Figure 27**). Sporadic juvenile polyps can be found in up to 1% of children and are not considered syndromic. The average age of patients at the time JPS is diagnosed is 18.5 years, and rectal bleeding is the most common symptom. Patients with JPS are at increased risk for colon, stomach, and small-bowel cancer. Individuals with mutations in the *SMAD4* gene can also have hereditary hemorrhagic telangiectasia.

Peutz-Jeghers Syndrome

PJS is caused by mutations in the *STK11* gene. Its incidence is approximately 1 in 200,000 live births. PJS hamartomas are found primarily in the small bowel but can also develop in the stomach and colon (**Figure 28**). PJS is also characterized by hyperpigmented mucocutaneous macules on the lips and buccal mucosa (**Figure 29**).

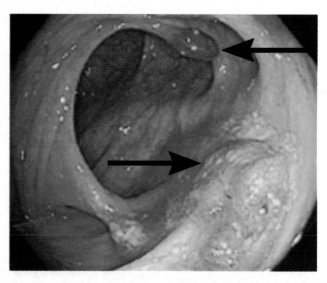

FIGURE 27. Juvenile polyps in the colon of a patient with juvenile polyposis syndrome, on endoscopy. Juvenile polyps can have an erythematous and waxy appearance.

Small bowel hamartomas develop at a young age in patients with PJS, and may present with intussusception, obstruction and bleeding. Patients with PJS have increased risk for cancer in the colon, stomach, small bowel, breast, ovary, cervix, uterus, testicles, lung, and pancreas.

PTEN Hamartoma Syndrome

Also known as Cowden syndrome, this syndrome is caused by germline mutations in the tumor suppressor gene *PTEN*. It is characterized by gastrointestinal hamartomas associated with a number of cancers, such as breast, thyroid, kidney, and colon cancer, as well as macrocephaly, esophageal glycogenic acanthosis, and dermatological manifestations. Colorectal cancer prevalence is estimated at 9% to 18%.

Serrated Polyposis Syndrome

Serrated polyposis syndrome is characterized by numerous serrated polyps in the colon. The definition is based on having any of the following:

- Five or more serrated polyps proximal to the sigmoid colon, with two or more greater than 10 mm in size

- Any number of serrated polyps in patients with first-degree relatives with serrated polyposis syndrome

- More than 20 serrated polyps throughout the colon

Estimates suggest that the prevalence of serrated polyposis syndrome is between 0.3% and 0.6%. Risk for colon cancer in patients with this syndrome is increased, and smoking appears to be a risk factor. Colonoscopy is recommended every 1 to 3 years with removal of all polyps greater than 5 mm in size. Surgery may be considered if the polyps cannot be managed endoscopically. No extracolonic manifestations have been noted in serrated polyposis syndrome. The genetic basis of the syndrome is unknown.

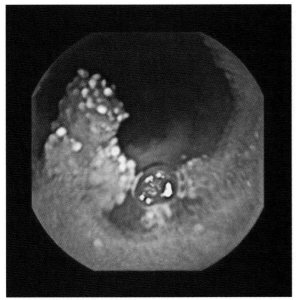

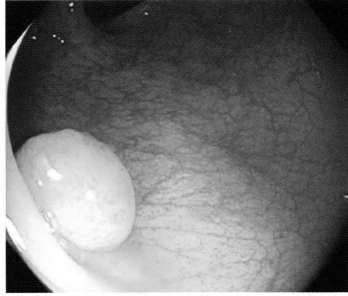

FIGURE 28. Peutz-Jeghers syndrome (PJS) polyps. Capsule endoscopy showing a PJS hamartomatous polyp in the small intestine (*left*); polyps in the small intestine can cause bleeding and/or obstructions. Colonoscopy showing a hamartomatous polyp in the colon of a patient with PJS (*right*).

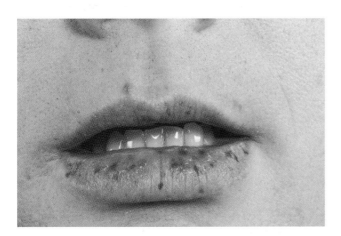

FIGURE 29. Peutz-Jeghers syndrome is associated with multiple hamartomatous polyps in the gastrointestinal tract and distinctive mucocutaneous pigmentations. The pigmented lesions occur most commonly on the lips and perioral region but can also occur on the nose, perianal area, and genitals.

KEY POINTS

- Lynch syndrome is caused by germline mutations in the mismatch repair genes and carries a lifetime risk for colorectal cancer of 50% to 80%.

- Syndromes that predispose persons to multiple adenomatous polyps in the colon include familial adenomatous polyposis, *MutYH*-associated polyposis, and polymerase proofreading-associated polyposis.

- Hamartomatous polyposis syndromes are associated with increased risk for multiple cancers, including colon cancer.

Disorders of the Liver

Approach to the Patient with Abnormal Liver Chemistry Studies

Basic metabolic panels commonly include liver chemistry tests. Liver chemistry tests are often abnormal (10% to 20% of the time); therefore, it is important to take a systematic approach to their evaluation. The patterns of the elevations of liver tests can be used to group causes into categories; however, these patterns are not specific. Elevations of aspartate aminotransferase (AST) and alanine aminotransferase (ALT) levels represent hepatic parenchymal inflammation. Elevated ALT levels are more specific for hepatic inflammation because AST is also found in other tissues such as heart and muscle.

Elevations in alkaline phosphatase (ALP) and bilirubin levels result from inflammation of the biliary tree or bile flow abnormalities. ALP is also produced in bone and placenta and high levels are seen in pregnancy. Elevation of ALP and other liver chemistries typically reflects liver injury. Fractionation of ALP levels can be performed to determine the source of elevation. Bilirubin can be divided into conjugated and unconjugated forms. Elevation of conjugated bilirubin reflects a liver disorder, whereas elevation of unconjugated bilirubin is seen in hematological disease or in benign alterations of bilirubin conjugation, such as Gilbert syndrome.

The prothrombin time and serum albumin levels reflect the synthetic function of the liver. Albumin levels are decreased in the setting of malnourishment, the nephrotic syndrome, acute inflammation, and protein-losing enteropathies. Prothrombin time can be prolonged in vitamin K deficiency, warfarin therapy, coagulopathy of liver disease, inherited or acquired factor deficiency, and the antiphospholipid antibody syndrome. In patients with abnormal liver enzyme levels, thrombocytopenia may be a clue to the presence of portal hypertension.

The relative levels and severity of elevations of AST, ALT, and ALP provide clues about the cause of the liver inflammation (**Table 26**). The duration of abnormal liver tests is also important in evaluating the causes of liver injury. Acute liver inflammation is defined as less than 6 months in duration, whereas chronic hepatitis is defined as elevated liver chemistries of greater than 6 months' duration.

Abdominal imaging can be helpful in the assessment of a patient with abnormal liver tests. Abdominal ultrasonography may show increased echogenicity, consistent with fatty infiltration of the liver, as well as nodularity of the liver seen in the setting of cirrhosis. Cross-sectional imaging may show findings of fatty infiltration of the liver as well as changes of cirrhosis. Noninvasive assessments of hepatic fibrosis are becoming more frequently used. Ultrasound-based transient elastography and magnetic resonance (MR) elastography measure tissue stiffness. Tissue stiffness correlates with stages of hepatic fibrosis, although high stiffness values may also

occur with hepatic congestion, infiltrative disorders, and bile duct obstruction.

KEY POINTS

- Elevations of aspartate aminotransferase and alanine aminotransferase levels represent hepatic parenchymal inflammation; alanine aminotransferase levels are more specific for hepatic inflammation.

- Elevations in alkaline phosphatase and bilirubin levels result from inflammation of the biliary tree or bile flow abnormalities.

- The prothrombin time and serum albumin levels reflect the synthetic function of the liver.

Viral Hepatitis

Hepatitis A

Hepatitis A virus (HAV) is an RNA virus that causes acute hepatitis mediated by the host immune response. HAV infection is a self-limited illness, but atypical forms exist, including a relapsing, remitting infection with cholestatic features and,

TABLE 26.	Typical Liver Chemistry Studies in Common Hepatobiliary Disorders				
Disease	**AST**	**ALT**	**ALP**	**Bilirubin**	**Other Features**
Acute viral hepatitis	↑↑↑	↑↑↑	Normal to ↑	Normal to ↑↑↑	Exposure history, fatigue, nausea
Chronic viral hepatitis	↑	↑↑	Normal to ↑	↑ if advanced	History of exposure to infected blood or body fluids
Nonalcoholic steatohepatitis	↑	↑	Normal to ↑	Normal	Metabolic syndrome
Alcoholic hepatitis	↑↑	Normal or ↑	↑	Normal to ↑↑↑	Excess alcohol intake
Acute autoimmune hepatitis	↑↑↑	↑↑↑	Normal to ↑	Normal to ↑↑	Autoantibodies
Chronic autoimmune hepatitis	↑	↑↑	Normal to ↑	Normal	Autoantibodies
Wilson disease	↑	↑	Low	↑ and often unconjugated	Hemolysis if acute, neurologic symptoms if chronic
α$_1$-Antitrypsin deficiency	↑	↑	Normal	↑ if advanced	May have pulmonary disease
Hemochromatosis	Normal	Normal	Normal	Normal	Joint symptoms, family history, other organ involvement
Primary biliary cholangitis	↑	↑	↑↑↑	↑ if advanced	Female, sicca symptoms, antimitochondrial antibody
Primary sclerosing cholangitis	↑	↑	↑↑↑	↑ if advanced or dominant stricture is present	Ulcerative colitis, abnormal cholangiogram
Large duct obstruction	↑ (↑↑ if acute)	↑ (↑↑ if acute)	↑↑	↑↑	Pain if acute, dilated ducts on imaging
Infiltrative liver disease	↑	↑	↑↑↑	Normal	Features of malignancy, sarcoid, amyloid, or mycobacterial or fungal infection
Hepatic ischemia	↑↑↑	↑↑↑	Normal	Normal	AST >5000 U/L, history of hypotension
Celiac disease	Normal or ↑	Normal or ↑	Normal or ↑	Normal	Usually other features of celiac disease

ALP = alkaline phosphatase; ALT = alanine aminotransferase; AST = aspartate aminotransferase.

rarely, acute liver failure. HAV is transmitted by the fecal-oral route. Risk factors include international travel, contacts with household members with HAV infection, men who have sex with men, and exposure to day care or institutionalized settings. The incidence of HAV infection declined dramatically after introduction of the HAV vaccination (see MKSAP 18 Infectious Diseases). Mortality is rare but may be increased in patients with preexisting chronic liver disease. The incubation period for HAV is 15 to 50 days. A prodrome of malaise, nausea, vomiting, fever, and right-upper-quadrant pain is followed by development of jaundice, with physical examination findings of jaundice and hepatomegaly. HAV can be transmitted during the prodrome stage and up to 1 week after development of jaundice. Laboratory studies may show aminotransferase levels greater than 1000 U/L and total bilirubin level of 10 mg/dL (171 μmol/L) or higher, mostly direct (conjugated). A positive test for IgM antibodies to HAV is suggestive of acute illness, although false positives may occur in the setting of other viral infections. The presence of IgG antibodies to HAV indicates previous infection or vaccination and provides immunity from reinfection. Treatment is supportive, and 90% of patients or more recover fully within 3 to 6 months of infection. Postexposure vaccination is sufficient for immunocompetent patients, and HAV immunoglobulin can be administered to immunocompromised patients.

Hepatitis B

Hepatitis B virus (HBV) is a DNA virus affecting 240 million persons worldwide and 2.2 million in the United States. See MKSAP 18 General Internal Medicine for HBV vaccination strategies. HBV can be transmitted vertically, through sexual exposure, percutaneously, or by close person-to-person contact. The risk for developing chronic HBV infection differs by age. Newborns acquiring HBV have the highest risk (90%), whereas adults have an approximately 5% risk. Testing for HBV is recommended in individuals with risk factors (**Table 27**).

HBV infection presents as acute hepatitis in a minority of patients. Approximately 30% of adults may develop jaundice as a result of acute infection with aminotransferase levels as high as 3000 U/L and nonspecific symptoms including malaise, nausea, and right-upper-quadrant pain. Acute liver failure (ALF) develops in approximately 0.5% of patients. Typically, adult patients recover within 1 to 4 months. Chronic HBV infection is diagnosed after 6 months in patients with persistent hepatitis B surface antigen (HBsAg) detected in serum.

Interpretation of HBV serologies is shown in **Table 28**. There are four phases of chronic HBV infection: immune tolerant, immune active, immune control, and reactivation (**Figure 30**). Patients who have acquired HBV through vertical transmission remain in the immune-tolerant phase for the first two to three decades. This stage does not require treatment except in specific cases (patients older than 40 years with an HBV DNA level of at least 1 million IU/mL and significant inflammation or fibrosis).

Patients transition to hepatitis B e antigen (HBeAg)–positive, immune-active hepatitis later in life. Hallmarks of the immune-active phase include elevated ALT levels, an HBV DNA level of at least 20,000 IU/mL, and a positive HBeAg test. Moderate to severe inflammation can occur, fibrosis can progress, and treatment is warranted in this phase.

Spontaneous seroconversion to the immune-control (inactive) phase with a loss of HBeAg and development of anti-HBe occurs at a rate of 10% per year. To be considered inactive, the ALT level must be normal and the HBV DNA level must be 2000 IU/mL or lower when measured every 3 to 4 months for 1 year.

Approximately 60% to 80% of cases remain in the inactive phase, but up to 20% can revert to the HBeAg-positive, immune-active phase. In addition, the HBeAg-negative reactivation phase can develop in 10% to 30% of cases; this phase is marked by fluctuating elevations in ALT levels and an HBV DNA level that is low but at least 2000 IU/mL, accompanied by ongoing inflammation and fibrosis that require treatment. Not all patients progress through each one of these phases or in sequence.

TABLE 27.	Risk Factors Requiring Testing for Hepatitis B Virus
Individuals born or raised in regions with high rates of hepatitis B virus infection, including Asia, Africa, the South Pacific, European Mediterranean countries, Eastern Europe, most of South America, Honduras, Guatemala, and the Middle East (except Israel and Cyprus)	
U.S.-born persons not vaccinated as infants whose parents were born in endemic areas	
Household or sexual contact with hepatitis B surface antigen-positive persons	
Intravenous drug use	
Multiple sex partners or history of sexually transmitted infection	
Men who have sex with men	
History of incarceration	
History of hepatitis C virus or HIV infection	
Hemodialysis	
Pregnancy	
Elevated aminotransferase levels of unknown cause	

TABLE 28.	Interpretation of Hepatitis B Virus Test Results						
Clinical Scenario	**HBsAg**	**Anti-HBs**	**IgM anti-HBc**	**IgG anti-HBc**	**HBeAg**	**Anti-HBe**	**HBV DNA (IU/mL)**
Acute hepatitis B; occasionally reactivation of chronic hepatitis B	+	−	+	−	+	−	>20,000
Resolved previous infection	−	+	−	+	−	+/−	Undetected
Immunity due to previous vaccination	−	+	−	−	−	−	Undetected
False positive anti-HBc or resolved previous infection	−	−	−	+	−	−	Undetected
Immune-tolerant chronic hepatitis B (perinatally acquired, age <30 years)	+	−	−	+	+	−	>1 million
Inactive chronic hepatitis B	+	−	−	+	−	+	<10,000
HBeAg-positive immune-active chronic hepatitis B	+	−	−	+	+	−	>10,000
HBeAg-negative immune-reactive chronic hepatitis B	+	−	−	+	−	+	>10,000

Anti-HBc = hepatitis B core antibody; anti-HBe = hepatitis B e antibody; anti-HBs = hepatitis B surface antibody; HBeAg = hepatitis B e antigen; HBsAg = hepatitis B surface antigen; HBV = hepatitis B virus.

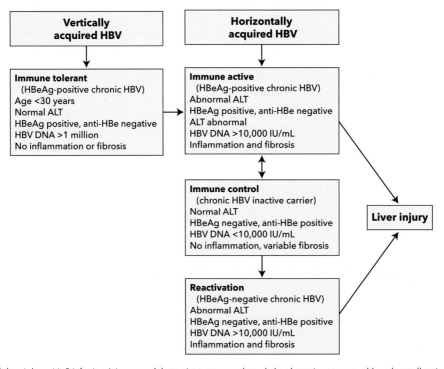

FIGURE 30. Phases of chronic hepatitis B infection. It is assumed that patients progress through the phases in sequence, although not all patients develop HBeAg-negative chronic hepatitis B, and only patients with vertical transmission of hepatitis B have a clinically recognized immune-tolerant phase. All phases have positive HBsAg, negative anti-HBs, and positive IgG anti-HBc.

ALT = alanine aminotransferase; anti-HBc = hepatitis B core antibody; anti-HBe = hepatitis B e antibody; anti-HBs = hepatitis B surface antibody; HBeAg = hepatitis B e antigen; HBsAg = hepatitis B surface antigen; HBV = hepatitis B virus; HBV DNA = hepatitis B virus DNA.

Risk factors for the development of cirrhosis and hepatocellular carcinoma in patients with chronic HBV infection are listed in **Table 29**.

Treatment is advised for patients with acute liver failure, infection in the immune-active phase or reactivation phase, and cirrhosis, and in immunosuppressed patients. Treatment thresholds in chronic immune-active or reactivation HBV infection are an ALT level at least twice the upper limit of normal and an HBV DNA level of at least 20,000 IU/mL (HBeAg-positive, immune-active phase), or an HBV DNA level of at least 2000 IU/mL (HBeAg-negative, reactivation phase). First-line treatment is entecavir or tenofovir. Lamivudine, adefovir, and telbivudine are less commonly used due to resistance. Pegylated interferon can be used for 48 weeks in patients with

TABLE 29. Risk Factors for Developing Cirrhosis or Hepatocellular Carcinoma in Patients with Chronic Hepatitis B Virus Infection

Age older than 40 years
Hepatitis B virus DNA level >2000 IU/mL
Elevated alanine aminotransferase level
Genotype C infection
Heavy alcohol use
Development of hepatitis B e antigen–negative reactivation phase of chronic hepatitis B virus infection
HIV infection
Hepatitis C virus or hepatitis D virus infection

high ALT levels, low HBV DNA levels, and without cirrhosis. Candidates for interferon are those who have a desire for finite therapy, are not pregnant, and do not have significant psychiatric disease, cardiac disease, seizure disorder, cytopenia, or autoimmune disease.

Treatment goals for patients in the HBeAg-positive, immune-active phase are HBeAg loss and anti-HBe seroconversion, which should be followed by an additional 12 months of treatment. Goals of treatment in the HBeAg-negative, reactivation phase are HBV DNA suppression and ALT normalization; oral antiviral agents are generally continued indefinitely. Patients with cirrhosis should continue oral antiviral medications indefinitely. HBsAg seroconversion rarely occurs with oral antiviral treatment and, therefore, is not a goal of treatment. Regression of fibrosis and even of cirrhosis can occur with treatment.

Prophylactic oral antiviral therapy should be given to patients who are HBsAg-positive or isolated core antibody-positive and receiving B-cell depleting therapy (for example, rituximab, or ofatumumab), prednisone (≥10 mg/d for at least 4 weeks), or anthracycline derivatives. Patients undergoing therapy with tumor necrosis factor-α or tyrosine kinase inhibitors should be considered for prophylaxis.

Rarely, patients with HBV infection develop polyarteritis nodosa or cryoglobulinemia, which should prompt treatment with oral antiviral therapy. Membranous glomerulonephritis is a rare extrahepatic association.

The survival rate after liver transplantation for end-stage liver disease from HBV infection is greater than 90% at 1 year. Recurrence of HBV infection in transplant recipients is prevented with HBV immunoglobulin and/or oral antiviral therapy.

The prognosis for untreated individuals with HBV infection worsens with age, particularly with age older than 40 years. Approximately 40% of deaths in HBV-infected persons older than age 40 years are related to hepatocellular carcinoma or decompensated cirrhosis. The following characteristics are associated with an increased risk for hepatocellular carcinoma in patients with HBV infection and are indications for surveillance with ultrasound or cross-sectional imaging every 6 months: (1) cirrhosis; (2) Asian descent plus male sex plus age older than 40 years; (3) Asian descent plus female sex plus age older than 50 years; (4) sub-Saharan African descent plus age older than 20 years; (5) persistent inflammatory activity (defined as an elevated ALT level and HBV DNA levels greater than 10,000 IU/mL for at least a few years); and (6) a family history of hepatocellular carcinoma.

Hepatitis C

Worldwide, 130 to 150 million individuals are infected with hepatitis C virus (HCV), with 2.7 to 3.9 million individuals with HCV infection in the United States. HCV is most commonly transmitted through intravenous or intranasal drug use, blood transfusions before 1992, or sexual intercourse. The efficiency of the virus' spread through vaginal intercourse is low. Individuals born between 1945 and 1965 require one-time HCV testing, as the prevalence is nearly 3% in this group and these individuals account for 75% of cases of HCV infection. Patients with risk factors should be tested (**Table 30**).

Acute HCV infection is asymptomatic in most patients. Jaundice, nausea, right-upper-quadrant pain, dark urine, and acholic stools can occur in the symptomatic cases. Evaluation of suspected acute infection includes HCV antibody and RNA tests. The HCV RNA test becomes positive first, and the HCV antibody test becomes positive within 1 to 3 months. HCV antibody seroconversion within 12 weeks in the presence of an initial positive HCV RNA test confirms an acute HCV infection. Infection that clears spontaneously, usually within 6 months, is more common in patients with symptoms, high ALT levels, female sex, younger age, and the *IL-28 CC* genotype. Monitoring HCV RNA quantification for clearance for 6 months is recommended in patients with acute infection.

TABLE 30. Conditions Requiring Testing for Hepatitis C Virus

Birth year 1945-1965
Injection-drug use or intranasal illicit-drug use (ever)
Long-term hemodialysis (ever)
Percutaneous/parenteral exposures in an unregulated setting (nonsterile technique)
Needlesticks, sharps, or mucosal exposure to hepatitis C virus-infected blood
Children born to women infected with hepatitis C virus
Receipt of blood or blood-components transfusion or organ transplantation before 1992
Receipt of clotting-factor concentrates produced before 1987
History of incarceration
HIV infection
Sexually active persons about to start preexposure prophylaxis for HIV
Undiagnosed chronic liver disease
Elevated alanine aminotransferase level
Living organ donors, before donation

HCV results in chronic infection in 60% to 80% of patients, with up to 30% progressing to cirrhosis over two to three decades. Patients with cirrhosis have a 2% to 4% risk per year for developing hepatocellular carcinoma.

The first step in the diagnosis of chronic HCV infection is HCV antibody testing, and if positive, a HCV RNA quantification. Patients with positive HCV antibody and RNA tests have active infection, and a genotype test should be performed. Asymptomatic patients with a positive HCV antibody and a negative HCV RNA test, and without recent exposure to HCV, do not have active infection and generally do not require further testing.

All patients infected with HCV should be tested for HBV and HIV because of the potential shared routes of transmission. HBV testing should include HBsAg to assess for active infection (followed by HBV DNA if positive) and antibodies to hepatitis B antigens (anti-HBs and anti-HBc) to assess for past infection. Susceptible patients should receive HBV vaccination. HBV reactivation can be seen during treatment of HCV infection with direct-acting antiviral therapy. Patients who test positive for HBsAg with detectable HBV DNA and who do not meet standard HBV treatment criteria should undergo HBV DNA monitoring approximately every 4 weeks until 12 weeks after completion of treatment for HCV infection, or they can be treated with oral HBV therapy prophylactically.

Patients with chronic HCV infection require a fibrosis assessment with a transient or MRI elastography or liver biopsy, unless they have a documented short duration of disease, decompensated cirrhosis, or a radiologic diagnosis of cirrhosis.

All patients infected with HCV should be considered for treatment unless there are significant life-limiting comorbidities or major barriers to adherence to treatment.

Treatment regimens include a combination of direct-acting antivirals, using different mechanisms to prevent viral reproduction (**Table 31**). Regimens are chosen based on genotype, previous treatment experience and response, and fibrosis status. Patients whose infection does not respond to newer regimens are generally managed by a hepatologist or infectious disease specialist because resistance-associated substitution–guided retreatment may be necessary. Patients with decompensated cirrhosis should see a hepatologist before treatment and be considered for liver transplantation. Post–liver transplantation recurrence of HCV infection is universal in treatment-naïve patients. Success rates of HCV treatment after liver transplantation are excellent.

Cure is defined by the absence of HCV RNA in blood 12 weeks after completion of treatment. HCV antibodies remain positive indefinitely and should not be rechecked. Patients can become reinfected after new exposures, and HCV RNA testing is appropriate to identify new infection. Cure rates exceed 90% in the majority of patients. Virologic cure reduces the risk for progression to cirrhosis, complications of cirrhosis, hepatocellular carcinoma, and liver-related mortality. Patients with stage F3 fibrosis or cirrhosis require ongoing surveillance for hepatocellular carcinoma even after virologic cure. Patients with cryoglobulinemic vasculitis and non–Hodgkin lymphoma are more likely to experience remission when HCV is eradicated.

Hepatitis D

Hepatitis D virus (HDV) is a defective RNA virus that requires HBV for human infection. HDV is endemic in the Mediterranean basin and Pacific islands and uncommon in Western countries. The diagnosis of HDV infection is made through detection of HDV IgG. The clinical course can range from inactive disease to progressive liver disease (in the case of simultaneous HBV-HDV coinfection) to fulminant hepatitis in HDV superinfection. Patients infected with HDV with evidence of progressive liver disease should receive treatment with pegylated interferon for 12 months; cure rates are 25% to 45%.

Hepatitis E

Hepatitis E virus (HEV) is an RNA virus with worldwide distribution. There are four different genotypes: genotypes 1 and 2 are more common in developing countries and are transmitted by the fecal-oral route through contaminated water; genotypes 3 and 4 are more common in developed countries where transmission occurs through contaminated food, mostly pork or deer meat. In developing countries, HEV infection generally occurs in young adults and can occur in large epidemics. In developed countries, HEV generally affects males older than age 40 years. The incubation period is 2 to 5 weeks. Approximately 50% of cases are asymptomatic. Symptoms of HEV infection are jaundice, malaise, nausea, vomiting, anorexia, and right-upper-quadrant pain. Aminotransferase levels are usually elevated to 1000 to 3000 U/L. Diagnosis relies on detection of HEV IgM or RNA. Treatment is supportive, and recovery is expected within 4 to 6 weeks. HEV infection should be considered in patients with an unknown cause of acute hepatitis and in immunocompromised patients with chronic hepatitis. Solid-organ transplant recipients with chronic hepatitis E have response rates of 70% with ribavirin treatment.

TABLE 31. Treatment Regimens for Hepatitis C Virus Infection
Drug Treatment Regimens
Grazoprevir[a] + elbasvir[b]
Paritaprevir[a] + ombitasvir[b] + dasabuvir[c]
Simeprevir[a] + sofosbuvir[d]
Daclatasvir[b] + sofosbuvir[d]
Ledipasvir[b] + sofosbuvir[d]
Velpatasvir[b] + sofosbuvir[d]
[a]Drug class: NS3/4A protease inhibitor (-previr)
[b]Drug class: NS5A inhibitor (-asvir)
[c]NS5B non-nucleoside polymerase inhibitor (-buvir)
[d]NS5B nucleotide polymerase inhibitor (-buvir)

Other Viruses

Other viruses can causes hepatitis, including Epstein-Barr virus (EBV), cytomegalovirus (CMV), herpes simplex virus (HSV), varicella zoster virus, and parvovirus. Approximately 90% of EBV-infected individuals have mild hepatitis, occasionally developing jaundice and elevated ALP levels. Diagnostic testing includes heterophile antibody testing or checking EBV serologies, which may demonstrate a positive viral-capsid antigen IgM. Treatment is supportive.

CMV can cause a syndrome that mimics EBV-related mononucleosis. CMV infection can cause mild aminotransferase elevations. Diagnosis is made with CMV serologies in the immunocompetent host. Treatment is supportive, and spontaneous recovery is the norm. CMV infection in solid-organ transplant recipients can cause CMV syndrome, marked by fever and myelosuppression, or tissue-invasive CMV infection involving the gastrointestinal tract, liver, lungs, and retina. Treatment with intravenous ganciclovir is required in immunocompromised hosts. Without treatment, CMV infection carries a high mortality rate in immunocompromised hosts.

HSV-caused hepatitis in women in the third trimester of pregnancy manifests with fever, altered mental status, right-upper-quadrant pain, hepatomegaly, and a presentation similar to sepsis. Aminotransferase levels are commonly elevated to 5000 U/L or higher with a disproportionately low bilirubin level, accompanied by coagulopathy. Diagnosis can be confirmed with polymerase chain reaction testing for HSV (when available) or a liver biopsy showing intranuclear inclusions, multinucleated giant cells, and coagulative necrosis with minimal inflammation. Intravenous acyclovir is the treatment of choice. The case fatality rate is approximately 80% in untreated patients.

In adults, primary varicella zoster virus is a very rare cause of acute hepatitis. Primary infection in organ transplant recipients can cause acute liver failure. Diagnosis in immunocompromised patients requires a biopsy of the skin or of the affected organ. Treatment is intravenous acyclovir.

Parvovirus B19 can result in transient elevation of aminotransferase levels but has also been associated with fulminant hepatic failure in very rare instances.

Other viruses associated with elevated liver chemistries include human herpes virus 6, 7, and 8, as well as adenoviruses.

KEY POINTS

- Treatment of hepatitis A virus infection is supportive, and 90% of patients or more recover fully within 3 to 6 months of infection.

- Treatment of hepatitis B virus infection is advised for patients with acute liver failure, infection in the immune-active phase or the reactivation phase, cirrhosis, and in immunosuppressed patients.

- Individuals born between 1945 and 1965 require one-time testing for hepatitis C virus.

- Up to 95% of patients with hepatitis C virus infection can be cured with direct-acting antiviral agents.

Autoimmune Hepatitis

Autoimmune hepatitis is a chronic inflammatory hepatitis that is four times more common in women than in men and can be associated with other autoimmune diseases (most commonly autoimmune thyroiditis, synovitis, or ulcerative colitis). It can affect individuals at any age but most commonly occurs in middle-aged adults. The presentation of autoimmune hepatitis can vary from asymptomatic elevation of transaminase levels to extrahepatic symptoms such as myalgia and malaise to acute liver failure. Diagnosis is made based on laboratory results (including positive antinuclear and smooth-muscle antibodies and elevated IgG levels), exclusion of other diagnoses (such as Wilson disease, viral hepatitis, and drug-induced liver injury), and histologic findings on liver biopsy.

Treatment includes prednisone and azathioprine for most patients. For uncomplicated autoimmune hepatitis without cirrhosis, budesonide can be considered in place of prednisone, but its role is not established. Prednisone monotherapy is less preferable due to adverse effects. Azathioprine requires monitoring for cytopenia. Typically, biochemical response occurs within 3 to 8 months for the 85% of patients whose disease responds to standard treatment. Histologic response can lag by many months. Duration of treatment should be 2 to 3 years before consideration of withdrawal. A liver biopsy is recommended to determine histologic response before consideration of drug withdrawal. High rates of relapse after discontinuation of treatment underscore the need for serial monitoring of liver tests. Patients with a severe acute form of autoimmune hepatitis presenting with jaundice should be managed by a hepatologist, and patients with features of acute liver failure require urgent transfer to a transplant center.

KEY POINTS

- Diagnosis of autoimmune hepatitis is made based on the presence of elevated aminotransferase levels, positive antinuclear antibody and smooth-muscle antibody, elevated levels of IgG, and compatible findings on liver biopsy.

- Wilson disease, viral hepatitis, and drug-induced liver injury need to be excluded before making the diagnosis of autoimmune hepatitis.

Alcohol-Induced Liver Disease

Alcohol-induced liver disease is the second most common reason for liver transplantation in the United States. Alcohol injury to the liver may take the form of steatosis, steatohepatitis, or severe steatohepatitis, also known as alcoholic hepatitis. Approximately 25% of heavy drinkers develop cirrhosis. History of alcohol use is the most important component in making the diagnosis, although not all patients are forthcoming about alcohol use. See MKSAP 18 General Internal Medicine for more information about screening for alcohol abuse. Most patients with alcoholic liver disease have consumed more than

100 g of alcohol daily for 20 years. The Alcoholic Liver Disease/Nonalcoholic Fatty Liver Disease Index score (www.mayoclinic.org/medical-professionals/model-end-stage-liver-disease/alcoholic-liver-disease-nonalcoholic-fatty-liver-disease-index) can be helpful in distinguishing alcoholic liver disease from nonalcoholic fatty liver disease. It includes the following variables: AST, ALT, mean corpuscular volume, age, height, weight, and sex. Physical examination may show evidence of hepatomegaly in patients with steatosis or steatohepatitis. In patients with alcoholic hepatitis or cirrhosis, findings of advanced liver disease may be present, including muscle wasting, scleral icterus, jaundice, spider angiomata, gynecomastia, left hepatic lobe hypertrophy, testicular atrophy, or palmar erythema. Laboratory evaluation of alcohol-related liver disease may show an elevated mean corpuscular volume, AST:ALT ratio greater than 2, elevated γ-glutamyl transferase level, and in advanced cases, elevated INR and thrombocytopenia.

Manifestations of alcoholic hepatitis include fever, jaundice, tender hepatomegaly, and leukocytosis. Ultrasound or cross-sectional imaging may reveal evidence of steatosis, cirrhosis, and findings consistent with portal hypertension. The diagnosis is most often made clinically, with liver biopsy reserved for cases with diagnostic uncertainty. Severity of alcoholic hepatitis is determined by the Maddrey discriminant function (MDF) score, which is calculated as follows:

$$\text{MDF score} = 4.6 \text{ (prothrombin time [s]} - \text{control prothrombin time [s])} + \text{total bilirubin (mg/dL)}$$

In severe cases, as defined by an MDF score of 32 or greater or the presence of hepatic encephalopathy, treatment with prednisolone is recommended by the American College of Gastroenterology (ACG) guideline. The STOPAH trial showed a trend toward improvement in 28-day mortality with the use of prednisolone, but results were not statistically significant. However, a meta-analysis of randomized studies (including the STOPAH study) showed that glucocorticoids were effective in reducing short-term mortality by 46%. Pentoxifylline can be used in patients with contraindications to steroids, including active infection, gastrointestinal bleeding, or kidney failure, but data supporting its benefit are inconclusive. Pentoxifylline is not effective in patients whose symptoms do not respond to prednisone. The ACG guideline makes a conditional recommendation against the use of pentoxifylline for patients with severe alcoholic hepatitis based on a low level of evidence. Due to risk for infection, prednisolone should be discontinued if the bilirubin level does not decrease by day 7. If the bilirubin level decreases, treatment should be continued for 28 days. Nonsevere alcoholic hepatitis (MDF score <32) requires supportive measures and should not be treated with prednisolone or pentoxifylline. All patients require assessment for nutritional deficiencies, thiamine replacement, and alcohol treatment with a goal of abstinence.

Alcoholic cirrhosis can be diagnosed on clinical and radiologic grounds in patients with obvious evidence of portal hypertension and a history of consistent alcohol intake. Occasionally a liver biopsy is necessary in cases with diagnostic ambiguity. In patients who drink alcohol, inflammation of the liver increases stiffness, making transient and MR elastography inaccurate. Nutritional assessments and alcohol treatment are required. Alcohol abstinence can result in significant stabilization of liver function and reversal of portal hypertension. Liver transplantation is reserved for appropriate candidates who are abstinent from alcohol for approximately 6 months.

KEY POINTS

- The Alcoholic Liver Disease/Nonalcoholic Fatty Liver Disease Index score can be helpful in distinguishing alcoholic liver disease from nonalcoholic fatty liver disease.
- Manifestations of alcoholic hepatitis include fever, jaundice, tender hepatomegaly, and leukocytosis.
- Severity of alcoholic hepatitis is determined by the Maddrey discriminant function score; patients with a score of 32 or greater or with hepatic encephalopathy may be considered for prednisone therapy.

Drug-Induced Liver Injury

Drug-induced liver injury encompasses a spectrum of liver injury and can be induced by many medications. Prescription, over-the-counter, and herbal medications have been implicated. Acetaminophen is the most recognized medication to have intrinsic hepatotoxicity, and its pattern of liver injury is easily recognizable. People who chronically drink alcohol can develop acetaminophen hepatotoxicity even when taking therapeutic doses of acetaminophen. The early recognition of acetaminophen-induced liver injury is critical so that N-acetylcysteine can be administered promptly to prevent liver failure.

Antibiotic (particularly amoxicillin-clavulanate) and antiepileptic medications (phenytoin and valproate) are among the most common medications associated with drug-induced liver injury, representing 60% of cases. The most common drugs that cause acute liver failure in the United States are antituberculosis drugs, sulfa-containing antimicrobial agents, and antifungal agents. The pattern of liver test abnormalities and histological injury can be unpredictable. Some medications, such as amoxicillin-clavulanate, can cause a cholestatic hepatitis, whereas others, such as erythromycin, can cause differing patterns of liver pathology. Patients should be asked about exposure within the past 6 months to medications, both prescription and nonprescription as well as herbal and dietary supplements. Withdrawal of the potentially offending drug with resolution of liver injury supports the diagnosis. Re-exposure to the drug to demonstrate recurrence is not advisable, due to the risk of severe hepatitis upon rechallenge.

Jaundice that occurs in the setting of cholestatic drug reactions can take months to resolve. An elevated bilirubin level in the setting of increased hepatic transaminases greater than three times the upper limit of normal is associated with mortality rates as high as 14%. Until resolution occurs, there is potential for progression to liver failure and a need for liver transplantation.

KEY POINTS

- Acetaminophen, antibiotics (particularly amoxicillin-clavulanate), and antiepileptic agents (phenytoin and valproate) are the most common causes of drug-induced liver injury.
- Liver injury typically resolves after discontinuation of the offending drug.

Acute Liver Failure

Acute liver failure is defined as the onset of hepatic encephalopathy and a prolonged prothrombin time within 26 weeks of occurrence of jaundice or other symptoms of liver inflammation in the absence of chronic liver disease. The most common cause of acute liver failure in the United States is acetaminophen overdose. Other widely recognized causes are presented in **Table 32**. The diagnosis requires immediate referral to a liver transplant center.

Patients with acute liver failure require careful monitoring of mental status because progressive hepatic encephalopathy can result in cerebral edema (see Hepatic Encephalopathy). Kidney injury is common, and continuous renal replacement therapy is better tolerated than intermittent hemodialysis. Patients with acute liver failure are at risk for hypoglycemia and infection.

Specific treatment is based on the cause: *N*-acetylcysteine is used for acetaminophen intoxication; antiviral medications for HBV infection and herpes simplex hepatitis; penicillin G for *Amanita* mushroom poisoning; and delivery of the fetus for acute fatty liver of pregnancy. Prompt treatment is crucial. For example, mortality rates for acetaminophen intoxication are lowest when *N*-acetylcysteine is administered within 12 hours of ingestion.

TABLE 32.	Causes of Acute Liver Failure
Acetaminophen	
Hepatitis A virus	
Herpes simplex virus	
Autoimmune hepatitis	
Other medications (antituberculosis drugs, sulfa-containing antimicrobial agents, antifungal agents, and herbal supplements)	
Hepatitis B virus	
Amanita phalloides mushrooms	
Acute fatty liver of pregnancy	

KEY POINTS

- The most common cause of acute liver failure in the United States is acetaminophen overdose.
- The diagnosis of acute liver failure requires immediate referral to a liver transplant center.

Metabolic Liver Diseases

Nonalcoholic Fatty Liver Disease

Nonalcoholic fatty liver disease (NAFLD) is the most common cause of liver disease in the world. Some 30% of the U.S. population may be affected by this condition. Most patients with NAFLD do not have liver inflammation. In these patients, the presence of fat in the liver without inflammation or fibrosis is considered a benign condition. Patients who have fatty liver with inflammation (nonalcoholic steatohepatitis [NASH]) have progressive disease that can lead to fibrosis and cirrhosis. NAFLD usually develops due to the metabolic syndrome, leading to triglyceride accumulation within the liver. The mechanisms by which patients with NAFLD develop NASH are not fully understood. Metabolic, genetic, and environmental factors likely play a role. Patients with NAFLD are often diagnosed by abdominal imaging. Ultrasound, CT, and MRI can detect the presence of hepatic fat. Symptoms of NAFLD are nonspecific and include fatigue and vague right-upper-quadrant abdominal pain. NASH is characterized by inflammation, risk for progressive fibrosis, and development of cirrhosis. NASH may affect 5% of the U.S. population. Mildly elevated hepatic transaminases are common in NASH. Unrecognized NASH is likely a major cause of cryptogenic cirrhosis.

There are no tests that can diagnose NASH as a cause of chronically elevated liver chemistries. Patients with elevated liver chemistries, a negative serological evaluation for alternative causes, clinical features of the metabolic syndrome, and characteristic abdominal imaging are presumed to have NASH. Low titers of autoantibodies are observed in 20% of patients with NAFLD. The NAFLD fibrosis score (www.nafldscore.com) uses clinical data to identify patients at risk for severe disease. Transient elastography can be used to determine whether patients with NASH have developed significant hepatic fibrosis. Liver biopsy is indicated when the diagnosis is in doubt, or if the presence of hepatic fibrosis cannot otherwise be determined.

The management of NAFLD is focused on weight loss through diet and lifestyle modification. No specific diet for NAFLD is recommended, although carbohydrate-restricted diets may result in greater reduction in liver fat than other diets. Bariatric surgery and concomitant weight loss results in improvement of inflammation and fibrosis associated with NAFLD. No drugs have been approved by the FDA for the treatment of NAFLD. Cardiovascular disease is the leading cause of death in patients with NASH, and therapy with statins should be considered.

α_1-Antitrypsin Deficiency

α_1-Antitrypsin deficiency is an autosomal recessive genetic disorder that results in accumulation of a variant protein in the liver. Homozygosity for this condition may result in liver injury and eventual cirrhosis. The hepatic accumulation of α_1-antitrypsin results in decreased circulating α_1-antitrypsin, leading to lung disease. Supplemental α_1-antitrypsin prevents progressive lung injury but does not affect the progression of cirrhosis. Patients with heterozygosity for α_1-antitrypsin deficiency are at increased risk for liver injury in the setting of other liver diseases, including viral hepatitis or fatty liver disease. Liver transplantation is required to treat liver failure resulting from α_1-antitrypsin deficiency.

Hereditary Hemochromatosis

Hereditary hemochromatosis is a condition characterized by excessive accumulation of iron in the liver due to a mutation in the genes that control the synthesis of hepcidin. Several genetic conditions can cause clinically significant iron overload; hereditary hemochromatosis typically results from homozygosity of the *C282Y* polymorphism of the *HFE* gene. Cirrhosis can develop in untreated patients with hereditary hemochromatosis and is associated with an increased risk for hepatocellular carcinoma.

Elevated transferrin saturation and elevated serum ferritin levels can suggest a diagnosis of hereditary hemochromatosis; transferrin saturation is recommended as the initial diagnostic test. Elevations in either test can be seen in other liver diseases, so confirmation of the diagnosis requires genetic testing.

Removal of excessive iron, usually by phlebotomy, effectively prevents the development of cirrhosis. Cirrhosis may be clinically apparent. If it is not apparent based on imaging or physical examination findings, it should be suspected in all patients with hereditary hemochromatosis who have a serum ferritin level greater than 1000 ng/mL (1000 µg/L). Confirmation of cirrhosis is important because surveillance for hepatocellular cancer is recommended in these patients. Patients with cirrhosis should undergo iron-lowering therapy to stabilize liver disease and to prevent other organ manifestations of iron overload. Liver failure resulting from hereditary hemochromatosis is treated by liver transplantation.

First-degree relatives of patients with hereditary hemochromatosis should be screened with iron studies as well as testing for the *HFE* gene mutation. Children of affected patients can be reassured that they do not have hemochromatosis if the other parent is tested for the *HFE* gene mutation and has a normal genotype, as this would mean that the children are obligate heterozygotes.

Hemochromatosis is discussed further in MKSAP 18 Hematology and Oncology.

Wilson Disease

Wilson disease is a rare autosomal recessive disorder that causes accumulation of copper in the liver. The accumulation of copper can result in sudden liver failure and the need for emergent liver transplantation, especially in younger patients. Unexplained liver disease or liver failure in any patient younger than age 40 years should prompt an investigation for Wilson disease, although older patients with Wilson disease have also been described.

Decompensated Wilson disease presents with Coombs-negative hemolytic anemia due to the sudden release of copper from hepatocytes. Laboratory findings include high levels of urinary copper and low levels of ceruloplasmin and ALP. Neurological changes can be seen in patients with Wilson disease (tremor, early-onset Parkinson disease, dystonia). Kayser-Fleischer rings can be seen on slit-lamp examination of patients with Wilson disease and neurologic findings. Histological changes on liver biopsy can be nonspecific, although levels of hepatic copper are typically high. Genetic testing for mutations in the *ATP7B* gene confirms Wilson disease. H

Treatment is lifelong and involves administration of copper chelators. Trientine is preferred over penicillamine due to a lower rate of adverse effects. Zinc supplements can be administered to decrease the intestinal absorption of copper.

KEY POINTS

- Nonalcoholic fatty liver disease is the commonest cause of liver disease in the world.
- Management of nonalcoholic liver disease is focused on weight loss through dietary and lifestyle modification.
- α_1-Antitrypsin deficiency is an autosomal recessive genetic disorder that results in accumulation of a variant protein in the liver; homozygosity can result in liver injury and cirrhosis.
- Hereditary hemochromatosis is a condition characterized by excessive iron absorption that results in accumulation of iron in the liver and the development of cirrhosis.
- Wilson disease is a rare autosomal recessive disorder that causes accumulation of copper in the liver.

Cholestatic Liver Disease

Primary Biliary Cholangitis

Primary biliary cholangitis (PBC), previously termed primary biliary cirrhosis, is an autoimmune disease affecting the small and medium bile ducts with a female to male predominance of 9 to 1. It is more common in individuals of European descent. PBC can present with fatigue and pruritus, but many patients are asymptomatic, with the diagnosis suggested by elevated ALP levels. Diagnosis does not require liver biopsy when the ALP is at least 1.5 times the upper limit of normal and antimitochondrial antibody testing is positive. In patients with negative antimitochondrial antibody test results and strong suspicion for PBC, a liver biopsy is necessary. Transient or MRI elastography can be used for fibrosis staging.

The initial treatment is ursodeoxycholic acid. Response to treatment is defined by improvement of ALP level to less than 1.67 times the upper limit of normal. Patients whose disease does not respond to ursodeoxycholic acid should receive obeticholic acid. Dose reductions are required for obeticholic acid use in patients with decompensated cirrhosis to avoid worsening liver failure. Ursodeoxycholic acid treatment results in histologic improvement, better survival rates, and diminished need for liver transplantation. Patients who present with normal bilirubin and albumin levels and respond to treatment have a life expectancy similar to that of individuals without PBC.

PBC is associated with other autoimmune conditions, particularly autoimmune thyroid disease. Therefore, in patients with PBC, thyroid-stimulating hormone level should be checked on a yearly basis. In patients with a PBC score of 4.1 or greater (www.mayoclinic.org/medical-professionals/model-end-stage-liver-disease/updated-natural-history-model-for-primary-biliary-cirrhosis), upper endoscopy is indicated to assess for esophageal varices. First-degree relatives of patients with PBC, especially women, should be screened by checking their ALP level periodically. Patients with advanced disease should be managed like other patients with cirrhosis and portal hypertension (see Complications of Advanced Liver Disease). Liver transplant outcomes for patients with PBC are excellent, with a 1-year survival rate greater than 90% and a recurrence rate of approximately 20% at 5 years after liver transplantation.

Primary Sclerosing Cholangitis

Primary sclerosing cholangitis (PSC) is an autoimmune fibro-inflammatory disease of the large bile ducts, but it can also affect the small bile ducts (small-duct PSC). It is more common in men than in women, which is unique among the autoimmune liver diseases. PSC is associated with inflammatory bowel disease (IBD) in about 85% of cases; up to 7.5% of patients with ulcerative colitis have PSC. All patients with PSC and without known IBD should have a colonoscopy at the time of PSC diagnosis. Patients with concomitant IBD may have a unique PSC-IBD phenotype, characterized by rectal sparing, mild pancolitis, and backwash ileitis; this carries a higher risk for colon cancer, requiring colonoscopy with surveillance biopsies every 1 to 2 years, as well as a higher risk for pouchitis after total colectomy. The diagnosis of PSC can be made non-invasively through MR cholangiopancreatography (MRCP) (**Figure 31**). Endoscopic retrograde cholangiopancreatography (ERCP) should be considered in patients with jaundice, worsening pruritus, bacterial cholangitis, or a dominant stricture or bile duct mass seen on MRCP. Diagnosis of PSC does not usually require liver biopsy; small-duct PSC, which cannot be diagnosed by MRCP, is an exception.

PSC often requires liver transplantation and has the highest case-based mortality rate among the autoimmune liver diseases. Median transplant-free survival for patients with PSC is 12 years. There is no current medical therapy for PSC. ERCP to dilate strictures and remove stones is used in symptomatic patients.

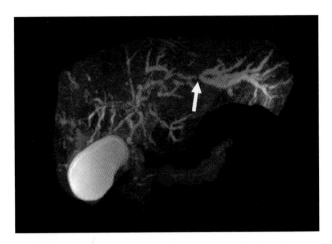

FIGURE 31. Magnetic resonance cholangiopancreatography showing multifocal intra- and extrahepatic bile-duct stricturing with a dominant left-lobe stricture (*arrow*) and upstream bile-duct dilation consistent with the diagnosis of primary sclerosing cholangitis.

Patients with PSC have a 15% lifetime risk for cholangiocarcinoma. Yearly MRCP and measurement of the carbohydrate 19-9 level is recommended for cholangiocarcinoma surveillance. The incidence of cholangiocarcinoma is highest in the first 2 years after diagnosis of PSC is made.

Liver transplantation should be considered for patients with decompensated cirrhosis, recurrent bacterial cholangitis, and hilar cholangiocarcinoma. Transplant outcomes for patients with PSC are excellent, with 1-year survival rates of at least 90% and recurrence rates of approximately 20% at 5 years after liver transplantation.

KEY POINTS

- In patients with primary biliary cholangitis, ursodeoxycholic acid treatment results in histologic improvement, better survival rates, and diminished need to for liver transplantation.

- Primary sclerosing cholangitis is associated with inflammatory bowel disease in about 85% of cases; these patients have an increased risk for colorectal cancer and require surveillance colonoscopy every 1 to 2 years.

- Primary sclerosing cholangitis often requires liver transplantation and has the highest case-based mortality rate among the autoimmune liver diseases.

Determining Prognosis

The Child-Turcotte-Pugh (CTP) score (**Table 33**) and Model for End-Stage Liver Disease (MELD) score are prognostic in patients with cirrhosis. The 1-year survival rates for patients with CTP class A, B, and C cirrhosis are 100%, 80%, and 45%, respectively.

The MELD formula includes bilirubin level, INR, and creatinine level, and is accurate in predicting 3-month mortality. Another version of the MELD score, the MELD-Na

TABLE 33. Child-Turcotte-Pugh Score[a]

	1 Point	2 Points	3 Points
Encephalopathy	None	Grade I-II	Grade III-IV
Ascites	None	Mild/moderate	Severe
Bilirubin	<2 mg/dL (34.2 µmol/L)	2-3 mg/dL (34.2-51.3 µmol/L)	>3 mg/dL (51.3 µmol/L)
Albumin	>3.5 g/dL (35 g/L)	2.8-3.5 g/dL (28-35 g/L)	<2.8 g/dL (28 g/L)
Prothrombin time/INR	<4 s/<1.7	4-6 s/1.7-2.3	>6 s/>2.3

[a]5-6 points = Child-Turcotte-Pugh class A; 7-9 points = Child-Turcotte-Pugh class B; 10-15 points = Child-Turcotte-Pugh class C.

CONT.

(https://optn.transplant.hrsa.gov/resources/allocation-calculators/meld-calculator/), adds sodium to the formula. The MELD score has been the basis for liver transplant allocation since 2002. In 2016, the allocation system was changed to include the MELD-Na score, which was found to be a better predictive model for 3-month mortality.

The MELD score can estimate postoperative mortality in patients with cirrhosis (www.mayoclinic.org/medical-professionals/model-end-stage-liver-disease/post-operative-mortality-risk-patients-cirrhosis). **H**

KEY POINT

- The Model for End-Stage Liver Disease-sodium formula accurately predicts 3-month mortality and is used for liver transplant allocation.

Complications of Advanced Liver Disease

Patients with chronic liver disease from any cause are at risk for the development of cirrhosis. Uncomplicated cirrhosis is referred to as "compensated cirrhosis" and may be asymptomatic or associated with nonspecific symptoms. Decompensated cirrhosis includes patients with complications such as ascites, jaundice, hepatocellular carcinoma, hepatorenal syndrome, variceal hemorrhage, spontaneous bacterial peritonitis, and hepatic encephalopathy.

Portal Hypertension

Portal venous hypertension develops in the setting of advanced cirrhosis due to obstruction of blood flow caused by intrahepatic fibrosis, the development of regenerating liver nodules, and increased intrahepatic vascular resistance. Prehepatic causes, including portal vein thrombosis, and posthepatic causes, such as Budd-Chiari syndrome, can also result in portal hypertension in the absence of cirrhosis. Hypersplenism, often also associated with thrombocytopenia, further increases flow within the portal vein, exacerbating portal hypertension. Complications of portal hypertension include gastroesophageal varices, ascites, and hepatic encephalopathy due to poor hepatic clearance of absorbed nitrogenous compounds from the intestines. These complications of portal hypertension herald a high rate of further complications and mortality, leading to consideration for liver transplantation.

Esophageal Varices

Esophageal varices are enlarged vessels within the lumen of the lower esophagus that provide extrahepatic pathways of blood flow from the portal circulation to the systemic circulation. Over time, esophageal varices enlarge and may spontaneously rupture, leading to bleeding and possible death. The mortality rate for acute variceal hemorrhage has been significantly reduced with treatment. Upper endoscopy should be performed on all patients with cirrhosis to assess for the presence of varices. Management of varices in patients with cirrhosis depends on size of the varix and whether the cirrhosis is compensated (**Table 34**).

See Gastrointestinal Bleeding for discussion of management and secondary prophylaxis of variceal hemorrhage.

Gastric Varices and Portal Hypertensive Gastropathy

Gastric varices are seen in as many as 20% of patients with cirrhosis and are responsible for 10% to 30% of variceal

TABLE 34. Management of Esophageal Varices in Patients with Cirrhosis

Findings	Management
No varices	Repeat upper endoscopy in 3 years (unless decompensation occurs)
Small varices (<5 mm)	Repeat upper endoscopy in 2 years (unless decompensation occurs)
Small varices with red wale marks (erythematous raised areas)	Initiate nonselective β-blocker therapy (propranolol, nadolol, or carvedilol)
Large varices (>5 mm)	Initiate nonselective β-blocker therapy or endoscopic variceal ligation
Varices in patients unable to tolerate β-blockers	Endoscopic variceal ligation

hemorrhage. Varices that extend from the esophagus into the cardia of the stomach are treated with band ligation, like esophageal varices. Varices of the gastric fundus, or isolated varices in other parts of the stomach, are not treated with band ligation. Bleeding varices in these areas should be treated with hemodynamic resuscitation, antibiotic therapy, and octreotide. Cyanoacrylate glue injection can be injected into bleeding gastric varices but is not FDA-approved for this indication. A transjugular intrahepatic portosystemic shunt (TIPS) should be considered for bleeding from gastric varices. Splenic vein thrombosis can cause isolated gastric varices and is treated with splenectomy.

Hepatic Encephalopathy

Hepatic encephalopathy is characterized by brain dysfunction ranging from minimal abnormalities to frank coma. It occurs due to insufficient hepatic function and porto-systemic shunting of blood caused by portal hypertension or vascular shunting. The development of hepatic encephalopathy can be spontaneous or precipitated by other conditions such as infection, sedating medications, volume depletion, or gastrointestinal bleeding, and heralds worsening of liver function.

Minimal manifestations of hepatic encephalopathy can be detected on neuropsychiatric testing, although overt changes of hepatic encephalopathy, ranging from personality changes to frank coma, are common in the setting of advanced cirrhosis (**Table 35**). Asterixis, a flapping hand tremor, is typically present in middle stages of hepatic encephalopathy. Asterixis is typically absent in subclinical stages of hepatic encephalopathy and is lost as patients progress to later stages of hepatic encephalopathy, including coma.

Patients with hepatic encephalopathy should be monitored in an ICU. Diminishing consciousness should prompt consideration of intubation because airway-protective reflexes can be lost in the advanced stage of hepatic encephalopathy. Measures to reduce intracranial hypertension include elevation of the head of the bed and increasing serum osmolality with mannitol infusions.

The treatment of hepatic encephalopathy is multifaceted. Precipitating causes, such as infection or gastrointestinal bleeding, should be promptly treated. The nonabsorbed disaccharide lactulose is typically administered to decrease absorption of nitrogenous substances. If a suboptimal response is seen with lactulose therapy, rifaximin can be administered to alter bacterial flora in the intestinal lumen. While rifaximin is better tolerated than lactulose, it is more expensive. Initial treatment with lactulose is preferred.

Ascites

Ascites occurs in 50% of patients within 10 years of diagnosis of cirrhosis and is the most common complication of cirrhosis. The finding of a fluid wave on physical examination can detect ascites; other findings are less reliable. Ultrasound is useful for identifying the presence of ascites. When ascites is first detected, diagnostic paracentesis should be performed. The serum-ascites albumin gradient is measured by subtracting the level of albumin in the ascitic fluid from a concurrent serum albumin measurement:

$$\text{serum-ascites albumin gradient = serum albumin}$$
$$\text{– ascites albumin}$$

Total protein levels in ascitic fluid also assist in determining the cause of the ascites. The differential diagnosis of ascites is presented in **Table 36**.

Cirrhosis is the cause in 85% of patients with ascites. The management of ascites involves a sodium-restricted diet (<2 g/d) and diuretic therapy, typically with spironolactone and furosemide. Kidney function and electrolyte levels are typically checked 7 to 10 days after changes to diuretic regimens.

Serial paracenteses can be performed if ascites does not resolve with sodium restriction and diuretic therapy. If more than 5 L of ascitic fluid is removed at one time, supplemental 25% albumin, at a dose of 7 to 9 g/L of ascitic fluid removed, should be administered to prevent circulatory dysfunction after paracentesis.

Patients with ascites should discontinue ACE inhibitors and NSAIDs. TIPS or intermittent paracentesis can be considered in patients with refractory ascites and a low MELD score. Indwelling drains in ascites due to portal hypertension are associated with high rates of complications and are not recommended.

Spontaneous Bacterial Peritonitis

Spontaneous bacterial peritonitis (SBP) is an infection of ascitic fluid in the setting of portal hypertension. SBP has a

TABLE 35.	Hepatic Encephalopathy Classification	
Severity of Encephalopathy	**Description**	**Findings**
Minimal	Detected only on neuropsychiatric testing	Few or absent clinical manifestations
Grade 1	Mild lack of awareness, sleep disturbances	Oriented to time and place, but with psychomotor slowing
Grade 2	Lethargic, disoriented, and with personality change	Disoriented to time, with asterixis
Grade 3	Somnolence, confusion, and significant disorientation	Disoriented to time, place, and situation, with asterixis
Grade 4	Coma	Lack of response even to painful stimuli

Adapted with permission from Vilstrup H, Amodio P, Bajaj J, Cordoba J, Ferenci P, Mullen KD, et al. Hepatic encephalopathy in chronic liver disease: 2014 practice guideline by the American Association for the Study of Liver Diseases and the European Association for the Study of the Liver. Hepatology. 2014;60:715-35. [PMID: 25042402] doi:10.1002/hep.27210.

TABLE 36. Characteristics of Ascites

	SAAG	Ascitic Fluid Total Protein Level	Other Characteristics
Cirrhosis	High[a]	Low[c]	Clear, straw-colored
Heart failure	High[a]	High[d]	—
Chylous ascites	Low[b] or high[a]	High[d]	High triglycerides SAAG can be high if caused by portal hypertension SAAG is low if caused by lymphatic disruption
Tuberculosis	Low[b]	High[d]	Peritoneal biopsy may be required to confirm diagnosis of tuberculosis
Malignancy	Low[b]	High[d]	Positive cytology
Nephrotic syndrome	Low[b]	Low[c]	Proteinuria and edema

SAAG = serum-ascites albumin gradient.

[a]≥1.1 g/dL (11 g/L)

[b]<1.1 g/dL (11 g/L)

[c]<2.5 g/dL (25 g/L)

[d]≥2.5 g/dL (25 g/L)

CONT.

high mortality rate, and patients who develop SBP should be considered for liver transplantation. SBP can present with fever, abdominal pain, and kidney disease, but its presence should be considered in any patient with ascites who experiences a decline in condition. Patients with very low total protein levels in their ascitic fluid (<1.5 g/dL [15 g/L]) in conjunction with hyponatremia, kidney dysfunction, or CTP class B or C cirrhosis are at high risk for development of SBP and should be given long-term primary prophylaxis with a fluoroquinolone antibiotic (for example, norfloxacin or ciprofloxacin).

The diagnosis of SBP is established by an ascitic-fluid neutrophil count of 250/μL or higher on diagnostic paracentesis. Bacterial culture of ascitic fluid should also be obtained. Prompt initiation of therapy with a third-generation cephalosporin (for example, cefotaxime) is the initial treatment of SBP. If patients have kidney dysfunction, or significant hepatic dysfunction as measured by a serum bilirubin level greater than 4 mg/dL (68 μmol/L), adjunctive therapy with albumin (1.5 g/kg body weight on day 1, as well as 1 g/kg on day 3) should be administered; such treatment has a demonstrated survival benefit.

Follow-up paracentesis to demonstrate improvement in inflammation can be performed if clinical improvement is not obvious. Indefinite secondary prophylactic therapy should be offered to patients after resolution of SBP and typically consists of once-daily fluoroquinolone therapy.

Hepatorenal Syndrome

Hepatorenal syndrome (HRS) occurs in the setting of portal hypertension and results from a reduction in renal blood flow during simultaneous dilatation of the splanchnic vasculature. Most patients who develop HRS have cirrhosis, although alcoholic hepatitis and acute liver failure are also associated with this syndrome. Type 1 HRS is characterized by a rise in serum

creatinine of at least 0.3 mg/dL (26.5 μmol/L) and/or ≥50% from baseline within 48 hours, bland urinalysis, normal kidney ultrasound, and exclusion of other causes of acute kidney injury. Often patients also have low fractional excretion of sodium and oliguria. Type 2 HRS is characterized by a more gradual decline in kidney function associated with refractory ascites.

Serum creatinine level is one of the most important predictors of death in patients with cirrhosis, and a rapid rise should prompt evaluation for infections and causes of hypovolemia.

Treatment of HRS involves withdrawal of diuretics, volume expansion, with intravenous albumin, and vasoconstrictors. Treatment may also include midodrine and octreotide with intravenous albumin to raise mean arterial pressure and improve kidney perfusion. Hemodialysis while awaiting liver transplantation may be required for patients whose kidney function does not improve with therapy.

Hepatopulmonary Syndrome

Hepatopulmonary syndrome is characterized by dilation of intrapulmonary vessels in patients with portal hypertension, resulting in right-to-left shunting of blood and hypoxemia. Features of hepatopulmonary syndrome include orthodeoxia (worsening oxygen saturation while upright) and platypnea (worsening sense of dyspnea when upright). The diagnosis should be suspected in patients with portal hypertension who have symptoms of dyspnea and evidence of hypoxia. Findings of intrapulmonary shunting with agitated saline administration during echocardiography confirm the diagnosis. Macroaggregated albumin perfusion studies can also aid in diagnosis. Hepatopulmonary syndrome is initially treated with supplemental oxygen, but it is uniformly fatal without liver transplantation.

Portopulmonary Hypertension

Patients with cirrhosis and portal hypertension who present with dyspnea on exertion should be suspected of having portopulmonary hypertension. While less common than hepatopulmonary syndrome, portopulmonary hypertension is a complication of advanced cirrhosis with a high mortality rate. Echocardiography demonstrates right ventricular systolic pressures greater than 50 mm Hg, which should prompt right-heart catheterization to confirm the diagnosis. Although portopulmonary hypertension was formerly considered a contraindication to liver transplantation, patients with preserved right ventricular function who can attain a mean pulmonary artery pressure of less than 35 mm Hg with the use of vasodilator therapies can benefit from liver transplantation. Prostacyclin analogues, phosphodiesterase inhibitors, and endothelin receptor antagonists have been used to successfully treat portopulmonary hypertension.

KEY POINTS

- Upper endoscopy should be performed on all patients with cirrhosis to assess for the presence of varices; primary prophylaxis to prevent bleeding includes nonselective β-blocker therapy (propranolol, nadolol, or carvedilol) or endoscopic variceal ligation.

- Precipitating causes of hepatic encephalopathy may include infection, sedating medications, volume depletion, or gastrointestinal bleeding; treatment involves addressing the precipitating cause and lactulose.

- **HVC** Ultrasound is the most effective means of ascertaining the presence of ascites; the serum–ascites albumin gradient and total protein levels in ascitic fluid assist in determining the cause of ascites.

- The management of ascites involves a sodium-restricted diet and diuretic therapy with spironolactone.

- An ascitic-fluid neutrophil count of 250/µL or greater confirms the diagnosis of spontaneous bacterial peritonitis; patients who develop this condition have a high mortality rate and should be considered for liver transplantation.

- Hepatopulmonary syndrome should be suspected in patients with portal hypertension who have symptoms of dyspnea and evidence of hypoxia; the diagnosis is confirmed by demonstrating intrapulmonary shunting with agitated saline administration during echocardiography.

Health Care Maintenance in Patients with Chronic Liver Disease

Patients with chronic liver disease are at risk for severe complications if they develop acute hepatitis and should be vaccinated against HAV and HBV if they are not immune. Nonresponse to vaccinations is more common in patients with cirrhosis, and postvaccination immunity should be assessed. Patients with chronic liver disease should receive annual influenza vaccination and recommended pneumococcal vaccinations. Other vaccinations should be given based on current recommendations (see MKSAP 18 General Internal Medicine).

Patients with cirrhosis should be counseled to avoid the use of alcohol. Sedating medications such as opiates and benzodiazepines should be avoided because they can precipitate symptoms of hepatic encephalopathy. Raw shellfish can transmit *Vibrio vulnificus*, which can be fatal in patients with cirrhosis; therefore, patients with cirrhosis should be counseled to avoid the consumption of raw shellfish.

Patients with cirrhosis should be screened for osteoporosis. Cholestasis results in decreased absorption of vitamin D, and all causes of cirrhosis can be associated with osteoporosis. The cause of osteoporosis in patients with cirrhosis is multifactorial and is associated with jaundice, hypogonadism, and decreased levels of insulin-like growth factor that are common in cirrhosis. Patients with osteoporosis should be treated with bisphosphonates. Patients with esophageal varices should receive intravenous rather than oral bisphosphonates. Patients with identified osteopenia should be treated with supplemental calcium plus vitamin D. Weight-bearing exercise should be encouraged in all patients with cirrhosis.

Protein-calorie malnutrition is common in patients with cirrhosis. Protein consumption is essential to prevent the catabolic effects of chronic liver disease. Daily protein intake of 1.5 g/kg body weight should be administered to patients with chronic liver disease.

Medications that are metabolized by the liver may require dosage adjustments depending on the severity of the cirrhosis. Patients with advanced cirrhosis (CTP class B or C) often require dosage adjustments, whereas patients with well-compensated cirrhosis (CTP class A) may not.

KEY POINTS

- Patients with cirrhosis should avoid alcohol, sedating drugs including opioids, and raw shellfish.

- Patients with cirrhosis should be screened for osteoporosis; confirmed osteoporosis should be treated with either oral or intervenous bisphosphonates.

- Patients with chronic liver disease should be vaccinated against hepatitis A and B viruses and should receive annual influenza vaccination and recommended pneumococcal vaccinations.

Hepatic Tumors, Cysts, and Abscesses

Benign liver masses are typically discovered incidentally on abdominal imaging. These findings are usually asymptomatic, with the exception of liver abscesses or lesions greater than 5 cm in size. Most liver lesions can be characterized and diagnosed noninvasively with CT or MRI. Percutaneous fine-needle aspiration of lesions is reserved for cases in which imaging is nondiagnostic and in which the information obtained will prompt a change in management. Risks associated with liver biopsy, including a 1% risk for serious complication, such as bleeding or perforation, and a 1-in-10,000 risk for death, need to be considered.

Hepatic Cysts

Hepatic cysts are a common radiological finding on abdominal imaging. Simple cysts are smooth with thin walls and anechoic features on ultrasonography. Patients with polycystic liver disease or autosomal dominant polycystic kidney disease can present with numerous liver cysts. Asymptomatic cysts are benign and require no follow-up. Large cysts, rarely presenting with abdominal pain, can be treated with surgical defenestration or, when surgery is contraindicated, with cyst aspiration and sclerotherapy. Rarely, polycystic liver disease with extensive cystic liver involvement may lead to portal hypertension and/or malnutrition. Obstruction of the portal vein or inferior vena cava can occur due to mass effect. Options for management include surgery, and if that is not technically feasible, liver transplantation. Cystadenomas with thick, irregular walls can be distinguished from simple cysts by ultrasonography; they require surgical resection due to risk for malignancy.

Hepatic Adenomas

Hepatic adenomas are rare liver neoplasms. Despite the benign nature of these lesions, adenomas that are greater than 5 cm in size have potential for risk for hemorrhage or malignant transformation. Hepatic adenomas are associated with oral contraception use and occur eight times more frequently in women than in men. Other risk factors include androgen treatment, type 1 and 3 glycogen storage disease, and obesity. Increasingly, hepatic adenoma is an incidental finding on abdominal ultrasound, CT, or MRI. Hepatic adenomas can be differentiated from focal nodular hyperplasia using MRI with gadobenate dimeglumine or gadoxetate disodium contrast. Biopsy is indicated when there is diagnostic uncertainty but may increase the risk for bleeding; therefore, it should only be performed if the diagnosis will result in a meaningful change in management. Hepatic adenomas 5 cm in size or smaller can be managed with serial imaging every 6 months for a 2-year period. For patients with hepatic adenomas larger than 5 cm in size, the risk for hemorrhage or malignant transformation is elevated and surgical resection should be considered.

Oral contraceptives should be discontinued in all patients with hepatic adenomas with follow-up CT or MRI at 6- to 12-month intervals to confirm stability or regression in the size of the lesion. The duration of surveillance depends on subsequent imaging findings. Biopsy to risk-stratify hepatic adenomas can be considered on a case-by-case basis. Hepatic adenomas with β-catenin activation are at higher risk for malignant transformation into hepatocellular carcinoma. Men with hepatic adenomas are at increased risk for malignant transformation, and resection is recommended.

Focal Nodular Hyperplasia

Focal nodular hyperplasia is the most common benign liver tumor and a frequent incidental finding. It is caused by a congenital arterial anomaly leading to a focal area of regeneration that can cause the formation of a stellate scar seen on CT or MRI. CT or MRI with and without contrast is recommended to confirm the diagnosis. Focal nodular hyperplasia does not have malignant potential or a risk for bleeding and does not require follow-up. In women with focal nodular hyperplasia who continue to use oral contraceptives, there is limited evidence to recommend liver ultrasonography every 2 to 3 years to assess for growth. MRI with a hepatobiliary contrast agent can be used to distinguish between focal nodular hyperplasia and hepatic adenomas.

Hepatic Hemangiomas

Hepatic hemangiomas are common and more frequent in women. Up to 20% of affected patients have multiple hemangiomas. In most cases, symptoms that might be ascribed to hemangioma are due to other causes. Kasabach-Merritt syndrome is a rare syndrome that develops with particularly large hemangiomas that develop consumptive coagulopathy with thrombocytopenia and sometimes disseminated intravascular coagulation. Hemangiomas do not have potential for malignancy, and spontaneous bleeding is rare. The diagnosis should be confirmed with MRI or CT with contrast, which typically shows peripheral nodular enhancement and progressive centripetal fill-in. Biopsies should be avoided due to bleeding risk. Hepatic hemangiomas are benign lesions that do not require intervention or follow-up except in the rare instance when they cause symptoms.

Hepatic Abscesses
Pyogenic Liver Abscesses

Pyogenic liver abscesses are complications of biliary tract infections or portal venous spread of intra-abdominal infections such as diverticulitis. Patients with pyogenic liver abscesses present with fever, right-upper-quadrant abdominal pain, and malaise. Liver abscesses are typically polymicrobial, and the diagnosis is confirmed by radiologically guided aspiration. Small abscesses (<3 cm) can be successfully treated by administration of broad-spectrum antibiotics. Larger abscesses are treated by aspiration or longer-term percutaneous tube drainage in addition to broad-spectrum antibiotics. The success of radiologically guided aspiration and tube drainage has resulted in only rare need for surgical excision of pyogenic hepatic abscesses.

Amebic Liver Abscesses

Amebic abscesses of the liver are found in developing areas of the world or in migrants from countries in which amebiasis is

CONT.

endemic. Intestinal infection with amoebae can result in invasion of the portal vein and migration to the liver. Typical symptoms of amebic liver abscesses include right-upper-quadrant abdominal pain and fever. Hepatic imaging and serological testing make the diagnosis of amebic liver abscess. Treatment of the hepatic infection with metronidazole or tinidazole should be accompanied by eradication of the coexistent intestinal infection with paromomycin. ◧

Hepatocellular Carcinoma

Hepatocellular carcinoma is the most common liver tumor arising in patients with cirrhosis, the fifth most common cause of cancer worldwide, and the second most common cause of cancer-related deaths worldwide. Approximately 85% of patients with hepatocellular carcinoma have cirrhosis.

Patients with cirrhosis, regardless of the cause, require surveillance liver ultrasound with or without α-fetoprotein measurement every 6 months, which leads to early diagnosis, increased rate of curative treatment, and improved 3-year survival rates. Patients with HBV infection can develop hepatocellular carcinoma even in the absence of cirrhosis; therefore, surveillance for hepatocellular carcinoma is recommended even in the absence of cirrhosis in individuals at high risk (individuals with HBV who are from sub-Saharan Africa and older than age 20 years, Asian men older than age 40 years, and Asian women older than age 50 years). The diagnosis of hepatocellular carcinoma can usually be made without biopsy using multiphase contrast-enhanced CT or MRI in patients with cirrhosis and a lesion at least 1 cm in size. Biopsy may be needed for lesions that are large, growing, or indeterminant on imaging.

Many specialty societies have issued guidelines for the management of hepatocellular carcinoma. Patients with CTP class A cirrhosis, without significant portal hypertension or jaundice, and a singular lesion 5 cm in size or smaller should be considered for resection. Liver transplantation should be considered in patients with hepatocellular carcinoma within the Milan criteria and with portal hypertension or jaundice. The Milan criteria are as follows: up to three liver lesions 3 cm in size or smaller or one lesion 5 cm in size or smaller, without macrovascular invasion, and without extrahepatic spread. Patients who are not surgical or liver transplantation candidates should be considered for locoregional therapy in the absence of macrovascular invasion (tumor thrombus) or extrahepatic spread. Locoregional therapies include radiofrequency ablation, microwave ablation, transarterial chemoembolization, and transarterial radioembolization. Decisions about locoregional therapy are increasingly made through multidisciplinary tumor boards. Sorafenib is used for advanced hepatocellular carcinoma, which includes cases with macrovascular invasion or extrahepatic spread. In 2017, the FDA approved two drugs for second-line therapy: regorafenib, an oral multi-kinase inhibitor, and nivolumab, an intravenous humanized monoclonal antibody against the programmed cell death receptor.

KEY POINTS

- Asymptomatic hepatic cysts are benign and require no follow-up. **HVC**

- Focal nodular hyperplasia, a common incidental finding, does not have malignant potential or a risk for bleeding, and does not require follow-up. **HVC**

- Hepatic adenomas 5 cm in size or smaller can be managed with serial imaging; hepatic adenomas larger than 5 cm in size should be considered for surgical resection.

- Patients with cirrhosis and high-risk patients with hepatitis B virus infection require hepatocellular carcinoma surveillance using liver ultrasound with or without α-fetoprotein measurement every 6 months.

Liver Transplantation

Referral for liver transplantation is indicated in patients whose MELD score is 15 or greater because liver transplantation provides a survival advantage in these patients. Patients with decompensated cirrhosis, including ascites, esophageal variceal bleeding, hepatic encephalopathy, jaundice, or hepatocellular carcinoma, should also be considered for referral. Patients should generally abstain from alcohol for at least 6 months, although transplant centers may differ in their requirements for sobriety duration and chemical-dependency treatment. Other factors important in candidate selection are adequate social support, adherence to treatment, and absence of significant cardiopulmonary, psychiatric, and active infectious diseases.

Appropriate candidates are placed on the national waiting list, with the highest priority given to patients with acute liver failure and high MELD-Na scores. In some conditions, the most common being hepatocellular carcinoma, exception points are added to the MELD score, resulting in increased scores every 3 months. Other conditions eligible for MELD exception points include portopulmonary hypertension, hepatopulmonary syndrome, familial amyloidotic polyneuropathy, primary hyperoxaluria, cystic fibrosis, and cholangiocarcinoma.

The average 1- and 5-year survival rates after liver transplantation are 92% and 75% to 85%, respectively. Recipients require lifelong immunosuppression, most commonly using tacrolimus, and less often, cyclosporine. Both drugs are metabolized by cytochrome P450 3A isozymes and pose a risk for drug-drug interactions. Recipients are at increased risk for developing diabetes, hypertension, hyperlipidemia, chronic kidney disease, and malignancy secondary to immunosuppressive medications. ◧

KEY POINT

- Referral to a transplant center is indicated for patients with acute liver failure or for patients with cirrhosis with a Model for End-Stage Liver Disease score of 15 or greater or decompensated cirrhosis.

Pregnancy-Related Liver Diseases

During pregnancy, physiological changes occur that mimic chronic liver disease. Altered hormonal states and increasing circulatory volume can lead to lower-extremity edema, palmar erythema, and spider angiomata.

In pregnant women with preexisting chronic liver disease, HBV and HCV can be transmitted to the newborn. There are no specific steps that can be taken to eliminate the risk for vertical transmission of HCV; however, vertical transmission is relatively rare, with less than 5% of women with HCV viremia transmitting the virus to their children.

HBV carries a higher risk for vertical transmission. Among women with replicating HBV infection, the vertical transmission rate can be as high as 90%. Pregnant women with an HBV DNA level greater than 200,000 IU/mL between gestational weeks 24 and 28 should start oral antiviral treatment to prevent vertical transmission. Oral antiviral agents approved in pregnancy include lamivudine, telbivudine, and tenofovir. Breastfeeding is not contraindicated during treatment. Passive immunization with HBV immune globulin and active HBV vaccination should be administered to newborns within 12 hours of delivery. These measures can reduce vertical transmission rates by 95%. Administration of antiviral medications in the third trimester to pregnant women with high HBV viremia can further reduce the risk for vertical transmission.

Women with autoimmune hepatitis who become pregnant typically continue the use of prednisone and/or azathioprine, which are generally felt to be safe during pregnancy.

Several diseases of the liver are unique to pregnancy and can affect the health of both the mother and fetus. During the first trimester, hyperemesis gravidarum occurs when prolonged, intractable vomiting results in fluid and electrolyte abnormalities. Elevated hepatic transaminase levels are seen in up to 50% of cases of hyperemesis gravidarum, but jaundice is rare. Laboratory abnormalities typically resolve when vomiting abates. Pyridoxine and antiemetic medications can resolve symptoms of hyperemesis gravidarum.

Intrahepatic cholestasis of pregnancy is presumed to result from cholestatic effects of increased levels of pregnancy-related hormones. Increased risk for this condition can be seen in women of South American descent, twin pregnancies, and in women with a history of liver disease. Intrahepatic cholestasis of pregnancy typically presents in the second to third trimesters of pregnancy. Symptoms include pruritus in most patients and jaundice in 10% to 25% of patients. Serum bile acid levels are elevated and help to establish the diagnosis. Fetal complications, including placental insufficiency, premature labor, and sudden fetal death, are more common in intrahepatic cholestasis of pregnancy. Ursodeoxycholic acid produces relief of pruritus and improves fetal outcomes. Increased fetal mortality is noted to occur late in gestation. Delivery is typically induced at 36 to 38 weeks of gestation in women with proven disease.

The most serious pregnancy-related liver diseases occur in the third trimester of pregnancy and are associated with high rates of maternal and fetal mortality. In these conditions, the only definitive therapy is delivery of the fetus. HELLP (Hemolysis, Elevated Liver enzymes, and Low Platelets) syndrome is a severe complication of preeclampsia. HELLP typically presents with nonspecific symptoms such as abdominal pain, nausea with vomiting, pruritus, and jaundice. Rates of maternal and fetal morbidity and mortality are high. Patients with HELLP syndrome should, therefore, be managed in high-risk obstetrical units. Blood pressure, fluid and electrolytes, kidney function, and coagulopathy may require careful management in the perinatal state. Although delivery is the definitive therapy for HELLP syndrome, the maternal condition may continue to worsen in the immediate postpartum period. Resolution is typically seen within days after delivery. Rarely, liver transplantation may be required if liver recovery is not seen. HELLP can reoccur in as many as 25% of subsequent pregnancies.

Acute fatty liver of pregnancy is a rare but serious condition that also occurs late in pregnancy. It presents with symptoms similar to those of HELLP syndrome. Indicators of liver failure, including hypoglycemia and coagulopathy, are often worse in acute fatty liver of pregnancy than in HELLP syndrome; both conditions require close monitoring to prevent adverse maternal and fetal outcomes. Acute fatty liver of pregnancy is a potential cause of acute liver failure. Affected patients may require transfer to a liver transplant center. Prompt delivery of the fetus once the diagnosis is recognized typically results in improvement of the mother's medical condition within 48 to 72 hours. Acute fatty liver of pregnancy can reoccur in subsequent pregnancies. It is also associated with long-chain 3-hydroxyacyl CoA dehydrogenase deficiency, and affected women and their offspring should be screened for this deficiency. H

KEY POINTS

- Measures to reduce vertical transmission of hepatitis B virus include administration of hepatitis B virus immune globulin to newborns and immediate vaccination of newborns.

- The most serious liver complications of pregnancy occur in the third trimester and include HELLP (Hemolysis, Elevated Liver enzymes, and Low Platelets) syndrome and acute fatty liver of pregnancy; both are managed in high-risk obstetrical units and with early delivery.

Vascular Diseases of the Liver

Portal Vein Thrombosis

Portal vein thrombosis is common in patients with decompensated cirrhosis and is a consequence of poor flow through the portal veins. The diagnosis is typically established by abdominal Doppler ultrasonography or contrast-enhanced CT or MRI. Hypercoagulable states are typically not present in patients with cirrhosis who develop portal vein thrombosis. Chronic portal vein thrombosis is typically asymptomatic and does not require anticoagulation therapy. Acute portal vein thrombosis can be symptomatic with the development of ascites or variceal hemorrhage. Anticoagulation can be considered if there is concern that portal vein thrombosis has extended into the superior mesenteric vein risking intestinal ischemia.

Budd-Chiari Syndrome

Budd-Chiari syndrome describes any disease process that obstructs the normal outflow of blood from the liver, usually as thrombosis of the hepatic veins. Causes vary, but it may occasionally be associated with hypercoagulable states such as in patients with a myeloproliferative neoplasm, pregnancy, oral contraceptive use, IBD, or inherited thrombophilias. Underlying malignancy, especially hepatocellular carcinoma, must be considered. Typical symptoms of Budd-Chiari syndrome include hepatomegaly, ascites, and right-upper-quadrant abdominal pain. Budd-Chiari syndrome is typically diagnosed by ultrasound with Doppler evaluation in the appropriate clinical setting. The caudate lobe of the liver is hypertrophied due to the presence of venous outflow channels distinct from the hepatic veins. Long-term anticoagulation is required in patients with Budd-Chiari syndrome, although bleeding risks are significant in patients with acute or chronic liver disease, portal hypertension, and esophageal varices. Angioplasty of the hepatic veins and/or TIPS placement can be used to reestablish adequate hepatic venous drainage. If liver failure develops, liver transplantation should be considered.

KEY POINTS

- Portal vein thrombosis is common in patients with decompensated cirrhosis and is a consequence of poor flow through the portal veins.
- The classic presentation of Budd-Chiari syndrome includes hepatomegaly, ascites, and right-upper-quadrant abdominal pain.

Disorders of the Gallbladder and Bile Ducts

Asymptomatic Gallstones

Gallstones can be characterized as either cholesterol stones or pigment stones, which are black or brown. Cholesterol stones are the result of supersaturation of the bile with cholesterol; they account for approximately 75% of cases in the United States. Risk factors for cholesterol cholelithiasis include older age, female sex (twice as likely as in men), American Indian ethnicity, Western diet, pregnancy, rapid weight loss, obesity, total parenteral nutrition, and drugs such as estrogen and somatostatin analogues. Black pigment stones, usually composed of

calcium bilirubinate, can form in patients with chronic hemolytic disease states, ineffective erythropoiesis, ileal disease such as Crohn disease, and cirrhosis. Brown pigment stones are composed of unconjugated bilirubin and varying amounts of other substances, such as cholesterol, but also contain bacteria. These are typically found in patients with biliary stasis and bacterial biliary infection, as can be seen in chronic biliary obstruction.

Gallstones are commonly discovered when patients undergo abdominal imaging for unrelated reasons. Ultrasound and CT can identify gallstones, whereas plain radiography identifies gallstones uncommonly.

Gallstones that are found incidentally do not typically cause any symptoms, and cholecystectomy is generally not recommended because most stones remain asymptomatic. Cholecystectomy is indicated in asymptomatic patients at high risk for gallbladder cancer, including patients with gallstones larger than 3 cm in size, porcelain gallbladder (intramural calcification of the gallbladder wall), gallbladder adenomas or polyps larger than 1 cm in size, or anomaly of pancreatic ductal drainage.

KEY POINT

- Gallstones that are found incidentally do not typically cause any symptoms, and cholecystectomy is generally not recommended because most stones remain asymptomatic. **HVC**

Biliary Colic

Biliary colic pain results from stimulation of the gallbladder in the presence of an obstructive cystic duct from gallstones or sludge. This pain is typically of relatively acute onset, is fairly severe and steady, and is located in the right upper quadrant or epigastrium. Pain may radiate to the right scapula and can be associated with nausea, vomiting, and diaphoresis, lasting 2 to 6 hours. This symptom complex may be precipitated by eating a fatty meal, which causes gallbladder contraction. Patients with unrelenting right-upper-quadrant or epigastric pain generally do not have biliary colic.

Patients with typical biliary colic symptoms and gallstones on imaging should undergo cholecystectomy, as the risk for complications from gallstones is approximately 2% to 3% per year. Complications include choledocholithiasis, cholangitis, and pancreatitis. Patients with atypical symptoms should be evaluated for other causes.

KEY POINT

- Patients with typical biliary colic symptoms and gallstones on imaging should undergo cholecystectomy.

Acute Cholecystitis

Acute cholecystitis develops in the setting of cystic-duct obstruction and gallbladder inflammation. In many patients,

CONT.

infection of the gallbladder ensues. Patients typically present with severe right-upper-quadrant or epigastric pain lasting longer than 6 hours, accompanied by fever and localized peritoneal signs in the right upper quadrant. A positive Murphy sign (arrested inspiration upon contact of the gallbladder wall with the examiner's fingers) may be seen on physical examination. Laboratory studies may show leukocytosis; liver chemistries are not usually elevated in uncomplicated acute cholecystitis. The diagnosis can be made by ultrasonography showing gallbladder wall thickening and/or edema and a sonographic Murphy sign. A hepatobiliary iminodiacetic acid scan can be used when the diagnosis is unclear, such as when symptoms suggest cholecystitis but the sonogram is normal.

Treatment includes pain control, intravenous antibiotics with gram-negative and anaerobic coverage (monotherapy with a β-lactam or β-lactamase, or combination therapy with a third-generation cephalosporin plus metronidazole), and cholecystectomy. Timing of cholecystectomy depends on the patient's surgical risk and response to antibiotics. An emergency operation is necessary in cases of suspected gallbladder perforation or emphysematous cholecystitis (infection of the gallbladder wall with gas-forming organisms such as *Clostridium perfringens*). For patients with low surgical risk, cholecystectomy, preferably laparoscopic, should be performed during the initial hospitalization. Patients who are deemed high-risk for surgery and who respond to antibiotics can be reassessed at a later time to determine if their surgical risk has decreased. In patients who are not good candidates for cholecystectomy and do not respond to antibiotics, percutaneous cholecystostomy tube or endoscopic drainage can be pursued. H

KEY POINTS

HVC
- The diagnosis of acute cholecystitis can be made by ultrasonography showing gallbladder wall thickening and/or edema and sonographic Murphy sign.
- Treatment of acute cholecystitis includes pain control, intravenous antibiotics with gram-negative and anaerobic coverage, and cholecystectomy during the initial hospitalization in good candidates for surgery.

Acalculous Cholecystitis

Acalculous cholecystitis typically occurs in critically ill patients and is a result of gallbladder ischemia that can be complicated by enteric bacterial infection. Risk factors for this condition include cardiac and aortic surgery, sepsis, burns, and vasculitis. The presentation depends on whether the patient is alert or sedated and mechanically ventilated. In alert patients, the presentation is pain, as seen in cholecystitis related to gallstones. In sedated or mechanically ventilated patients, it may present with leukocytosis, jaundice, and sepsis. The diagnosis is made using ultrasonography, which may show gallbladder wall thickening, pericholecystic fluid, gallbladder distention,

or gallbladder-wall pneumatosis in the absence of calculi. In this setting, the gallbladder may not be visualized on a hepatobiliary iminodiacetic acid scan.

Treatment consists of empiric intravenous antibiotics to cover enteric bacteria and cholecystectomy. A cholecystostomy tube may be needed if the patient is unstable or a poor candidate for surgery. The role of endoscopic gallbladder drainage is evolving. The mortality rate for untreated acalculous cholecystitis is as high as 75%. H

KEY POINTS
- Acalculous cholecystitis typically occurs in critically ill patients and is a result of gallbladder ischemia that can be complicated by enteric bacterial infection.
- Left untreated, the mortality rate for acalculous cholecystitis is as high as 75%.

Functional Gallbladder Disorder

The Rome 4 criteria for gallbladder disorders suggest that evaluation for functional gallbladder disorder is appropriate in patients with typical biliary pain in the absence of gallstones or structural pathology. Typical biliary pain is located in the epigastrium and/or right upper quadrant; is intermittent; lasts ≥30 minutes; crescendos and then plateaus; is severe enough to interrupt normal activities or results in an emergency department visit; and is not relieved by bowel movements, positional changes, or acid suppression. Supportive features include a gallbladder ejection fraction of less than 40% measured by cholecystokinin-stimulated cholescintigraphy and normal liver chemistry tests and pancreatic enzymes. Other causes of upper abdominal discomfort, including functional dyspepsia, peptic ulcer disease, and angina, should be carefully considered. Gallstones should be excluded by transabdominal ultrasonography. Endoscopic ultrasonography may be helpful if the transabdominal ultrasound is normal. If no other cause of pain is found and the gallbladder ejection fraction is less than 40%, cholecystectomy can be considered. The data supporting cholecystokinin-stimulated cholescintigraphy is poor. In clinical practice, it is not uncommon to see patients who have met these criteria and undergo cholecystectomy, but continue to have the same upper-abdominal symptoms postoperatively.

Common Bile Duct Stones and Cholangitis

Stones in the common bile duct are a leading cause of obstructive jaundice. Complications in patients with common bile duct stones are more common than in those with gallstones, but 20% of patients spontaneously pass the stones, and less than 50% of patients develop symptoms. Symptomatic common bile duct stones present with jaundice, abdominal pain, or pruritus due to obstruction of bile flow. Abdominal imaging, including CT, ultrasonography, or magnetic resonance cholangiopancreatography (MRCP), can detect dilation of extrahepatic and intrahepatic bile ducts, indicating the presence of stones. Endoscopic retrograde cholangiopancreatography (ERCP) is the preferred therapeutic method for relieving obstruction of the common bile duct by stones.

The presence of cholangitis is heralded by the onset of the Charcot triad (fever, jaundice, and right-upper-quadrant abdominal pain) or Reynold pentad (Charcot triad plus hypotension and altered mental status). Cholangitis is potentially life-threatening, and antibiotic therapy targeting gram-negative *Enterobacteriaceae* should be administered. Identified common bile duct stones should be removed urgently with ERCP in patients with cholangitis, after which elective cholecystectomy should be performed within 6 weeks to reduce the risk for complications. In patients who are not surgical candidates, endoscopic sphincterotomy can be performed to facilitate the passage of additional common bile duct stones.

> **KEY POINTS**
>
> - Endoscopic retrograde cholangiopancreatography is the preferred therapeutic method for relieving obstruction due to a common bile duct stone.
> - Cholangitis (heralded by the onset of fever, jaundice, and right-upper-quadrant abdominal pain) is potentially life-threatening; antibiotic therapy targeting gram-negative *Enterobacteriaceae* should be administered, and identified common bile duct stones should be removed urgently.

Gallbladder Polyps

Gallbladder polyps, usually incidental findings, can be seen on 1% to 5% of gallbladder ultrasounds. They can be neoplastic, such as an adenoma, or nonneoplastic, such as cholesterol polyps or adenomyomas. The best predictor of a malignant or premalignant lesion is size of the gallbladder polyp, with polyps greater than 1 cm in size being more likely to be neoplastic. Gallbladder polyps associated with gallbladder stones or primary sclerosing cholangitis are also more likely to be neoplastic. Management of gallbladder polyps is outlined in **Figure 32**.

> **KEY POINT**
>
> - Gallbladder polyps greater than 1 cm in size and those associated with gallbladder stones or primary sclerosing cholangitis are more likely to be neoplastic.

Gallbladder Cancer

Gallbladder cancer is the most common biliary cancer in the United States, but it is rare, with 3700 new cases per year. Risk factors include female sex, ethnicity or race (American Indian, Alaskan native, black), cholelithiasis, gallbladder polyps, porcelain gallbladder, anomalous pancreaticobiliary junction, and obesity. The gallbladder serves as a reservoir for *Salmonella typhi* in chronically infected patients, and patients with this organism are at higher risk for gallbladder cancer.

Presenting symptoms may include right-upper-quadrant pain, nausea, vomiting, weight loss, or jaundice in advanced cancers, and biliary colic in early cancers. Gallbladder cancer should be suspected if an enhancing gallbladder mass is seen on CT or MRI.

Early gallbladder cancer is most commonly diagnosed incidentally at the time of cholecystectomy performed for biliary colic. Incidental tumors found to invade the lamina propria (stage T1a) do not require further treatment, whereas more advanced lesions require extended cholecystectomy.

The treatment of choice for gallbladder cancer is surgery. Treatment for unresectable disease can include chemotherapy with or without radiation, or palliative care.

Prophylactic cholecystectomy is recommended for patients with an anomalous pancreaticobiliary junction, gallbladder polyps 1 cm in size or larger, or gallbladder polyp(s) in the presence of biliary colic or gallstones; it is also recommended for patients with primary sclerosing cholangitis and a gallbladder polyp larger than 8 mm in size. Prophylactic cholecystectomy can be considered for porcelain gallbladder or for gallstones larger than 3 cm in size.

Cholangiocarcinoma

Cholangiocarcinoma, although rare, is an increasingly recognized malignancy. It is classified as (1) intrahepatic—seen in the smaller bile ducts entirely within the liver parenchyma; (2) hilar—most commonly arising from confluence of right and left hepatic ducts (Klatskin tumor); or (3) distal—arising distal to the cystic-duct entrance. Risk factors include primary sclerosing cholangitis, choledochal cysts, liver flukes (*Opisthorchis*), exposure to thorium dioxide (contrast medium), and hepatolithiasis. Symptoms vary with tumor location and may include jaundice, pain in the right upper quadrant, and constitutional symptoms.

Intrahepatic, hilar, and distal cholangiocarcinomas can occur in patients without liver disease. Intrahepatic

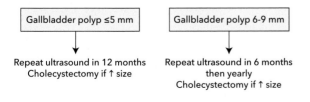

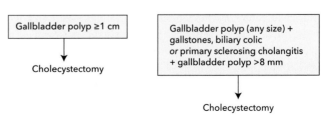

FIGURE 32. Management of gallbladder polyps.

cholangiocarcinoma can complicate cirrhosis, and hilar cholangiocarcinoma can complicate primary sclerosing cholangitis.

Diagnosis of intrahepatic cholangiocarcinoma requires imaging with CT or MRI, and usually a biopsy. An elevated CA 19-9 level is supportive but insufficient for diagnosis. First-line therapy for intrahepatic cholangiocarcinoma is resection. Locoregional and/or systemic chemotherapy are appropriate for patients who are not candidates for resection.

Diagnosis of hilar cholangiocarcinoma can be challenging and is made by a combination of MRCP and ERCP. During ERCP, bile-duct brushings should be obtained for cytologic examination and fluorescence in situ hybridization testing. The latter test uses DNA probes to evaluate for gain or loss of chromosomes or loci, which are often present in biliary cancer. An elevated CA 19-9 level is supportive, but repeat ERCP is often required every 2 to 3 months to make the diagnosis. First-line therapy for hilar cholangiocarcinoma is resection. Patients with obstructive jaundice may require ERCP with stent placement to allow for biliary drainage. Patients with unresectable hilar cholangiocarcinoma smaller than 3 cm in size and without extrahepatic spread can be evaluated for liver transplantation at select centers with neoadjuvant chemoradiation protocols. However, percutaneous or transluminal biopsy of hilar cholangiocarcinoma excludes a patient for liver transplantation due to the risk for tumor seeding.

The preferred treatment for distal cholangiocarcinoma is a Whipple resection.

Metastatic cholangiocarcinoma of any variety should be treated with gemcitabine-cisplatin.

The 5-year survival rate for patients with cholangiocarcinoma (excluding liver transplant recipients), including those who undergo resection, is 20% to 30%.

> **KEY POINTS**
> - Resection is first-line treatment for cholangiocarcinoma.
> - Selected patients with unresectable hilar cholangiocarcinoma smaller than 3 cm in size and without extrahepatic spread may be candidates for liver transplantation.

Gastrointestinal Bleeding

Overview

In the United States, gastrointestinal bleeding is a common gastrointestinal cause of hospitalization. Upper gastrointestinal bleeding (UGIB) is defined as bleeding from the esophagus, stomach, or duodenum. The mortality rate for patients with UGIB varies from 2% to 10% but is usually due to other factors related to comorbid diseases. Lower gastrointestinal bleeding (LGIB) occurs from the colon or anorectum. It is less common, typically less severe, and has a lower mortality rate than UGIB. Small-bowel bleeding, formerly called obscure gastrointestinal

bleeding, is bleeding that does not appear to originate from the upper or lower gastrointestinal tract; it is relatively uncommon.

> **KEY POINT**
> - Upper gastrointestinal bleeding is more common, more severe, and has a higher mortality rate than lower gastrointestinal bleeding.

Upper Gastrointestinal Bleeding

UGIB can present in various ways, including hematemesis, "coffee-ground" emesis, melena, or hematochezia. Hematemesis is vomiting of bright red blood or clots. Coffee-ground emesis is the vomiting of dark, digested blood. Melena is black, tarry stool with a distinctive odor. Hematochezia is the passage of fresh blood or clots from the rectum.

Causes

Common causes of UGIB include peptic ulcer disease, gastroesophageal varices, and Mallory-Weiss tear. Peptic ulcer disease is the most common cause (50%), with most gastroduodenal ulcers caused by *Helicobacter pylori* or NSAID use. Erosive esophagitis is a common endoscopic finding but only rarely causes clinically important UGIB. Therefore, in a patient with UGIB and erosive esophagitis, alternative causes for the bleeding should be excluded.

Bleeding gastroesophageal varices typically occur in the distal esophagus or proximal stomach in individuals with advanced liver disease. Bleeding risk of varices is proportional to varix size.

A Mallory-Weiss tear consists of a mucosal disruption at the gastroesophageal junction and typically forms after repeated episodes of severe vomiting or retching.

Less common causes of UGIB include Cameron erosions, Dieulafoy lesion, gastric antral vascular ectasia, aortoenteric fistula, hemosuccus pancreaticus, hemobilia, and upper gastrointestinal tumors (**Table 37**).

Evaluation

The initial step in the approach to UGIB is a risk assessment to determine the severity of UGIB. This risk assessment includes the measurement of vital signs and reviewing patient factors. Tachycardia (pulse rate >100/min), hypotension (systolic blood pressure <100 mm Hg), age older than 60 years, and major comorbid medical conditions are all associated with increased risk for rebleeding and death.

Findings of stigmata of chronic liver disease suggest a possible variceal source of bleeding.

Management

Patients with altered mental status, massive hematemesis, or an increased risk for aspiration should undergo endotracheal intubation. Hemoglobin levels should be measured. A restrictive transfusion strategy is recommended and initiated when

TABLE 37. Less Common Causes of Upper Gastrointestinal Bleeding

Lesion	Pathogenesis	Presentation	Treatment
Cameron erosion	Mechanical trauma to mucosal folds of hiatal hernia	Typically chronic GI bleeding presenting as iron deficiency anemia	Includes medical therapy with PPI and iron, and surgical repair of hiatal hernia
Dieulafoy lesion	Dilated, aberrant submucosal vessel	Included in differential diagnosis of recurrent, often massive bleeding without clear source	Endoscopic
Gastric antral vascular ectasia	Most idiopathic; associated with cirrhosis and systemic sclerosis	Acute bleeding or iron deficiency anemia	Endoscopic
Aortoenteric fistula	Direct communication between aorta and GI tract	"Herald" bleed followed by massive exsanguination	Surgical
Hemosuccus pancreaticus	Erosion of pancreatic pseudocyst or tumor into a vessel with bleeding into pancreatic duct	Upper GI bleeding in setting of pancreatic disease	Mesenteric angiography with coil embolization
Hemobilia	Bleeding from the hepatobiliary tract often caused by arteriobiliary fistula from trauma or liver biopsy	Triad of jaundice, biliary colic, and GI bleeding	Angiography or surgical
Upper GI tumors	Benign or malignant neoplasms	Slow or massive hemorrhage	Palliative radiographic and endoscopy for malignant tumors, surgical resection for benign tumors

GI = gastrointestinal; PPI = proton pump inhibitor.

CONT.

the hemoglobin level is below 7 g/dL (70 g/L) in hemodynamically stable patients without preexisting cardiovascular disease. Patients with hypotension due to severe, ongoing UGIB and those with concomitant cardiovascular disease should be transfused before the hemoglobin level decreases below 7 g/dL (70 g/L) to prevent the decreases below 7 g/dL (70 g/L) that may occur with fluid resuscitation alone.

For variceal bleeding, resuscitative measures need to be initiated with the goal of hemodynamic stabilization. Two large-bore peripheral intravenous catheters (minimum 18

gauge) are required with initiation of crystalloid fluids, either normal saline or lactated Ringer solution, to maintain adequate blood pressure. See Disorders of the Liver for discussion of variceal bleeding, including prophylaxis.

Pre-endoscopic Care

Intravenous proton pump inhibitor (PPI) therapy initiated before endoscopy decreases high-risk endoscopic stigmata seen (**Figure 33** and **Figure 34**) but does not influence outcome. Octreotide and antibiotics should be initiated if variceal

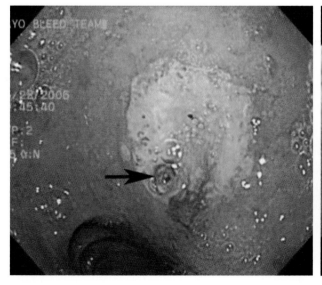
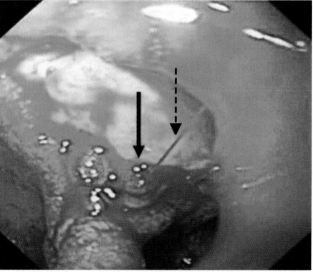

FIGURE 33. *Left*: Duodenal ulcer with nonbleeding visible vessel (*arrow*) that is at high risk for rebleeding and must be treated endoscopically. *Right*: Active arterial spurting (*dotted arrow*) from a duodenal ulcer (*solid arrow*). This lesion is at the highest risk for rebleeding and must be treated endoscopically.

Courtesy of Louis M. Wong Kee Song, MD, Mayo Clinic.

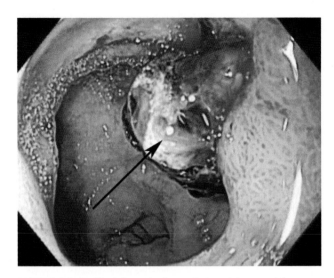

FIGURE 34. Duodenal ulcer with adherent clot (*arrow*) that is at risk for rebleeding. This can be treated medically or by clot removal and endoscopic therapy in addition to standard medical therapy.

Courtesy of Louis M. Wong Kee Song, MD, Mayo Clinic.

CONT.

hemorrhage is suspected. Intravenous erythromycin given before endoscopy improves gastric visualization and decreases the need for repeat endoscopy, but it should be administered only when requested by the endoscopist, not routinely. Nasogastric tube lavage is not required, as it has shown no evidence of clinical benefit.

Vitamin K and 4-factor prothrombin complex concentrate should be administered to patients on anticoagulation with a supratherapeutic INR. The risk for continued bleeding on anticoagulation therapy should be weighed against the risk associated with stopping therapy. Furthermore, endoscopy should not be delayed for anticoagulation reversal unless the INR is greater than 3.0.

Decisions regarding discontinuing antiplatelet therapy are based on whether the therapy is for primary or secondary prophylaxis. If aspirin is being taken for primary prophylaxis, then it should be discontinued because the risk for recurrent bleeding outweighs the benefit. Aspirin for secondary prophylaxis can be discontinued for 3 days but needs to be promptly resumed when hemostasis is secure. Decisions regarding discontinuing clopidogrel and other antiplatelet agents should be made in conjunction with a cardiologist.

Patients with hemodynamic instability or active bleeding (hematemesis or recurrent large-volume hematochezia) should be admitted to an ICU for resuscitation. Other patients can be admitted to a regular hospital ward. Several decision rules and predictive models have been developed to identify patients who are at low risk for recurrent or life-threatening UGIB. The modified Glasgow-Blatchford bleeding score is calculated using the blood urea nitrogen level, hemoglobin level, systolic blood pressure, and pulse rate. It predicts the need for clinical intervention, rebleeding, and mortality. Patients at low risk according to the modified

Glasgow-Blatchford score may be considered for early discharge or outpatient treatment.

Endoscopic Evaluation and Treatment

Upper endoscopy is the primary diagnostic modality for evaluating UGIB. For patients hospitalized with UGIB, endoscopy should be performed within 24 hours of resuscitation; in those with rapid bleeding or suspected variceal hemorrhage, it should be done more emergently. The possibility of aortoenteric fistula should always be considered in patients who have had previous aortic graft surgery and who present with gastrointestinal bleeding because aortoenteric fistula is life-threatening, with a mortality rate of 50% even with surgical intervention. When there is a high degree of suspicion for an aortoenteric fistula, CT with intravenous contrast should be performed before endoscopy or other types of gastrointestinal evaluation.

Endoscopy can determine the cause of bleeding and helps to risk-stratify the patient. Lesions at high risk for recurrent bleeding that require endoscopic treatment include: actively bleeding peptic ulcers, ulcers with nonbleeding visible vessels (see Figure 33), and ulcers with adherent clots (see Figure 34). An adherent clot should be irrigated with the intention of removing the clot; if clot removal is successful, the ulcer is then considered low-risk for rebleeding. Lesions at low risk for rebleeding (clean-based ulcers, ulcers with pigmented spots, and Mallory-Weiss tears) do not require endoscopic treatment (**Figure 35**). Most Mallory-Weiss tears (**Figure 36**) stop bleeding spontaneously. Endoscopic techniques such as injection therapy, thermal devices, and endoclips can be used for actively bleeding tears.

The initial therapy for acute esophageal variceal hemorrhage (**Figure 37**) is resuscitation in an ICU with the goal of maintaining hemodynamic stability and a hemoglobin of 7 g/dL (70 g/L). Overtransfusion can precipitate variceal rebleeding due to increased portal pressure.

The most effective approach for control of acute variceal hemorrhage is combined therapy with octreotide (somatostatin analog) and endoscopic therapy. Octreotide decreases splanchnic blood flow and lowers portal pressure; it should be initiated before endoscopic evaluation and continued for 3 to 5 days after variceal hemorrhage. Endoscopic variceal ligation within 12 hours of presentation is the endoscopic treatment of choice for hemostasis of active variceal hemorrhage, with a success rate of 90%. Subsequent endoscopy with further band ligation as needed to obliterate varices should be performed every 2 to 4 weeks.

Patients who develop variceal hemorrhage are at high risk for infection, such as pneumonia and urinary tract infection, and nearly 50% of patients with cirrhosis who are hospitalized with UGIB have a bacterial infection. Rates of rebleeding and death are reduced with prophylactic antibiotics (such as ceftriaxone or quinolone). Initiation of antibiotics at the time of hospitalization is recommended in all patients with cirrhosis and gastrointestinal bleeding, and antibiotic therapy should continue for 7 days after variceal hemorrhage, even in the absence of ascites.

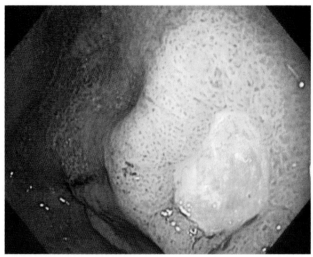
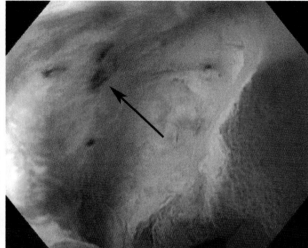

FIGURE 35. Ulcers at low risk for rebleeding, for which endoscopic therapy is not indicated. *Left*: Clean-based gastric ulcer with no blood vessels, pigmented spots/protuberances, or clots noted in the base. *Right*: Nonprotuberant pigmented spot (*arrow*) in a duodenal ulcer bed.

Courtesy of Louis M. Wong Kee Song, MD, Mayo Clinic.

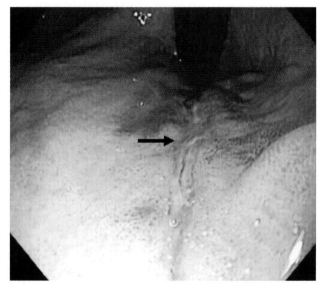

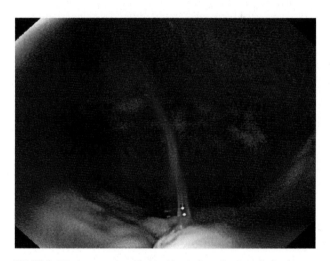

FIGURE 37. Acute esophageal variceal hemorrhage. A varix in the distal esophagus is seen spurting bright red blood.

FIGURE 36. Mallory-Weiss tear. A superficial linear mucosal tear (*arrow*) seen on endoscopic retroflexion in the proximal stomach.

Courtesy of Louis M. Wong Kee Song, MD, Mayo Clinic.

Postendoscopic Care

Patients with low-risk stigmata (see Figure 35) can be fed within 24 hours of endoscopy, receive once-daily oral PPI therapy, and be discharged from the hospital. Patients with high-risk lesions and those with adherent clots requiring endoscopic treatment should receive intravenous PPI therapy for 72 hours to decrease risk for rebleeding and remain in the hospital for this interval.

Nonselective β-blocker therapy (propranolol, nadolol, or carvedilol) should be initiated in addition to endoscopic band ligation for secondary prophylaxis of variceal hemorrhage. The dosage of β-blockers should be increased as tolerated to obtain a resting pulse rate of 55 to 60/min.

If bleeding recurs, endoscopic therapy should be repeated, but routine second-look endoscopy is not recommended. Interventional radiology or surgery is reserved for cases of rebleeding despite endoscopic treatment. For variceal bleeding, placement of a transjugular intrahepatic portocaval shunt is reserved for bleeding that is not controlled by drug and endoscopic therapy.

When hemostasis is secure, antithrombotic agents can be restarted while continuing high-dose oral PPI therapy twice daily. Patients with idiopathic peptic ulcer disease, unrelated to NSAID use or *Helicobacter pylori* infection, should continue once-daily oral PPI therapy indefinitely because of the high risk for recurrent bleeding.

For discussion of management of peptic ulcer disease, see Disorders of the Stomach and Duodenum. ∎

KEY POINTS

- The most common causes of upper gastrointestinal bleeding include peptic ulcer disease, gastroesophageal varices, and Mallory-Weiss tear.

- Tachycardia (pulse rate >100/min), hypotension (systolic blood pressure <100 mm Hg), age older than 60 years, and major comorbid medical conditions are all associated with increased risk for rebleeding and death in patients with upper gastrointestinal bleeding.

- Upper endoscopy is the primary diagnostic modality for evaluating upper gastrointestinal bleeding.

- Management of an ulcer depends on the endoscopic appearance and risk for rebleeding.

Lower Gastrointestinal Bleeding

Twenty percent of all cases of gastrointestinal bleeding originate in the colon or rectum. Most cases of LGIB stop spontaneously and have good outcomes; however, higher rates of morbidity and mortality are seen in older patients and in those with comorbid conditions. Patients with LGIB usually present with sudden onset of hematochezia (maroon or red blood per rectum). Occasionally, bleeding from the cecum or right colon may appear black and tarry, like melena. LGIB may present with additional symptoms of pain, diarrhea, or change in bowel movements.

Causes

The most common cause of minor LGIB is hemorrhoidal bleeding. Hemorrhoidal bleeding is usually characterized by a small volume of bright red blood and does not cause hemodynamic instability or significant volume loss (see Disorders of the Small and Large Bowel for discussion of hemorrhoids). Causes of severe LGIB that may lead to clinical instability include diverticular bleeding, colonic angiodysplasia, postpolypectomy bleeding, Dieulafoy lesion, solitary rectal ulcer syndrome, rectal varices, or malignancy (**Table 38**). Fifteen percent

TABLE 38. Causes of Severe Lower Gastrointestinal Bleeding

Diverticulosis
Aortoenteric fistula
Colonic or rectal varices
Dieulafoy lesions
Neoplasm
Colitis
Ischemic
Inflammatory bowel disease
Infectious
Intussusception
Meckel diverticulum
Angiodysplasia

of patients with a presumed lower gastrointestinal source of bleeding are found to have an upper gastrointestinal source.

Diverticular bleeding is arterial, usually painless, occurs in the neck or dome of a diverticulum, and stops spontaneously in 75% of cases. In patients with diverticulosis, the risk for bleeding is estimated at 0.5 per 1000 person-years. For further discussion of diverticular disease, see Disorders of the Small and Large Bowel.

Angiodysplasia, also known as angiectasia or arteriovenous malformation, can occur throughout the colon but is most common in the right colon. Elderly patients and patients on anticoagulation therapy are at highest risk.

Postpolypectomy bleeding can occur immediately after polyp removal or days or weeks later. Risk is increased in patients with polyps larger than 2 cm in size, with polyps located in the right colon, and with resumption of antithrombotic therapy.

Patients with ischemic colitis usually present with severe abdominal pain, often out of proportion to physical findings. Diarrhea, abdominal pain, and hematochezia can occur with inflammatory bowel disease and infectious colitis. LGIB from a colon malignancy may be painless or associated with obstructive symptoms. Patients with cardiac disease, such as valve dysfunction or dilated cardiomyopathy, are at risk for acquired von Willebrand disease and gastrointestinal bleeding.

Evaluation

An initial patient assessment and hemodynamic resuscitation should be performed simultaneously. The timing and quality of any previous colonoscopy should be assessed, as should whether or not polypectomy or biopsies were performed. The patient's medication history, especially use and dosing of antithrombotic agents, should be assessed, as well as personal history, risk factors for liver disease, other comorbidities, and recent illness.

Management

Resuscitation goals for patients with LGIB should be normalization of blood pressure and heart rate, as well as the transfusion of packed red blood cells if needed to maintain the hemoglobin level above 7 g/dL (70 g/L), with a threshold of 9 g/dL (90 g/L) in patients with massive bleeding, or when treatment may be delayed. Platelet transfusion to maintain counts above 50,000 cells/µL (50×10^9/L) is recommended in patients with active bleeding. The decision to discontinue or reverse anticoagulant agents should balance the risk of ongoing bleeding with the risk of thromboembolic events and often requires a multidisciplinary approach.

Colonoscopy is the initial diagnostic test in the majority of patients with LGIB and should be performed within 24 hours of presentation after adequate colon preparation in patients with significant bleeding. Colonoscopy identifies a source of LGIB in two thirds of patients. Hematochezia with

H CONT.

hemodynamic instability may indicate a rapid UGIB source, and upper endoscopy may be indicated.

Radiographic interventions should be considered in patients with ongoing bleeding who do not respond to resuscitation, patients who cannot tolerate colonoscopy or colon preparation, or patients in whom a source of bleeding is not identified endoscopically. Techniques include CT angiography, angiography, and, less frequently, tagged red blood cell scintigraphy.

Angiography with embolization is frequently used to stop persistent or recurrent diverticular bleeding because endoscopic approaches are limited due to the typical location of the vessel inside a thin-walled diverticulum. Surgical consultation is usually reserved for patients who do not respond to endoscopic or radiographic measures.

The risk for rebleeding is highest in patients with diverticular bleeding (9% to 47%) and angiodysplasia bleeding (37% to 64%). For prevention of recurrent LGIB, nonaspirin NSAIDs should be avoided, particularly after diverticular or angiodysplasia bleeding. The continued use of antiplatelet or anticoagulants needs to be weighed against the risk for rebleeding. Aspirin for secondary prevention in patients with high-risk cardiovascular disease should not be discontinued. Decisions about discontinuation of dual antiplatelet therapy in patients with an acute coronary syndrome or coronary stent placement should be made in conjunction with a cardiologist. Anticoagulation use for other medical indications should be resumed as soon as possible, within at least 7 days for most patients. H

KEY POINTS

- Patients with lower gastrointestinal bleeding usually present with sudden onset of hematochezia (maroon or red blood per rectum).
- Most cases of lower gastrointestinal bleeding stop spontaneously and have good outcomes; however, higher rates of morbidity and mortality are seen in older patients and in those with comorbid conditions.
- Colonoscopy identifies a source of lower gastrointestinal bleeding in two thirds of patients.

H Small-Bowel Bleeding

The term *small-bowel bleeding* is preferred to *obscure gastrointestinal bleeding* because in many clinical situations the cause of the bleeding can now be identified. Patients with small-bowel bleeding often have normal results on upper endoscopy and colonoscopy. Small-bowel bleeding can be characterized as overt or occult. In patients with visible bleeding (either melena or hematochezia), it is overt. In patients who present with anemia but no gross signs of bleeding, the bleeding is considered occult. It is estimated that 5% to 10% of gastrointestinal bleeding occurs between the ligament of Treitz and the ileocecal valve; this is also known as midgastrointestinal bleeding.

Causes

The likely underlying cause of small-bowel bleeding varies with patient age (**Table 39**). Patients younger than age 40 years are likely to have bleeding due to inflammatory bowel disease, Dieulafoy lesions, neoplasia (leiomyoma, carcinoid, lymphoma, or adenocarcinoma), Meckel diverticulum, or a polyposis syndrome. Patients older than age 40 years are likely to have bleeding due to angiodysplasia, Dieulafoy lesion, neoplasia, or NSAID-related ulcers. Angiodysplasia (**Figure 38**) is the most common cause of small-bowel bleeding. It is found in 40% of cases and is often seen in elderly patients. Rare causes of bleeding include Henoch-Schönlein purpura, small-bowel varices or portal hypertensive enteropathy, amyloidosis, blue rubber bleb nevus syndrome, hematobilia, aortoenteric fistula, and hemosuccus entericus.

Evaluation

A detailed medical history and physical examination are needed to narrow the differential diagnosis to a small-bowel source. Patients should be asked about NSAID use to evaluate for NSAID-induced small-bowel ulcers, aortic aneurysm

TABLE 39. Causes of Small-Bowel Gastrointestinal Bleeding

Differential Diagnosis	Patient Age (Years)	Clinical Clues
Angiodysplasia	>60	Intermittent, usually occult bleeding; may also occur in the colon
Peutz-Jeghers syndrome	<20	Perioral pigmentation, obstructive symptoms
Meckel diverticulum	20-60	Possible abdominal pain
Hemangioma	<20	Possible cutaneous hemangiomas
Malignancy	>50	Weight loss, abdominal pain
Hereditary hemorrhagic telangiectasia	>50	Mucocutaneous telangiectasias

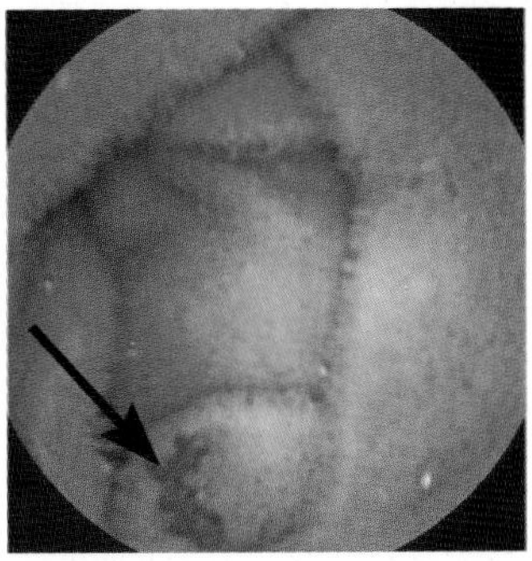

FIGURE 38. Capsule endoscopy image of angiodysplasia. The lesion (*arrow*) has a fernlike pattern and is red in color. Angiodysplasia can have no bleeding or active bleeding.

CONT.

repair (which raises concern for an aortoenteric fistula), necrotizing pancreatitis (which causes hemosuccus pancreaticus), or liver damage (such as trauma, tumor, or recent biopsy causing hemobilia). The presence of skin lesions may help determine an underlying diagnosis, including mucocutaneous telangiectasia (hereditary hemorrhagic telangiectasia, also known as Osler-Weber-Rendu syndrome [**Figure 39**]) or dermatitis herpetiformis (celiac disease).

If the bleeding source is not identified, but clinical suspicion suggests that the cause of the bleeding is discoverable by a conventional endoscopic examination, a second-look endoscopy or colonoscopy should be done. The diagnostic yield is up to 25% with this approach.

Angiography
Conventional angiography is a diagnostic and therapeutic test. However, it is limited to detecting bleeding at rates greater than 0.5 mL/min. Clinical predictors of successful angiography include hemodynamic instability and the need for transfusion of more than 5 units of blood. Potential complications of angiography include acute kidney injury, systemic embolism, hematoma, and vascular dissection or aneurysm.

CT angiography uses multiple phases of contrast enhancement, including arterial enhancement. It can identify bleeding at rates as low as 0.3 mL/min, but its usefulness is limited because the patient must have active bleeding to identify the location.

Technetium-Labeled Nuclear Scan
Technetium 99m–labeled red blood cell or sulfur colloid nuclear scans are able to detect bleeding rates between 0.1 to 0.4 mL/min. Their accuracy in identifying a source of bleeding varies, ranging from 24% to 91%, and they do not provide for therapeutic intervention. A nuclear scan is often done before angiography to confirm the presence of active bleeding.

Follow-up studies after a positive scan can include repeat endoscopy or angiography, both of which can offer more accurate localization and therapy.

Wireless Capsule Endoscopy
Capsule endoscopy employs a wireless capsule camera (**Figure 40**) that is swallowed by the patient to take images of the small bowel. The images are transmitted to a radiofrequency receiver worn by the patient. Capsule endoscopy is the preferred test for evaluating stable patients for causes of small-bowel bleeding after normal results on upper endoscopy and colonoscopy. Capsule endoscopy is able to visualize the entire small bowel in up to 90% of cases, with a diagnostic yield as high as 83%. Limitations of capsule endoscopy include the inability for therapeutic intervention and difficulty with localization of the lesion. The primary complication is possibility of capsule retention due to obstruction or strictures. The capsule can be retrieved by deep enteroscopy or surgery.

If there is continued concern for bleeding from the small bowel, specialized types of enteroscopy may be considered, including push, spiral, and balloon enteroscopy. These techniques allow visualization beyond the ligament of Treitz for diagnosis and the opportunity for therapeutic intervention. In general, the rates of complications are low, but complications can include perforation and in the case of balloon enteroscopy, ileus and pancreatitis.

Small-Bowel Imaging
Endoscopy has replaced imaging for the initial evaluation of suspected bleeding from the small bowel.

Barium-based examinations are no longer recommended for the evaluation of small-bowel bleeding because of low diagnostic yields. CT enterography is beneficial in diagnosing small-bowel masses and has shown a diagnostic yield of 40% for bleeding. Due to insufficient data, MR enterography is not recommended for the evaluation of small-bowel bleeding. However, it can be considered in patients younger than age 40 years, and it offers lower exposure to radiation than CT.

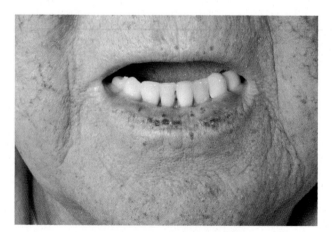

FIGURE 39. Hereditary hemorrhagic telangiectasia (Osler-Weber-Rendu syndrome) is a disorder of development of the vasculature characterized by telangiectases and arteriovenous malformations in specific locations. It is one of the most common monogenic disorders, but affected individuals are frequently not diagnosed. The most common features of the disorder—nosebleeds and telangiectases on the lips, hands, and oral mucosa—are often quite subtle.

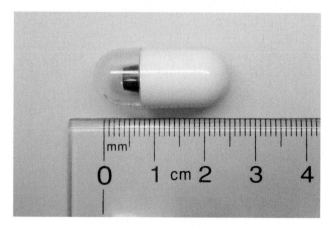

FIGURE 40. Endoscopy capsule.

Courtesy of Elizabeth Rajan, MD, Mayo Clinic.

Intraoperative Endoscopy

Intraoperative endoscopy occurring during laparotomy is often a last resort because it is the most invasive modality available. The diagnostic yield for small-bowel bleeding has been reported in the range of 58% to 88%; however, its use should be reserved for patients in whom all other diagnostic modalities have failed.

Management

After achieving hemodynamic stabilization, therapy is guided by the underlying source of bleeding. Vascular lesions (angiodysplasia) should be treated with electrocautery, argon plasma coagulation, injection therapy, mechanical hemostasis (hemoclips or banding), or a combination of these techniques. Medical therapy for vascular lesions may require a somatostatin analog, such as octreotide. Hormonal therapy no longer has a role in the medical management of small-bowel bleeding.

Tumors or masses require surgical intervention, and if massive bleeding is present, embolization of the bleeding vessel may be needed with the assistance of interventional radiology.

Anemia should be treated with blood transfusion acutely if needed and iron supplementation. If a causative agent is identified, such as an NSAID, the agent should be stopped. Patients with angiodysplasia in the setting of aortic stenosis (known as Heyde syndrome) benefit from valve replacement surgery. While not FDA approved, thalidomide, which inhibits vascular endothelial growth factor, has shown some benefit in decreasing bleeding in patients with vascular malformations of the gut.

KEY POINTS

- Capsule endoscopy is the preferred test for evaluating stable patients for small-bowel bleeding after normal results on endoscopy and colonoscopy.
- After achieving hemodynamic stabilization, therapy for small-bowel bleeding is guided by the underlying source of bleeding.

Bibliography

Disorders of the Esophagus

Bowers SP. Esophageal motility disorders. Surg Clin North Am. 2015;95:467-82. [PMID: 25965124] doi:10.1016/j.suc.2015.02.003

Ganz RA. A review of new surgical and endoscopic therapies for gastroesophageal reflux disease. Gastroenterol Hepatol (N Y). 2016;12:424-31. [PMID: 27489524]

Gunasingam N, Perczuk A, Talbot M, Kaffes A, Saxena P. Update on therapeutic interventions for the management of achalasia. J Gastroenterol Hepatol. 2016;31:1422-8. [PMID: 27060999] doi:10.1111/jgh.13408

Katz PO, Gerson LB, Vela MF. Guidelines for the diagnosis and management of gastroesophageal reflux disease. Am J Gastroenterol. 2013;108:308-28; quiz 329. [PMID: 23419381] doi:10.1038/ajg.2012.444

Kavitt RT, Hirano I, Vaezi MF. Diagnosis and treatment of eosinophilic esophagitis in adults. Am J Med. 2016;129:924-34. [PMID: 27155108] doi:10.1016/j.amjmed.2016.04.024

Pandolfino JE, Kahrilas PJ; American Gastroenterological Association. AGA technical review on the clinical use of esophageal manometry. Gastroenterology. 2005;128:209-24. [PMID: 15633138]

Shaheen NJ, Falk GW, Iyer PG, Gerson LB; American College of Gastroenterology. ACG clinical guideline: diagnosis and management of Barrett's esophagus. Am J Gastroenterol. 2016;111:30-50; quiz 51. [PMID: 26526079] doi:10.1038/ajg.2015.322

Vaezi MF, Pandolfino JE, Vela MF. ACG clinical guideline: diagnosis and management of achalasia. Am J Gastroenterol. 2013;108:1238-49; quiz 1250. [PMID: 23877351] doi:10.1038/ajg.2013.196

Zerbib F, Roman S. Current therapeutic options for esophageal motor disorders as defined by the Chicago Classification. J Clin Gastroenterol. 2015;49:451-60. [PMID: 25844840] doi:10.1097/MCG.0000000000000317

Disorders of the Stomach and Duodenum

American Cancer Society. Cancer facts & figures 2016. Atlanta: American Cancer Society; 2016.

Berg P, McCallum R. Dumping Syndrome: A Review of the Current Concepts of Pathophysiology, Diagnosis, and Treatment. Dig Dis Sci. 2016;61:11-8. [PMID: 26396002] doi:10.1007/s10620-015-3839-x

Camilleri M, Parkman HP, Shafi MA, Abell TL, Gerson L; American College of Gastroenterology. Clinical guideline: management of gastroparesis. Am J Gastroenterol. 2013;108:18-37; quiz 38. [PMID: 23147521] doi:10.1038/ajg.2012.373

Chey WD, Leontiadis GI, Howden CW, Moss SF. ACG clinical guideline: treatment of Helicobacter pylori infection. Am J Gastroenterol. 2017;112:212-239. [PMID: 28071659] doi:10.1038/ajg.2016.563

Evans JA, Chandrasekhara V, Chathadi KV, Decker GA, Early DS, Fisher DA, et al; ASGE Standards of Practice Committee. The role of endoscopy in the management of premalignant and malignant conditions of the stomach. Gastrointest Endosc. 2015;82:1-8. [PMID: 25935705] doi:10.1016/j.gie.2015.03.1967

Ingle SB, Hinge Ingle CR. Eosinophilic gastroenteritis: an unusual type of gastroenteritis. World J Gastroenterol. 2013;19:5061-6. [PMID: 23964139] doi:10.3748/wjg.v19.i31.5061

Laine L. Clinical Practice. Upper gastrointestinal bleeding due to a peptic ulcer. N Engl J Med. 2016;374:2367-76. [PMID: 27305194] doi:10.1056/NEJMcp1514257

Lanza FL, Chan FK, Quigley EM; Practice Parameters Committee of the American College of Gastroenterology. Guidelines for prevention of NSAID-related ulcer complications. Am J Gastroenterol. 2009;104:728-38. [PMID: 19240698] doi:10.1038/ajg.2009.115

Moayyedi PM, Lacy BE, Andrews CN, Enns RA, Howden CW, Vakil N. ACG and CAG Clinical guideline: management of dyspepsia. Am J Gastroenterol. 2017;112:988-1013. [PMID: 28631728] doi:10.1038/ajg.2017.154

Park JY, Lam-Himlin D, Vemulapalli R. Review of autoimmune metaplastic atrophic gastritis. Gastrointest Endosc. 2013;77:284-92. [PMID: 23199649] doi:10.1016/j.gie.2012.09.033

Stanghellini V, Chan FK, Hasler WL, Malagelada JR, Suzuki H, Tack J, et al. Gastroduodenal disorders. Gastroenterology. 2016;150:1380-92. [PMID: 27147122] doi:10.1053/j.gastro.2016.02.011

Syngal S, Brand RE, Church JM, Giardiello FM, Hampel HL, Burt RW; American College of Gastroenterology. ACG clinical guideline: genetic testing and management of hereditary gastrointestinal cancer syndromes. Am J Gastroenterol. 2015;110:223-62; quiz 263. [PMID: 25645574] doi:10.1038/ajg.2014.435

Talley NJ, Ford AC. Functional dyspepsia. N Engl J Med. 2015;373:1853-63. [PMID: 26535514] doi:10.1056/NEJMra1501505

Zong L, Chen P. Billroth I vs. Billroth II vs. Roux-en-Y following distal gastrectomy: a meta-analysis based on 15 studies. Hepatogastroenterology. 2011;58:1413-24. [PMID: 21937419] doi:10.5754/hge10567

Disorders of the Pancreas

Banks PA, Bollen TL, Dervenis C, Gooszen HG, Johnson CD, Sarr MG, et al; Acute Pancreatitis Classification Working Group. Classification of acute pancreatitis—2012: revision of the Atlanta classification and definitions by international consensus. Gut. 2013;62:102-11. [PMID: 23100216] doi:10.1136/gutjnl-2012-302779

Canto MI, Hruban RH, Fishman EK, Kamel IR, Schulick R, Zhang Z, et al; American Cancer of the Pancreas Screening (CAPS) Consortium. Frequent detection of pancreatic lesions in asymptomatic high-risk individuals. Gastroenterology. 2012;142:796-804; quiz e14-5. [PMID: 22245846] doi:10.1053/j.gastro.2012.01.005

Di MY, Liu H, Yang ZY, Bonis PA, Tang JL, Lau J. Prediction models of mortality in acute pancreatitis in adults: a systematic review. Ann Intern Med. 2016;165:482-490. [PMID: 27454310]

Elta GH, Enestvedt BK, Sauer BG, Marie Lennon A. ACG Clinical Guideline: Diagnosis and management of pancreatic cysts. Am J Gastroenterol. 2018 Feb 27. doi:10.1038/ajg.2018.14. [Epub ahead of print] [PMID: 29485131]

Khorana AA, Mangu PB, Berlin J, Engebretson A, Hong TS, Maitra A, et al. Potentially curable pancreatic cancer: American Society of Clinical Oncology clinical practice guideline. J Clin Oncol. 2016;34:2541-56. [PMID: 27247221] doi:10.1200/JCO.2016.67.5553

Kunz PL, Reidy-Lagunes D, Anthony LB, Bertino EM, Brendtro K, Chan JA, et al; North American Neuroendocrine Tumor Society. Consensus guidelines for the management and treatment of neuroendocrine tumors. Pancreas. 2013;42:557-77. [PMID: 23591432] doi:10.1097/MPA.0b013e31828e34a4

Majumder S, Chari ST. Chronic pancreatitis. Lancet. 2016;387:1957-66. [PMID: 26948434] doi:10.1016/S0140-6736(16)00097-0

Okano K, Oshima M, Yachida S, Kushida Y, Kato K, Kamada H, et al. Factors predicting survival and pathological subtype in patients with ampullary adenocarcinoma. J Surg Oncol. 2014;110:156-62. [PMID: 24619853] doi:10.1002/jso.23600

Okazaki K, Uchida K. Autoimmune Pancreatitis: the past, present, and future. Pancreas. 2015;44:1006-16. [PMID: 26355544] doi:10.1097/MPA.0000000000000382

Tenner S, Baillie J, DeWitt J, Vege SS; American College of Gastroenterology. American College of Gastroenterology guideline: management of acute pancreatitis. Am J Gastroenterol. 2013;108:1400-15; 1416. [PMID: 23896955] doi:10.1038/ajg.2013.218

Vaughn VM, Shuster D, Rogers MAM, Mann J, Conte ML, Saint S, et al. Early versus delayed feeding in patients with acute pancreatitis: a systematic review. Ann Intern Med. 2017;166:883-892. [PMID: 28505667]

Disorders of the Small and Large Bowel

Brandt LJ, Feuerstadt P, Longstreth GF, Boley SJ; American College of Gastroenterology. ACG clinical guideline: epidemiology, risk factors, patterns of presentation, diagnosis, and management of colon ischemia (CI). Am J Gastroenterol. 2015 Jan;110(1):18-44; quiz 45. doi: 10.1038/ajg.2014.395. [PMID: 25559486]

Brenner DM, Shah M. Chronic constipation. Gastroenterol Clin North Am. 2016 Jun;45(2):205-16. doi: 10.1016/j.gtc.2016.02.013. [PMID: 27261894]

Clair DG, Beach JM. Mesenteric ischemia. N Engl J Med. 2016 Mar 10; 374(10):959-68. [PMID: 26962730]

Downey L, Houten R, Murch S, et al.; Guideline Development Group. Recognition, assessment, and management of coeliac disease: summary of updated NICE guidance. BMJ. 2015 Sep 2;351:h4513. doi: 10.1136/bmj.h4513. [PMID: 26333593]

Ford AC, Moayyedi P, Lacy BE, et al.; Task Force on the Management of Functional Bowel Disorders. American College of Gastroenterology monograph on the management of irritable bowel syndrome and chronic idiopathic constipation. Am J Gastroenterol. 2014 Aug;109 Suppl 1:S2-26; quiz S27. [PMID: 25091148]

Freeman A, Menees S. Fecal incontinence and pelvic floor dysfunction in women: a review. Gastroenterol Clin North Am. 2016 Jun;45(2):217-37. [PMID: 27261895]

Keefer L, Drossman DA, Guthrie E, et al. Centrally mediated disorders of gastrointestinal pain. Gastroenterology. 2016 Feb 19. pii: S0016-5085(16)00225-0. [PMID: 27144628]

Kornbluth A, Sachar DB; Practice Parameters Committee of the American College of Gastroenterology. Ulcerative colitis practice guidelines in adults: American College of Gastroenterology, Practice Parameters Committee. Am J Gastroenterol. 2010 Mar;105(3):501-23; quiz 524. Erratum in: Am J Gastroenterol. 2010 Mar;105(3):500. [PMID: 20068560]

Leeds IL, Fang SH. Anal cancer and intraepithelial neoplasia screening: a review. World J Gastrointest Surg. 2016 Jan 27;8(1):41-51. [PMID: 26843912]

Lichtenstein GR, Hanauer SB, Sandborn WJ; Practice Parameters Committee of American College of Gastroenterology. Management of Crohn's disease in adults. Am J Gastroenterol. 2009 Feb;104(2):465-83; quiz 464, 484. [PMID: 19174807]

Mearin F, Lacy BE, Chang L, et al. Bowel disorders. Gastroenterology. 2016 Feb 18. pii: S0016-5085(16)00222-5. [PMID: 27144627]

Nikaki K, Gupte GL. Assessment of intestinal malabsorption. Best Pract Res Clin Gastroenterol. 2016 Apr;30(2):225-35. [PMID: 27086687]

Pardi DS, Tremaine WJ, Carrasco-Labra A. American Gastroenterological Association Institute technical review on the medical management of microscopic colitis. Gastroenterology. 2016 Jan;150(1):247-274.e11. [PMID: 26584602]

Riddle MS, DuPont HL, Connor BA. ACG clinical guideline: diagnosis, treatment, and prevention of acute diarrheal infections in adults. Am J Gastroenterol. 2016 May;111(5):602-22. [PMID: 27068718]

Rubio-Tapia A, Hill ID, Kelly CP, et al; American College of Gastroenterology. ACG clinical guidelines: diagnosis and management of celiac disease. Am J Gastroenterol. 2013 May;108(5):656-76; quiz 677. [PMID: 23609613]

Schiller LR, Pardi DS, Spiller R, et al. Gastro 2013 APDW/WCOG Shanghai working party report: chronic diarrhea: definition, classification, diagnosis. J Gastroenterol Hepatol. 2014 Jan;29(1):6-25. [PMID: 24117999]

Shepherd SJ, Lomer MC, Gibson PR. Short-chain carbohydrates and functional gastrointestinal disorders. Am J Gastroenterol. 2013 May;108(5):707-17. [PMID: 23588241]

Tursi A, Papa A, Danese S. Review article: the pathophysiology and medical management of diverticulosis and diverticular disease of the colon. Aliment Pharmacol Ther. 2015 Sep;42(6):664-84. [PMID: 26202723]

Wald A, Bharucha AE, Cosman BC, Whitehead WE. ACG clinical guideline: management of benign anorectal disorders. Am J Gastroenterol. 2014 Aug;109(8):1141-57; (Quiz) 1058. [PMID: 25022811]

Colorectal Neoplasia

American Cancer Society. Colorectal Cancer Facts and Figures 2014-2016. Atlanta: American Cancer Society, 2014.

American Gastroenterology Association. AGA institute guidelines for colonoscopy surveillance after cancer resection: clinical decision tool. Gastroenterology. 2014 May;146(5):1413-4. [PMID: 24742563]

Bibbins-Domingo K; U.S. Preventive Services Task Force. Aspirin use for the primary prevention of cardiovascular disease and colorectal cancer: U.S. Preventive Services Task Force recommendation statement. Ann Intern Med. 2016 Jun 21;164(12):836-45. [PMID: 27064677]

Bouvard V, Loomis D, Guyton KZ, et al.; International Agency for Research on Cancer Monograph Working Group. Carcinogenicity of consumption of red and processed meat. Lancet Oncol. 2015 Dec;16(16):1599-600. [PMID: 26514947]

Giardiello FM, Allen JI, Axilbund JE, et al. Guidelines on genetic evaluation and management of Lynch syndrome: a consensus statement by the US Multi-Society Task Force on Colorectal Cancer. Dis Colon Rectum. 2014 Aug;57(8):1025-48. [PMID: 25003300]

Lieberman DA, Rex DK, Winawer SJ, et al.; United States Multi-Society Task Force on Colorectal Cancer. Guidelines for colonoscopy surveillance after screening and polypectomy: a consensus update by the US Multi-Society Task Force on Colorectal Cancer. Gastroenterology. 2012 Sep;143(3):844-57. [PMID: 22763141]

Provenzale D, Gupta S, Ahnen DJ, Bray T, Cannon JA, Cooper G, et al. Genetic/Familial High-Risk Assessment: Colorectal Version 1.2016, NCCN Clinical Practice Guidelines in Oncology. J Natl Compr Canc Netw. 2016;14:1010-30. [PMID: 27496117]

Rubenstein JH, Enns R, Heidelbaugh J, Barkun A; Clinical Guidelines Committee. American Gastroenterological Association Institute guideline on the diagnosis and management of Lynch Syndrome. Gastroenterology. 2015 Sep;149(3):777-82; quiz e16-7. [PMID: 26226577]

Syngal S, Brand RE, Church JM, et al.; American College of Gastroenterology. ACG clinical guideline: genetic testing and management of hereditary gastrointestinal cancer syndromes. Am J Gastroenterol. 2015 Feb;110(2):223-62; quiz 263. [PMID: 25645574]

Disorders of the Liver

AASLD-IDSA. Recommendations for testing, managing, and treating hepatitis C. https://www.hcvguidelines.org/. Accessed February 14, 2018.

Chalasani NP, Hayashi PH, Bonkovsky HL, Navarro VJ, Lee WM, Fontana RJ; Practice Parameters Committee of the American College of Gastroenterology. ACG clinical guideline: the diagnosis and management of idiosyncratic drug-induced liver injury. Am J Gastroenterol. 2014;109:950-66; quiz 967. [PMID: 24935270] doi:10.1038/ajg.2014.131

Chalasani N, Younossi Z, Lavine JE, Charlton M, Cusi K, Rinella M, et al. The diagnosis and management of nonalcoholic fatty liver disease: practice guidance from the American Association for the Study of Liver Diseases. Hepatology. 2017. [PMID: 28714183] doi:10.1002/hep.29367

European Association for the Study of the Liver. EASL clinical practice guidelines: autoimmune hepatitis. J Hepatol. 2015;63:971-1004. [PMID: 26341719] doi:10.1016/j.jhep.2015.06.030

Heimbach J, Kulik LM, Finn R, Sirlin CB, Abecassis M, Roberts LR, et al. AASLD guidelines for the treatment of hepatocellular carcinoma. Hepatology. 2017. [PMID: 28130846] doi:10.1002/hep.29086

Ilyas JA, Kanwal F. Primary prophylaxis of variceal bleeding. Gastroenterol Clin North Am. 2014;43:783-94. [PMID: 25440925] doi:10.1016/j.gtc.2014.08.008

Kamar N, Bendall R, Legrand-Abravanel F, Xia NS, Ijaz S, Izopet J, et al. Hepatitis E. Lancet. 2012;379:2477-88. [PMID: 22549046] doi:10.1016/S0140-6736(11)61849-7

Lindor KD, Gershwin ME, Poupon R, Kaplan M, Bergasa NV, Heathcote EJ; American Association for Study of Liver Diseases. Primary biliary cirrhosis. Hepatology. 2009;50:291-308. [PMID: 19554543] doi:10.1002/hep.22906

Lindor KD, Kowdley KV, Harrison ME; American College of Gastroenterology. ACG clinical guideline: primary sclerosing cholangitis. Am J Gastroenterol. 2015;110:646-59; quiz 660. [PMID: 25869391] doi:10.1038/ajg.2015.112

Radcke S, Dillon JF, Murray AL. A systematic review of the prevalence of mildly abnormal liver function tests and associated health outcomes. Eur J Gastroenterol Hepatol. 2015;27:1-7. [PMID: 25380394] doi:10.1097/MEG.0000000000000233

Singal AK, Bataller R, Ahn J, Kamath PS, Shah VH. ACG Clinical Guideline: Alcoholic Liver Disease. Am J Gastroenterol. 2018. [PMID: 29336434] doi:10.1038/ajg.2017.469

Terrault NA, Bzowej NH, Chang KM, Hwang JP, Jonas MM, Murad MH; American Association for the Study of Liver Diseases. AASLD guidelines for treatment of chronic hepatitis B. Hepatology. 2016;63:261-83. [PMID: 26566064] doi:10.1002/hep.28156

Thursz MR, Richardson P, Allison M, Austin A, Bowers M, Day CP, et al; STOPAH Trial. Prednisolone or pentoxifylline for alcoholic hepatitis. N Engl J Med. 2015;372:1619-28. [PMID: 25901427] doi:10.1056/NEJMoa1412278

Westbrook RH, Dusheiko G, Williamson C. Pregnancy and liver disease. J Hepatol. 2016;64:933-45. [PMID: 26658682] doi:10.1016/j.jhep.2015.11.030

Disorders of the Gallbladder and Bile Ducts

Cotton PB, Elta GH, Carter CR, Pasricha PJ, Corazziari ES. Rome IV. Gallbladder and sphincter of Oddi disorders. Gastroenterology. 2016. [PMID: 27144629] doi:10.1053/j.gastro.2016.02.033

European Association for the Study of the Liver (EASL). Clinical Practice Guidelines on the prevention, diagnosis and treatment of gallstones. J Hepatol. 2016;65:146-181. [PMID: 27085810] doi:10.1016/j.jhep.2016.03.005

Razumilava N, Gores GJ. Cholangiocarcinoma. Lancet. 2014;383:2168-79. [PMID: 24581682] doi:10.1016/S0140-6736(13)61903-0

Gastrointestinal Bleeding

Fisher L, Lee Krinsky M, Anderson MA, Appalaneni V, Banerjee S, Ben-Menachem T, et al; ASGE Standards of Practice Committee. The role of endoscopy in the management of obscure GI bleeding. Gastrointest Endosc. 2010;72:471-9. [PMID: 20801285] doi:10.1016/j.gie.2010.04.032

Gerson LB, Fidler JL, Cave DR, Leighton JA. ACG clinical guideline: diagnosis and management of small bowel bleeding. Am J Gastroenterol. 2015;110:1265-87; quiz 1288. [PMID: 26303132] doi:10.1038/ajg.2015.246

Laine L. Clinical practice. Upper gastrointestinal bleeding due to a peptic ulcer. N Engl J Med. 2016;374:2367-76. [PMID: 27305194] doi:10.1056/NEJMcp1514257

Laine L, Jensen DM. Management of patients with ulcer bleeding. Am J Gastroenterol. 2012;107:345-60; quiz 361. [PMID: 22310222] doi:10.1038/ajg.2011.480

Leighton JA. The role of endoscopic imaging of the small bowel in clinical practice. Am J Gastroenterol. 2011;106:27-36; quiz 37. [PMID: 20978483] doi:10.1038/ajg.2010.410

Liu K, Kaffes AJ. Review article: the diagnosis and investigation of obscure gastrointestinal bleeding. Aliment Pharmacol Ther. 2011;34:416-23. [PMID: 21692820] doi:10.1111/j.1365-2036.2011.04744.x

Strate LL, Gralnek IM. ACG clinical guideline: management of patients with acute lower gastrointestinal bleeding. Am J Gastroenterol. 2016;111:459-74. [PMID: 26925883] doi:10.1038/ajg.2016.41

Teshima CW. Small bowel endoscopy for obscure GI bleeding. Best Pract Res Clin Gastroenterol. 2012;26:247-61. [PMID: 22704568] doi:10.1016/j.bpg.2012.01.020

Villanueva C, Colomo A, Bosch A, Concepción M, Hernandez-Gea V, Aracil C, et al. Transfusion strategies for acute upper gastrointestinal bleeding. N Engl J Med. 2013;368:11-21. [PMID: 23281973] doi:10.1056/NEJMoa1211801

Gastroenterology and Hepatology Self-Assessment Test

This self-assessment test contains one-best-answer multiple-choice questions. Please read these directions carefully before answering the questions. Answers, critiques, and bibliographies immediately follow these multiple-choice questions. The American College of Physicians (ACP) is accredited by the Accreditation Council for Continuing Medical Education (ACCME) to provide continuing medical education for physicians.

The American College of Physicians designates MKSAP 18 Gastroenterology and Hepatology for a maximum of 22 *AMA PRA Category 1 Credits*™. Physicians should claim only the credit commensurate with the extent of their participation in the activity.

Successful completion of the CME activity, which includes participation in the evaluation component, enables the participant to earn up to 22 medical knowledge MOC points in the American Board of Internal Medicine's Maintenance of Certification (MOC) program. It is the CME activity provider's responsibility to submit participant completion information to ACCME for the purpose of granting MOC credit.

Earn Instantaneous CME Credits or MOC Points Online

Print subscribers can enter their answers online to earn instantaneous CME credits or MOC points. You can submit your answers using online answer sheets that are provided at mksap.acponline.org, where a record of your MKSAP 18 credits will be available. To earn CME credits or to apply for MOC points, you need to answer all of the questions in a test and earn a score of at least 50% correct (number of correct answers divided by the total number of questions). Please note that if you are applying for MOC points, you must also enter your birth date and ABIM candidate number.

Take either of the following approaches:

- Use the printed answer sheet at the back of this book to record your answers. Go to mksap.acponline.org, access the appropriate online answer sheet, transcribe your answers, and submit your test for instantaneous CME credits or MOC points. There is no additional fee for this service.

- Go to mksap.acponline.org, access the appropriate online answer sheet, directly enter your answers, and submit your test for instantaneous CME credits or MOC points. There is no additional fee for this service.

Earn CME Credits or MOC Points by Mail or Fax

Pay a $20 processing fee per answer sheet and submit the printed answer sheet at the back of this book by mail or fax, as instructed on the answer sheet. Make sure you calculate your score and enter your birth date and ABIM candidate number, and fax the answer sheet to 215-351-2799 or mail the answer sheet to Member and Customer Service, American College of Physicians, 190 N. Independence Mall West, Philadelphia, PA 19106-1572, using the courtesy envelope provided in your MKSAP 18 slipcase. You will need your 10-digit order number and 8-digit ACP ID number, which are printed on your packing slip. Please allow 4 to 6 weeks for your score report to be emailed back to you. Be sure to include your email address for a response.

If you do not have a 10-digit order number and 8-digit ACP ID number, or if you need help creating a username and password to access the MKSAP 18 online answer sheets, go to mksap.acponline.org or email custserv@acponline.org.

CME credits and MOC points are available from the publication date of July 31, 2018, until July 31, 2021. You may submit your answer sheet or enter your answers online at any time during this period.

Directions

Each of the numbered items is followed by lettered answers. Select the ONE lettered answer that is BEST in each case.

Self-Assessment Test

Item 1

A 60-year-old woman is evaluated for persistent constipation symptoms of 2 years' duration. She has reflex sympathetic dystrophy syndrome involving the right arm and neck that began 3 years earlier and requires chronic opioid analgesic therapy. She reports passing two hard bowel movements per week. Trials of several fiber supplements caused severe bloating and abdominal distention without relieving symptoms. A trial of polyethylene glycol (PEG) has not been effective; the patient reports that her stool is soft, but she still has no more than two bowel movements per week. Adding bisacodyl caused severe abdominal cramping, prompting its discontinuation. Colonoscopy at the onset of constipation was unremarkable. In addition to PEG, her medications are gabapentin, hydrocodone, fentanyl patch, and a calcium supplement with vitamin D.

On physical examination, vital signs and other findings are normal.

Which of the following is the most appropriate treatment for her constipation?

(A) Add docusate sodium
(B) Add lactulose
(C) Increase PEG dosage
(D) Switch to naloxegol

Item 2

A 29-year-old woman is evaluated during a new-patient appointment. She was diagnosed with hepatitis B virus (HBV) infection 10 years ago; her mother had HBV infection, and it was presumed that the patient acquired the infection at birth. She reports feeling well. Her medical history is otherwise unremarkable and she takes no medication.

On physical examination, vital signs are normal, as is the remainder of the examination.

Laboratory studies are positive for hepatitis B surface antigen and positive for hepatitis B e antigen. The serum HBV DNA level is 20,000,000 IU/mL. Alanine aminotransferase and aspartate aminotransferase levels are within normal limits.

Which of the following is the most appropriate next step in management?

(A) Entecavir
(B) Hepatic ultrasonography
(C) Pegylated interferon
(D) Repeat liver chemistry tests in 6 months
(E) Tenofovir

Item 3

A 58-year-old man is counseled before undergoing colonoscopy and polypectomy in 10 days' time. A routine screening CT colonography showed two polyps in the descending colon, 10 mm and 8 mm in size. Two years earlier, he had an inferior wall myocardial infarction. His medications are low-dose aspirin, atorvastatin, metoprolol, and enalapril.

Which of the following is the most appropriate management of his aspirin therapy?

(A) Continue aspirin use until the day of the polypectomy; resume in 48 hours
(B) Discontinue aspirin use 7 days before the polypectomy; resume immediately after
(C) Discontinue aspirin use 7 days before the polypectomy; resume in 48 hours
(D) Do not discontinue aspirin

Item 4

A 48-year-old woman is evaluated at a follow-up appointment for elevated liver chemistry tests over the preceding 6 months. She reports no symptoms. She has type 2 diabetes mellitus and hypertension. Her family history is unremarkable. She drinks two glasses of wine one or two times per month. Her medications are metformin and lisinopril.

On physical examination, vital signs are normal; BMI is 31. No spider angiomata, palmar erythema, splenomegaly, abdominal distention, or lower-extremity edema is noted.

Laboratory studies:
Alkaline phosphatase	96 U/L
Alanine aminotransferase	85 U/L
Aspartate aminotransferase	74 U/L
Anti–smooth muscle antibody	Positive (1:20 titer)

Results of other studies, including hepatitis C antibody, hepatitis B surface antigen, iron saturation, α1-antitrypsin phenotype, tissue transglutaminase IgA antibody, antimitochondrial antibody, and IgG, are within normal limits.

On ultrasonography, the liver is hyperechoic and enlarged.

Which of the following is the most likely diagnosis?

(A) Antimitochondrial antibody–negative primary biliary cholangitis
(B) Autoimmune hepatitis
(C) Nonalcoholic fatty liver disease
(D) Primary sclerosing cholangitis

Item 5

A 75-year-old man is evaluated for progressive dysphagia of 8 months' duration for both solid food and water, and the necessity to induce vomiting several times each month to relieve his symptoms. He also has experienced chest pain and heartburn symptoms. He has lost approximately 6 kg (13 lb) of weight over the preceding 3 months and a total of 9 kg (20 lb) since his symptoms began. He has a long history of cigarette and alcohol use. His medical history and review of systems is otherwise negative. He has no travel history outside the northeastern United States. He takes no medication.

On physical examination, vital signs are normal; BMI is 23. He appears thin and tired. The remainder of the physical examination is unremarkable.

Upper endoscopic findings reveal retained saliva, liquid, and food in the esophagus without mechanical obstruction. Manometry demonstrates incomplete lower esophageal relaxation and aperistalsis.

Which of the following is the most likely diagnosis?

(A) Achalasia
(B) Chagas disease
(C) Eosinophilic esophagitis
(D) Pseudoachalasia

Item 6

A 35-year-old man is evaluated for a 1-year history of near-daily postprandial diarrhea, episodic abdominal cramping relieved with a bowel movement, and abdominal bloating. He is otherwise healthy, and his only medication is loperamide. This treatment has not been consistently effective in reducing diarrhea symptoms and has had no effect on the cramping and bloating, despite increased frequency of dosing.

Vital signs are normal. Diffuse tenderness to abdominal palpation is noted. Other physical examination findings are normal.

Stool testing for infection and celiac antibody testing are negative.

Colonoscopy findings are unremarkable.

Which of the following is the most appropriate treatment?

(A) Alosetron
(B) Linaclotide
(C) Low-FODMAP (Fermentable Oligosaccharides, Disaccharides, Monosaccharides, And Polyols) diet
(D) Lubiprostone

Item 7

A 52-year-old man is evaluated for dysphagia of 3 months' duration. He reports regurgitating undigested food soon after eating solid food, occasional coughing and choking after swallowing, and chronic halitosis. He reports no weight loss or chest pain. He drinks two beers weekly and does not smoke.

On physical examination, vital signs are normal; BMI is 25. The remainder of the examination, including abdominal examination, is unremarkable.

Which of the following is the most appropriate diagnostic test to perform next?

(A) Barium esophagography
(B) Esophageal manometry
(C) 24-Hour esophageal pH monitoring
(D) Upper endoscopy

Item 8

A 48-year-old woman is evaluated for shortness of breath of 6 weeks' duration. She has cirrhosis due to primary biliary cholangitis.

On physical examination, vital signs are normal. Spider nevi are present on the skin. The cardiopulmonary examination is normal. There is no edema. When the patient is

supine, oxygen saturation is 98% breathing ambient air, but oxygen saturation drops to 92% with standing.

A radiograph of the chest is normal.

Which of the following is the most appropriate diagnostic test?

(A) Bronchoscopy
(B) CT angiography
(C) Echocardiography with agitated saline
(D) Pulmonary function testing

Item 9

A 72-year-old woman is evaluated in the hospital for new-onset abdominal pain in the right upper quadrant and fever that developed abruptly on hospital day 5. She was hospitalized 5 days earlier for altered mental status. In the emergency department, she was found to be confused, hypotensive, and tachycardic. She was transferred to the ICU, where she was diagnosed and treated for urosepsis. Within 24 hours, she was hemodynamically stable and the sepsis syndrome resolved. She also has type 2 diabetes mellitus, hypertension, and hyperlipidemia. Her medications are insulin glargine, insulin aspart, lisinopril, atorvastatin, and piperacillin-tazobactam.

On physical examination, the patient is alert. Temperature is 38.2 °C (100.8 °F), blood pressure is 90/62 mm Hg, pulse rate is 110/min, and respiration rate is 20/min. Abdominal examination is notable for tenderness to palpation of the right upper quadrant. A soft palpable mass is felt in this area.

Laboratory studies show a leukocyte count of 20,000/µL (20 × 10^9/L) and a serum total bilirubin level of 5 g/dL (85.5 µmol/L).

Ultrasonography shows a distended gallbladder with wall thickening and pericholecystic fluid. No gallstones are seen and bile ducts are normal.

Which of the following is the most appropriate next step in management?

(A) Cholecystostomy tube placement
(B) Endoscopic retrograde cholangiopancreatography
(C) Hepatobiliary iminodiacetic acid scan
(D) MR cholangiopancreatography

Item 10

A 45-year-old man is evaluated for severe lower back and hip pain related to degenerative joint disease. His pain responds to naproxen, but he was hospitalized 6 months earlier for a bleeding gastric ulcer attributed to daily naproxen use. Naproxen was stopped, and twice-daily omeprazole was initiated at that time. Three months later, the ulcer had healed completely and omeprazole was discontinued. The patient's pain did not respond to trials of acetaminophen. He did not tolerate tramadol. The patient has no other medical problems and currently takes only acetaminophen.

Which of the following is the most appropriate treatment regimen?

(A) Celecoxib
(B) Celecoxib and omeprazole

(C) Ibuprofen and misoprostol

(D) Naproxen and ranitidine

Item 11

A 55-year-old woman is evaluated after screening colonoscopy showed three polyps at the rectosigmoid junction. The three polyps were 3 mm, 5 mm, and 6 mm in size. All three polyps were completely excised and pathology showed them to be hyperplastic. Colonoscopy preparation was excellent and the procedure was complete to the cecum. Family history is significant for colon cancer diagnosed in her paternal grandfather at age 80 years.

All physical examination findings, including vital signs, are normal.

When should this patient next undergo colonoscopy?

(A) 1 year

(B) 3 years

(C) 5 years

(D) 10 years

Item 12

A 62-year-old woman is evaluated in the emergency department for a 12-hour history of fever, dark urine, and abdominal pain in the right upper quadrant.

On physical examination, temperature is 39.7 °C (103.5 °F); other vital signs are normal. Her mental status is normal. Scleral icterus is noted. The abdomen is tender to palpation in the right upper quadrant.

Laboratory studies:

Hematocrit	36%
Leukocyte count	14,600/µL (14.6 × 10⁹/L)
Platelet count	350,000/µL (350 × 10⁹/L)
Alanine aminotransferase	453 U/L
Total bilirubin	3.5 mg/dL (59.9 µmol/L)

An abdominal ultrasound shows a stone in the common bile duct and intrahepatic biliary dilation. Gallbladder stones are also noted.

Antibiotic therapy is initiated.

Which of the following is the most appropriate next step in management?

(A) Cholecystectomy

(B) Endoscopic retrograde cholangiopancreatography

(C) MR cholangiopancreatography

(D) Percutaneous cholecystostomy

Item 13

A 30-year-old man is evaluated for ongoing symptoms of dysphagia. He was previously diagnosed with eosinophilic esophagitis on upper endoscopy and has completed an 8-week course of swallowed aerosolized fluticasone, which did not alleviate his symptoms. He takes no other medications.

On physical examination, vital signs are normal; BMI is 25. Other findings, including those of an abdominal examination, are unremarkable.

Upper endoscopy shows an area of high-grade stenosis in the distal esophagus.

Which of the following is the most appropriate treatment?

(A) Increase fluticasone

(B) Endoscopy with dilation

(C) Omeprazole

(D) Oral prednisone

Item 14

A 24-year-old man is evaluated in the emergency department for a 2-week history of worsening bloody diarrhea with up to 10 bloody bowel movements per day. He also reports increasing lower abdominal pain and distension and that stool frequency has decreased over the past day. He has extensive ulcerative colitis of 5 years' duration. His medications are infliximab and azathioprine.

On physical examination, the patient appears ill. Temperature is 38.3 °C (101 °F), blood pressure is 90/60 mm Hg, and pulse rate is 110/min; other vital signs are normal. The abdomen is distended with guarding. Bowel sounds are hypoactive.

Laboratory studies show a hemoglobin level of 10 g/dL (100 g/L), leukocyte count of 16,000/µL (16 × 10⁹/L), and blood urea nitrogen level of 26 mg/dL (9.3 mmol/L).

An abdominal radiograph is shown.

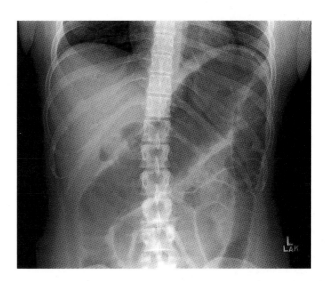

Which of the following is the most appropriate next step in management?

(A) Colectomy

(B) Colonoscopy

(C) CT of the abdomen

(D) Stool culture

Item 15

A 65-year-old woman is evaluated for watery, nonbloody diarrhea of 8 months' duration. She reports up to six bowel movements per day with nocturnal awakenings, but no abdominal pain, bloating, flatulence, or weight loss. Her last screening colonoscopy at age 60 years was normal. She has no personal or family history of colon cancer or polyps. She also has osteoarthritis, and her only medication is ibuprofen approximately three times weekly. The patient is not exposed to children and has no recent travel history or engagement in outdoor recreational activities.

On physical examination, vital signs are normal. The remainder of the physical examination, including abdominal examination, is normal.

Laboratory studies show hemoglobin, serum albumin, total IgA, and tissue transglutaminase IgA levels to be within normal limits.

Which of the following is the most likely diagnosis?

(A) *Giardia lamblia* infection
(B) Microscopic colitis
(C) Small intestinal bacterial overgrowth
(D) Ulcerative colitis

Item 16

A 78-year-old man is evaluated in the emergency department for worsening jaundice of 2 weeks' duration, dry mouth, dark urine, and light stools. He has also noticed swelling under his jaw bilaterally. He reports no abdominal pain or weight loss.

On physical examination, vital signs are normal. Swollen submandibular glands bilaterally and jaundice are noted.

Laboratory studies:

Alkaline phosphatase	180 U/L
Alanine aminotransferase	66 U/L
Aspartate aminotransferase	55 U/L
Total bilirubin	6.2 mg/dL (106.0 µmol/L)
Direct bilirubin	4.8 mg/dL (82.1 µmol/L)

A CT scan of the abdomen shows a narrowed pancreatic duct and enlargement of the pancreas parenchyma, described as a "sausage-shaped" pancreas, as well as findings consistent with retroperitoneal fibrosis. Endoscopic ultrasound–guided biopsy of the pancreas shows more than 10 IgG4-positive cells/hpf and no evidence of malignancy.

Which of the following is the most appropriate treatment?

(A) Azathioprine
(B) Endoscopic retrograde cholangiopancreatography with bile-duct stenting
(C) Pancreaticoduodenectomy
(D) Prednisone

Item 17

A 25-year-old woman is evaluated in the hospital for right-upper-quadrant abdominal pain, jaundice, and nausea of 10 days' duration. She is in her 35th week of pregnancy. Her only medication is a prenatal vitamin.

On physical examination, the patient is drowsy. Temperature is normal. Blood pressure is 95/60 mm Hg, pulse

rate is 108/min, and respiration rate is 22/min. Jaundice is apparent. Abdominal examination shows tenderness to palpation in the right upper quadrant. The uterus is of appropriate size for gestation.

Laboratory studies:

Hematocrit	34%
Leukocyte count	6000/µL (6×10^9/L)
Platelet count	155,000/µL (155×10^9/L)
INR	2.2
Alanine aminotransferase	115 U/L
Aspartate aminotransferase	130 U/L
Total bilirubin	6.2 mg/dL (106.0 µmol/L)
Glucose	55 mg/dL (3.1 µmol/L)

On abdominal ultrasonography, the liver is hyperechoic. Hepatic vasculature is patent, and there is no bile-duct dilation.

She is transferred to an ICU setting, and intravenous fluids with glucose are administered.

Which of the following is the most appropriate next step in management?

(A) Endoscopic retrograde cholangiopancreatography
(B) Immediate delivery of the fetus
(C) Lactulose
(D) Ursodeoxycholic acid

Item 18

A 65-year-old man is evaluated after a screening ultrasound for abdominal aortic aneurysm showed incidental gallbladder findings. He reports no symptoms. He continues to smoke cigarettes, 1 pack per day. He has no other medical problems and takes no medications.

On physical examination, vital signs are normal, as is the remainder of the examination.

The results of all laboratory studies, including a complete blood count and alkaline phosphatase, alanine aminotransferase, aspartate aminotransferase, and total bilirubin levels, are within normal limits.

The abdominal ultrasound shows numerous layering gallstones and an immobile 8-mm gallbladder polyp.

Which of the following is the most appropriate next step in management?

(A) Cholecystectomy
(B) MR cholangiopancreatography
(C) Repeat ultrasonography in 6 months
(D) Ursodeoxycholic acid

Item 19

A 60-year-old woman is evaluated 1 month after completing a 14-day course of *Helicobacter pylori* eradication therapy consisting of amoxicillin, clarithromycin, and omeprazole. Initial upper endoscopy before treatment showed patchy gastric erythema with no ulcers or erosions, and biopsies revealed *H. pylori* gastritis. Currently, she reports alleviated symptoms. She is otherwise healthy and takes no medication.

Which of the following is the most appropriate test to perform next?

(A) Serologic antibody testing for *H. pylori*
(B) Upper endoscopy with gastric biopsy
(C) Urea breath test
(D) No further testing

Item 20

A 36-year-old woman is evaluated 3 days after being hospitalized for gallstone pancreatitis. An abdominal ultrasound showed multiple gallstones in the gallbladder and a normal-diameter common bile duct. She was treated with intravenous hydration and pain medication. Over the course of 3 days, she tolerated eating and her pain subsided.

On physical examination, vital signs are normal; BMI is 32. Minimal tenderness to palpation is noted on abdominal examination. All other findings are unremarkable.

All laboratory studies have returned to baseline normal values.

Which of the following is the most appropriate treatment?

(A) Endoscopic retrograde cholangiopancreatography
(B) Laparoscopic cholecystectomy before discharge from the hospital
(C) Laparoscopic cholecystectomy 4 weeks after discharge from the hospital
(D) MR cholangiopancreatography
(E) Ursodeoxycholic acid

Item 21

A 48-year-old man is hospitalized with a fever and rigors. He has primary sclerosing cholangitis and ulcerative colitis. His only medication is mesalamine.

On physical examination, temperature is 38.6 °C (101.5 °F), blood pressure is 118/75 mm Hg, pulse rate is 95/min, and respiration rate is 18/min. Abdominal examination is notable for right-upper-quadrant tenderness to palpation. The remainder of the examination is normal.

Laboratory studies show a leukocyte count of 14,000/µL (14×10^9/L). Blood cultures are pending.

A 1-L bolus of intravenous normal saline is administered, and intravenous piperacillin-tazobactam is given.

Which of the following is the most appropriate test to perform next?

(A) CA 19-9 measurement
(B) Endoscopic retrograde cholangiopancreatography
(C) IgG4 measurement
(D) Percutaneous transhepatic biliary tube placement
(E) PET scan

Item 22

A 39-year-old woman is evaluated for fatigue, intermittent rectal bleeding, and abdominal pain over the past 2 months. She reports that the bleeding is not accompanied by anal pain or itching. She has experienced an unintentional 2.3-kg (5.1-lb) weight loss since her symptoms started. She has no personal or family history of colon cancer or other cancers. She takes no medication.

On physical examination, her pulse rate is 102/min; other vital signs are normal. BMI is 22. Abdominal examination reveals mild tenderness in the left lower quadrant with no rebound or guarding. Rectal examination shows no masses. Large, friable hemorrhoids are present.

Laboratory studies show a hemoglobin level of 10.5 g/dL (105 g/L) and a serum ferritin level of 5 ng/mL (5 µg/L).

Which of the following is the most appropriate next step in management?

(A) Anoscopy
(B) Colonoscopy
(C) Flexible sigmoidoscopy
(D) Topical hemorrhoid treatment

Item 23

A 52-year-old woman is evaluated for midabdominal pain and nausea. These symptoms worsen after eating large meals. The pain does not alleviate after bowel movements, and she reports frequent constipation. She has gained 2.3 kg (5.1 lb) over the past year. The pain began 1 year earlier, after she was hospitalized with an episode of gallstone pancreatitis for which she underwent laparoscopic cholecystectomy. After cholecystectomy, she had persistent abdominal pain. Over the next several weeks she had upper and lower endoscopies, a CT scan of the abdomen and pelvis, and multiple laboratory tests; all were normal. She states that the only thing that helps the pain is hydrocodone, but as the dose of hydrocodone has increased, so has her pain intensity.

On physical examination, vital signs are normal; BMI is 26. Tenderness to palpation in all quadrants is noted on abdominal examination. Other findings are unremarkable.

Which of the following is the most likely diagnosis?

(A) Chronic pancreatitis
(B) Distal intestinal obstruction syndrome
(C) Irritable bowel syndrome
(D) Narcotic bowel syndrome

Item 24

A 60-year-old man is evaluated for constant low-grade epigastric pain radiating to his back that worsens after he eats fatty foods. He has a 2-year history of chronic pancreatitis. The pain has progressively worsened over the preceding 6 months. His weight is stable. He has a normal bowel movement once every other day. He does not drink alcohol. He continues to smoke 2 packs of cigarettes per day as he has done for 30 years. The patient has a remote history of opioid abuse.

On physical examination, vital signs are normal. Abdominal examination shows tenderness to palpation in the epigastrium.

A contrast-enhanced CT scan of the abdomen shows calcifications throughout the pancreas with no pancreatic mass, no dilated pancreatic duct, and no cystic lesions.

Which of the following is the most appropriate initial treatment?

(A) Celiac plexus block

(B) NSAIDs, low-fat diet, and smoking cessation

(C) Oxycodone

(D) Pancreatic enzyme replacement therapy

Item 25

A 43-year-old man is evaluated for 4 days of fever and arthralgia, as well as a raised purple rash over his lower extremities of 1 week's duration. He is a current intravenous drug user. He has no other medical problems and takes no medications.

On physical examination, temperature is 37.8 °C (100 °F) and blood pressure is 132/85 mm Hg; other vital signs are normal. The large and small joints are tender to palpation without evidence of synovitis. The abdomen is not tender to palpation. The liver edge is palpable below the right costal margin. The skin findings are shown.

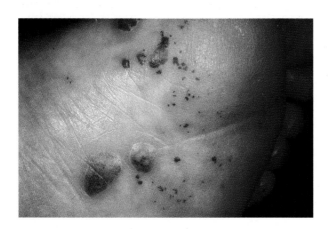

Laboratory studies:

Alanine aminotransferase	143 U/L
Aspartate aminotransferase	130 U/L
Total bilirubin	2.2 mg/dL (37.6 µmol/L)
Creatinine	1.0 mg/dL (88.4 µmol/L)
Hepatitis B surface antigen	Positive
IgM antibody to hepatitis B core antigen	Positive
Hepatitis B e antigen	Positive
HBV DNA	10,000,000 IU/mL
Hepatitis C antibody	Negative
HIV-1/HIV-2 antigen and antibody combination immunoassay	Negative
Cryoglobulin	Normal
Urinalysis	Normal

Which of the following is the most appropriate treatment?

(A) Entecavir

(B) Plasma exchange

(C) Prednisone and cyclophosphamide

(D) Sofosbuvir and ledipasvir

(E) Tenofovir, emtricitabine, and raltegravir

Item 26

A 34-year-old woman is evaluated 4 days after being hospitalized for severe epigastric abdominal pain associated with nausea and vomiting. At the time of hospitalization, her serum lipase level was 4650 U/L and an abdominal ultrasound examination showed cholelithiasis. She has taken nothing by mouth (NPO) since hospitalization and reports having no appetite. She is being treated with intravenous fluids and opioid pain medication. A CT scan of the abdomen and pelvis with contrast showed changes consistent with pancreatic necrosis. Her medical history is unremarkable and she took no medication before hospitalization.

On physical examination, temperature is 38 °C (100.4 °F), blood pressure is 130/70 mm Hg, pulse rate is 90/min, and respiration rate is 15/min. Abdominal examination shows tenderness in the epigastrium with no abdominal distention.

Which of the following is the most appropriate next step in management of her nutrition?

(A) Initiate enteral feeding

(B) Initiate total parenteral nutrition

(C) Maintain NPO status until cholecystectomy is performed

(D) Maintain NPO status until the lipase level normalizes

Item 27

A 55-year-old man is evaluated in the hospital for new-onset ascites. He has a history of cirrhosis due to hepatitis C viral infection. His only medication is propranolol.

On physical examination, pulse rate is 58/min; other vital signs are normal. The abdomen is soft and distended consistent with ascites.

Laboratory studies show a serum albumin level of 2.5 g/dL (25 g/L), serum total bilirubin level of 3.6 mg/dL (61.6 µmol/L), and serum creatinine level of 1.4 mg/dL (123.8 µmol/L).

Paracentesis with analysis of ascitic fluid shows a leukocyte count of 200/µL with 30% neutrophils, albumin level of 0.4 g/dL (4 g/L), and total protein level of 0.9 g/dL (9 g/L).

Which of the following is the most appropriate next step in management?

(A) Increase propranolol therapy

(B) Initiate albumin infusion

(C) Initiate ciprofloxacin therapy

(D) Initiate lisinopril therapy

Item 28

A 53-year-old woman is evaluated for an 8-month history of palpitations, tachycardia, lightheadedness, and sweating with explosive diarrhea and nausea within 15 to 30 minutes of eating. She has lost 6.8 kg (15 lb) during this time period and describes feeling better if she eats smaller portions. She reports no vomiting. Upper endoscopy performed 1 year earlier for refractory gastroesophageal reflux disease incidentally found a small gastrointestinal stromal tumor in her stomach, and she underwent a partial gastrectomy with gastrojejunostomy. Her only medication is omeprazole.

On physical examination, vital signs are normal; BMI is 28. Abdominal examination shows a well-healed scar with no abdominal pain on palpation and no organomegaly.

Which of the following is the most likely diagnosis?

(A) Dumping syndrome
(B) Gastroparesis
(C) Irritable bowel syndrome
(D) Small intestinal bacterial overgrowth

Item 29

A 35-year-old woman is evaluated for constipation. She reports passage of hard stool every 3 to 4 days and associated bloating. Her symptoms have been present for more than 10 years and have progressed gradually. Trials of over-the-counter fiber supplementation and polyethylene glycol worsened the bloating, prompting discontinuation. Senna tea was ineffective. Bisacodyl caused abdominal cramping. She is otherwise healthy and currently takes no medication.

On physical examination, vital signs and other findings are normal.

Which of the following is the most appropriate treatment?

(A) Lactulose
(B) Linaclotide
(C) Methylnaltrexone
(D) Rifaximin

Item 30

A 28-year-old woman is evaluated at 28 weeks' gestation. This is her first pregnancy. She has chronic hepatitis B virus (HBV) infection acquired through vertical transmission. The patient reports feeling well. Her only medication is a prenatal vitamin.

On physical examination, vital signs are normal. The uterus is enlarged, consistent with 28-week intrauterine gestation. No stigmata of chronic liver disease are noted.

Laboratory studies are positive for hepatitis B surface antigen and hepatitis B e antigen. The HBV DNA level is 300,000 IU/mL. The results of other studies, including alanine aminotransferase, aspartate aminotransferase, and total bilirubin levels, are within normal limits.

Which of the following is the most appropriate next step in management?

(A) Cesarean delivery at term
(B) HBV DNA measurement in 3 months
(C) Pegylated interferon
(D) Tenofovir

Item 31

A 60-year-old man is evaluated following the diagnosis of acute pancreatitis. Abdominal ultrasonography showed a normal gallbladder, biliary system, and liver, but the pancreas was not well visualized due to overlying loops of bowel. He reports decreased appetite, vague new back pain, and an unintentional 6.9-kg (15.2-lb) weight loss over the

preceding 6 months. He does not smoke or drink alcohol. He takes no medication.

On physical examination, vital signs are normal; BMI is 20. Abdominal examination shows a thin abdomen with tenderness to deep palpation in the epigastrium. No jaundice is noted.

Which of the following is the most appropriate next step in management?

(A) CT of the abdomen with contrast
(B) Endoscopic retrograde cholangiopancreatography
(C) Endoscopic ultrasound
(D) Clinical observation

Item 32

A 75-year-old man is evaluated after hospitalization for an episode of hematemesis. Upon admission, his INR was 2.5. Intravenous proton pump inhibitor therapy was initiated, and his warfarin was held. Endoscopy showed a large duodenal bulb ulcer with an actively bleeding visible vessel; endoscopic hemostasis was achieved. Vital signs have been normal for 24 hours after endoscopy. The patient also has hypertension and atrial fibrillation and a history of transient ischemic attack. His daily medications are warfarin, losartan, and metoprolol.

On physical examination, vital signs are normal; BMI is 32. Other than an irregularly irregular heart rhythm, the physical examination is normal.

Which of the following is the most appropriate management of the patient's warfarin therapy?

(A) Restart warfarin therapy now
(B) Restart warfarin therapy in 10 days
(C) Restart warfarin therapy in 30 days
(D) Hold warfarin therapy indefinitely

Item 33

A 32-year-old woman is evaluated for a 6-month history of loose stools, bloating, and a 3.2-kg (7-lb) weight loss. Her medical history is otherwise unremarkable. Her brother has type 1 diabetes mellitus, and her mother has autoimmune thyroid disease. She reports no other symptoms and takes no medication.

On physical examination, vital signs and other findings are normal; BMI is 19.

Laboratory studies:

Hemoglobin	11.0 g/dL (110 g/L)
Alanine aminotransferase	60 U/L
Aspartate aminotransferase	42 U/L
Total bilirubin	0.9 mg/dL (15.4 µmol/L)
Ferritin	6 ng/mL (6 µg/L)

Which of the following is the most appropriate test to perform next?

(A) Anti–gliadin IgA antibody
(B) Anti–*Saccharomyces cerevisiae* IgA antibody
(C) Anti–smooth muscle antibody
(D) Anti–tissue transglutaminase IgA antibody

Item 34

A 63-year-old woman is evaluated at a follow-up appointment after undergoing right hemicolectomy for colon cancer 1 year earlier. Her paternal grandfather had colon cancer diagnosed at age 75 years. She reports that she has been feeling well and takes no medication.

All physical examination findings, including vital signs, are normal.

When should this patient's next surveillance colonoscopy take place?

(A) Now
(B) In 1 year
(C) In 3 years
(D) In 5 years

Item 35

A 60-year-old man is evaluated for epigastric pain that occurs intermittently after eating. He was hospitalized twice in the preceding year for idiopathic recurrent acute pancreatitis. He is a former smoker and reports no alcohol use.

On physical examination, vital signs are normal, as is the remainder of the examination.

Contrast-enhanced CT of the abdomen shows a diffusely dilated main pancreatic duct with normal intrahepatic and extrahepatic bile ducts and a normal gallbladder. No tumor is seen in the pancreas or liver, and there is no peripancreatic inflammation or necrosis. Endoscopic ultrasonography confirms no evidence of a tumor or gallstone, but the main pancreatic duct appears dilated throughout the pancreas. Mucin is seen exuding from the ampulla of Vater during the endoscopy.

Which of the following is the most appropriate next step in management?

(A) Endoscopic ultrasonography in 1 year
(B) MRI of the abdomen in 1 year
(C) Oral prednisone
(D) Pancreatic resection

Item 36

A 36-year-old man is evaluated in the emergency department after passing three bowel movements of red to maroon–colored blood. He recently injured his knee playing soccer and has been taking ibuprofen three times a day for a week. He has no other relevant medical history and does not smoke or drink alcohol.

On physical examination, he is lightheaded but alert. His blood pressure is 80/60 mm Hg, pulse rate is 126/min, respiratory rate is 12/min, and oxygen saturation is 98% breathing ambient air. Cardiac examination shows tachycardia. Rectal examination shows maroon-colored stool. All other findings are unremarkable.

The patient's vital signs improve after he is given intravenous hydration.

Laboratory studies show a hemoglobin level of 9 g/dL (90 g/L) upon presentation. Six hours later, the hemoglobin level is 7.4 g/dL (74 g/L).

Which of the following is the most appropriate test to perform next?

(A) Angiography
(B) Capsule endoscopy
(C) Colonoscopy
(D) Upper endoscopy

Item 37

A 72-year-old woman is evaluated for a 3-month history of large-volume, watery, nonbloody diarrhea with mucus, which occurs even when she is fasting. She reports no abdominal pain or flushing but has experienced an unintentional 3-kg (6.6-lb) weight loss. She has never had a colonoscopy.

On physical examination, blood pressure is 100/50 mm Hg and pulse rate is 95/min; other vital signs and examination findings are normal.

Laboratory studies show a serum sodium level of 130 mEq/L (130 mmol/L) and a serum potassium level of 3.3 mEq/L (3.3 mmol/L). Hemoglobin and serum creatinine levels are within normal limits.

Which of the following types of diarrhea is most compatible with the patient's findings?

(A) Infectious
(B) Inflammatory
(C) Osmotic
(D) Secretory

Item 38

A 25-year-old woman is evaluated for a 1-month history of intermittent, loose, bloody bowel movements associated with pain in the left lower quadrant before defecation. The bleeding occurs with and without bowel movements. She reports no fever, chills, night sweats, arthralgia, eye pain, or rash. The patient works in a day care center and has not traveled or used antibiotics recently. She takes no medication.

On physical examination, vital signs are normal. The abdomen is scaphoid and soft, with suprapubic tenderness. The remainder of the physical examination is normal.

Stool testing for bacterial enteropathogens, including *Clostridium difficile*, is negative.

Colonoscopy results show patchy erythema and ulceration in the cecum, ascending colon, descending colon, and sigmoid colon with no involvement of the transverse colon or rectum. Mucosal biopsies of the involved mucosa reveal distorted and branching colonic crypts with lymphocytic and neutrophilic infiltration. Ileal examination is normal.

Which of the following is the most likely diagnosis?

(A) Crohn disease
(B) Giardiasis
(C) Microscopic colitis
(D) Ulcerative colitis

Item 39

A 55-year-old man is evaluated at a follow-up appointment 4 days after being diagnosed with acute sigmoid diverticulitis.

He is on day 4 of oral antibiotics and reports that his pain is almost gone. He has no other symptoms and has never had a colonoscopy. He takes no other medication.

His vital signs are normal. Abdominal examination is positive for minimal tenderness on deep palpation in the left lower quadrant without rebound or guarding.

The CT scan of the abdomen from the emergency department shows mild sigmoid diverticulitis with no abscess.

When should this patient undergo colonoscopy?

(A) Now
(B) In 1 to 2 months
(C) In 6 months
(D) In 12 months

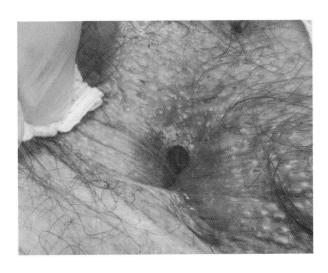

Item 40

A 65-year-old woman is reevaluated following an initial evaluation for anemia. Other than a gradually increasing sense of fatigue, she has no symptoms. Her only other medical problem is autoimmune thyroid disease, which is being treated with levothyroxine. Her last screening colonoscopy, done 4 years earlier, was normal.

Physical examination reveals normal vital signs. There is evidence of conjunctival rim pallor. The remainder of the examination, including thyroid and neurologic examinations, is normal.

At the time of her initial evaluation, laboratory studies showed a hemoglobin level of 10 g/dL (100 g/L) and mean corpuscular volume of 104 fL. Serum cobalamin and ferritin levels were low. An antiparietal cell antibody test was positive. Stool testing revealed no evidence of blood.

Which of the following is the most appropriate test to perform next?

(A) Capsule endoscopy
(B) Glucose hydrogen breath test
(C) Serum gastrin measurement
(D) Upper endoscopy

Item 41

A 28-year-old woman is evaluated for 2 weeks of intense rectal pain that occurs with most bowel movements. She also reports periodic rectal bleeding and occasional constipation symptoms that have worsened since a recent shoulder surgery. Over-the-counter hemorrhoid cream has not alleviated her symptoms. Family history includes colon cancer diagnosed in her grandmother at age 74 years. The patient's medications are acetaminophen with codeine and an over-the-counter stool softener as needed.

On physical examination, vital signs are normal. Rectal examination findings are shown (see top of next column).

Which of the following is the most appropriate next step in management?

(A) Anal botulinum toxin injection
(B) Flexible sigmoidoscopy

(C) Prednisone suppository
(D) Sitz baths and psyllium
(E) Topical hydrocortisone and lubiprostone

Item 42

A 25-year-old man is evaluated for worsening heartburn of 4 months' duration, despite treatment with twice-daily omeprazole. He has no pertinent personal or family medical history and takes no other medication.

On physical examination, vital signs and other findings are normal.

Upper endoscopy shows a normal esophagus with a normal gastroesophageal junction. The stomach has 30 small (<10 mm) sessile polyps seen in the fundus. The duodenum is normal. Pathology of a polyp shows it to be a fundic gland polyp.

Which of the following is the most appropriate next step in evaluation of this patient?

(A) Colonoscopy
(B) Gastrectomy
(C) Repeat upper endoscopy in 3 months
(D) No further evaluation

Item 43

A 44-year-old man is evaluated after his routine yearly follow-up for ulcerative colitis showed elevated liver chemistry test results. He was diagnosed with ulcerative colitis 5 years ago. He reports that he passes solid, formed stool every 1 to 2 days without abdominal pain. His only medication is mesalamine.

On physical examination, vital signs are normal; BMI is 26. Hepatomegaly and palmar erythema are noted.

Laboratory studies:

Alkaline phosphatase	412 U/L
Alanine aminotransferase	78 U/L
Aspartate aminotransferase	62 U/L
Total bilirubin	2 mg/dL (34.2 µmol/L)
Direct bilirubin	1.5 mg/dL (25.7 µmol/L)

A complete blood count and serum creatinine level are normal, and an antimitochondrial antibody titer is negative.

MR cholangiopancreatography shows hepatomegaly but is otherwise normal.

Liver biopsy is pending.

Which of the following is the most likely diagnosis?

(A) Antimitochondrial antibody–negative primary biliary cholangitis
(B) Drug-induced liver injury
(C) Nonalcoholic fatty liver disease
(D) Primary sclerosing cholangitis

Item 44

A 45-year-old man is evaluated for a 2-month history of a burning sensation starting in his stomach and radiating into his chest, usually occurring 4 to 5 times weekly. He says that he usually eats dinner late and then goes to sleep. He often wakes up with a sour taste in his mouth. He reports no dysphagia or unintentional weight loss. He takes no medication.

On physical examination, vital signs are normal; BMI is 34. The remainder of the examination, including abdominal examination, is unremarkable.

Which of the following is the most appropriate next step in management?

(A) Ambulatory pH testing
(B) Barium esophagography
(C) Empiric trial of a proton pump inhibitor
(D) Upper endoscopy

Item 45

A 45-year-old woman is evaluated during a routine follow-up appointment for cirrhosis due to primary biliary cholangitis. She has chronic symptoms of fatigue that are unchanged since her previous visits. She has no other new symptoms of advancing liver dysfunction, including no ascites, jaundice, or hepatic encephalopathy. A recent upper endoscopy showed small esophageal varices without red wale marks. Her only medication is ursodeoxycholic acid. She is up to date for her influenza, 23-valent polysaccharide pneumococcal, and hepatitis A and B immunizations.

On physical examination, vital signs are normal. Scattered spider angiomas are seen on her chest and upper back. The remainder of the examination is normal.

An abdominal ultrasound shows changes in the liver consistent with cirrhosis. No liver masses are seen.

Which of the following is the most appropriate intervention to perform next?

(A) Bone densitometry
(B) Colonoscopy
(C) Contrast-enhanced abdominal CT
(D) Herpes zoster immunization

Item 46

A 30-year-old man is evaluated after being hospitalized for an acute flare of extensive ulcerative colitis. He reports six to eight bloody bowel movements daily with prominent urgency and lower abdominal cramping for the past 2 weeks. He has been taking prednisone daily for 1 week. His only other medication is mesalamine.

On physical examination, vital signs are normal. Abdominal examination reveals lower abdominal tenderness. The abdomen is not distended and bowel sounds are normal. Blood is seen on digital rectal examination.

Hemoglobin level is 10 g/dL (100 g/L). He remains hemodynamically stable.

Which of the following is the most appropriate venous thromboembolism prophylaxis for this patient?

(A) Aspirin
(B) Graduated compression stockings
(C) Heparin
(D) Intermittent pneumatic compression
(E) Low-dose warfarin

Item 47

A 37-year-old man is evaluated during a follow-up appointment after resection of a well-differentiated adenocarcinoma of the ascending colon, which was diagnosed 1 month earlier. His family history is significant for endometrial cancer diagnosed in his mother at age 50 years and colon cancer diagnosed in his maternal grandfather at age 49 years. The patient reports that he has been feeling well and takes no medication.

All physical examination findings, including vital signs, are normal.

Which of the following is the most appropriate next step in management?

(A) Colonoscopy in 3 years
(B) Fecal immunochemical testing in 1 year
(C) Genetic counseling
(D) Upper endoscopy and capsule endoscopy

Item 48

A 35-year-old man is evaluated during a follow-up appointment for persistent heartburn with chronic cough. He has a 1-year history of gastroesophageal reflux disease and takes pantoprazole twice daily. He reports no nausea, vomiting, or dysphagia. Upper endoscopy performed 1 year earlier showed no abnormal findings.

His vital signs and physical examination are normal. Results of an ear, nose, and throat evaluation are noncontributory.

Which of the following is the most appropriate next diagnostic test?

(A) Ambulatory pH testing
(B) Barium esophagography
(C) Esophageal manometry
(D) Upper endoscopy

Item 49

A 55-year-old man is evaluated for ascites. He recently went to the emergency department, where paracentesis was performed. He was then discharged for outpatient follow-up. He has a history of cirrhosis due to nonalcoholic steatohepatitis and also has hypertension. Endoscopy 3 months earlier showed small varices without stigmata, making prophylaxis for esophageal variceal bleeding unnecessary. His only medication is lisinopril.

On physical examination, vital signs are normal; BMI is 28. Abdominal examination shows abdominal distention without tenderness.

Laboratory studies of the ascitic fluid show a leukocyte count of 80/µL with 20% neutrophils and protein level of 1.6 g/dL (16 g/L). Serum studies show a creatinine level of 1.3 mg/dL (114.9 µmol/L) and sodium level of 134 mEq/L (134 mmol/L).

An abdominal ultrasound from the emergency department shows changes consistent with cirrhosis. The portal vein and hepatic veins are patent with normal flow direction. A moderate amount of free-flowing ascites is seen.

In addition to initiating a sodium-restricted diet, which of the following is the most appropriate next step in management?

(A) Discontinue lisinopril
(B) Initiate free-water restriction
(C) Initiate propranolol
(D) Insert an indwelling drain into the peritoneal cavity

Item 50

A 30-year-old man is evaluated in the emergency department for the recent onset of confusion and jaundice of 6 weeks' duration. His medical history is unremarkable.

On physical examination, the patient is confused. His temperature is 36.9 °C (98.4 °F), blood pressure is 102/60 mm Hg, pulse rate is 115/min, and respiration rate is 22/min. Jaundice and asterixis are noted. No organomegaly is noted.

Laboratory studies:

Hematocrit	38%
Leukocyte count	11,000/µL (11×10^9/L)
Platelet count	350,000/µL (350×10^9/L)
INR	2.6
Alanine aminotransferase	200 U/L
Aspartate aminotransferase	150 U/L
Total bilirubin	18.6 mg/dL (318.1 µmol/L)
Creatinine	3.0 mg/dL (265.2 µmol/L)

On abdominal ultrasound, the liver appears normal with intact vasculature. No splenomegaly or dilation of bile ducts is noted.

Which of the following is the most appropriate next step in management?

(A) Administer fresh frozen plasma
(B) Initiate hemodialysis
(C) Perform endoscopic retrograde cholangiopancreatography
(D) Refer for liver transplantation

Item 51

A 21-year-old woman is evaluated for a 6-week history of frequent bowel movements (three times daily) with intermittent passage of small amounts of blood and mucus. She also reports suprapubic cramping pain that is relieved with passage of stool. She reports no fever, chills, nausea, vomiting, or weight loss. She is otherwise healthy and takes no medication.

On physical examination, vital signs are normal. The abdomen is scaphoid, with tenderness to palpation in the suprapubic area. Rectal examination is notable for a small amount of blood on the examining finger.

Laboratory studies show a normal complete blood count and C-reactive protein level. Stool testing for enteropathogens, including *Clostridium difficile*, is negative.

Results of colonoscopy show continuous, symmetric rectal and sigmoid inflammation characterized by erythema, edema, and friable mucosa. The remainder of the colonic mucosa and distal ileum is normal. Biopsy specimens from the rectum and sigmoid colon show evidence of mildly active chronic colitis.

Which of the following is the most appropriate treatment?

(A) Mesalamine enema
(B) Mesalamine suppository
(C) Oral mesalamine
(D) Oral mesalamine and mesalamine enema

Item 52

A 20-year-old man is evaluated for epigastric pain that has gradually increased in severity over 8 months. The pain worsens with eating and is not relieved by antacids. The patient reports no melena, diarrhea, or constipation. The patient's personal medical history is unremarkable and he takes no medication.

On physical examination, vital signs are normal. Epigastric tenderness to palpation is noted. Other findings are normal.

A complete blood count is normal.

Which of the following is the most appropriate next step in management?

(A) Initiation of omeprazole
(B) Stool antigen testing for *Helicobacter pylori*
(C) Ultrasonography of the right upper quadrant
(D) Upper endoscopy

Item 53

A 46-year-old man is evaluated for abdominal pain in the right upper quadrant and fever of 1 month's duration. He recently emigrated from Mexico. His medical history is unremarkable, and he takes no medication.

On physical examination, temperature is 37.7 °C (99.9 °F); other vital signs are normal. Abdominal examination shows tenderness to palpation of the right upper quadrant. No scleral icterus is noted. The remainder of the examination is normal.

An ultrasound of the liver shows a fluid-containing structure and complex wall consistent with hepatic abscess.

Laboratory studies show a leukocyte count of 10,600/μL (10.6 × 10⁹/L). Testing for *Entamoeba histolytica* IgG is positive.

Which of the following is the most appropriate treatment?

(A) Meropenem
(B) Metronidazole and paromomycin
(C) Percutaneous drainage of the abscess
(D) Surgical resection

Item 54

A 26-year-old woman is evaluated for a 2-month history of diarrhea characterized by two to three semibloody stools per day associated with cramping lower abdominal pain. She reports no fever, chills, nausea, vomiting, or weight loss. She has not traveled internationally. She takes no medication.

On physical examination, vital signs are normal. Abdominal examination shows left and right lower abdominal tenderness to palpation. Rectal examination is remarkable for bright red blood.

Stool testing for enteric pathogens is negative.

Results of colonoscopy show inflamed mucosa characterized by granularity, erythema, friability, and loss of vascular pattern that starts at the anorectal verge and extends proximally in a continuous and symmetric fashion to the splenic flexure where there is an abrupt transition from affected to normal mucosa. The terminal ileum is normal. Biopsy results for the inflamed mucosa reveal crypt abscesses along with distorted and branching colonic crypts.

Which of the following is the most likely diagnosis?

(A) Chronic *Entamoeba histolytica* infection
(B) Crohn colitis
(C) Cytomegalovirus infection
(D) Ulcerative colitis

Item 55

A 26-year-old woman is evaluated for the new onset of jaundice. She reports no fever or abdominal pain. Her medical history is unremarkable and she takes no medication.

On physical examination, vital signs are normal. Scleral icterus and psychomotor slowing are noted.

Laboratory studies:

Hemoglobin	10.2 g/dL (102 g/L)
Reticulocyte count	8% of total erythrocyte count
Alkaline phosphatase	26 U/L
Alanine aminotransferase	78 U/L
Aspartate aminotransferase	156 U/L
Total bilirubin	6.4 mg/dL (109.4 μmol/L)
Conjugated bilirubin	2.6 mg/dL (44.5 μmol/L)

Testing for hepatitis A, B, and C viral infections is negative for acute infection.

On abdominal ultrasonography, the liver is small and nodular. Splenomegaly is noted.

Which of the following is the most appropriate test to perform next?

(A) Antimitochondrial antibody test
(B) Hepatitis B virus DNA measurement
(C) Serum ceruloplasmin measurement
(D) Transferrin saturation measurement

Item 56

A 55-year-old man is evaluated for progressive dysphagia of 2 years' duration. He reports dysphagia to both solid food and liquids. He has cardiomyopathy, with an ejection fraction of 15%. His medications are pantoprazole, furosemide, valsartan, digoxin, metoprolol, low-dose aspirin, and amiodarone. He is unable to walk up two flights of stairs without stopping. He does not drink or smoke.

On physical examination, his blood pressure is 100/65 mm Hg, pulse rate is 90/min, and respiratory rate is 22/min; BMI is 32. His examination is remarkable for fine crackles at the lung bases posteriorly, a third heart sound, and 2+ pitting edema to the knees.

Upper endoscopy shows no masses. A barium esophagram is shown.

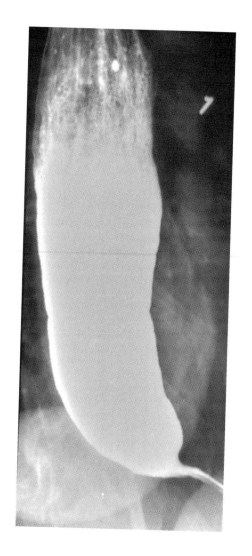

Which of the following is the most appropriate treatment?

(A) Botulinum toxin injection

(B) Calcium channel blockers

(C) Endoscopic pneumatic dilation

(D) Laparoscopic surgical myotomy

Item 57

A 56-year-old woman is evaluated for chest discomfort after meals occurring intermittently over the preceding month. She describes a sensation of heaviness on her chest, and says that she also notices this pain sometimes while walking up stairs. She reports no nausea, dysphagia, or reflux. She has been taking ranitidine with minimal relief of symptoms. She also takes atorvastatin for hyperlipidemia. She smokes half a pack of cigarettes daily.

On physical examination, her blood pressure is 140/90 mm Hg and other vital signs are normal; BMI is 34. The remainder of the examination, including abdominal examination, is unremarkable.

Which of the following is the most appropriate next step in management?

(A) Barium esophagography

(B) Electrocardiography

(C) Empiric trial of a proton pump inhibitor

(D) Upper endoscopy

Item 58

A 32-year-old woman is evaluated for arthralgia and jaundice. Three months earlier, she traveled to Mexico for a 2-week vacation and developed nausea, vomiting, abdominal pain, fever, and jaundice approximately 3 weeks after returning to the United States. Testing for hepatitis A virus IgM was positive, and she was treated with supportive measures. Her symptoms and jaundice resolved within 3 weeks. A few weeks later, jaundice reappeared along with arthralgia. The patient's medical history is otherwise unremarkable, and she takes no medication.

On physical examination, vital signs are normal; BMI is 27. Jaundice is noted. The remainder of the examination is unremarkable.

Laboratory studies:

Alkaline phosphatase	272 U/L
Alanine aminotransferase	775 U/L
Aspartate aminotransferase	672 U/L
Total bilirubin	5.8 mg/dL (99.2 µmol/L)

The results of other studies, including a complete blood count, INR, serum creatinine level, antinuclear antibody, anti–smooth muscle antibody, and total IgG level, are within normal limits.

Ultrasonography of the liver is normal.

Which of the following is the most likely diagnosis?

(A) Autoimmune hepatitis

(B) Leptospirosis

(C) Malaria

(D) Relapsing, remitting hepatitis A viral infection

Item 59

A 75-year-old woman with longstanding gastroesophageal reflux disease (GERD) comes to the office with concerns related to her new diagnosis of osteopenia. Her GERD is well controlled with once-daily pantoprazole, which she has taken without side effects for 1 year. She also takes calcium and vitamin D supplements. Other than her age, she has no additional risk factors for osteoporosis.

Her vital signs and the remainder of the physical examination are normal.

Which of the following is the most appropriate next step in management?

(A) Attempt to discontinue or reduce pantoprazole

(B) Continue pantoprazole at current dose

(C) Obtain an upper endoscopy

(D) Switch to ranitidine and metoclopramide

(E) Switch to sucralfate

Item 60

A 22-year-old woman is evaluated for intractable pruritus that keeps her awake at night. She is in her 25th week of pregnancy. Her medications are a prenatal vitamin and a folate supplement.

On physical examination, vital signs are normal. Scleral icterus is noted. Excoriations are seen on the arms, chest, abdomen, and legs.

Laboratory studies:

Hematocrit	35%
Platelet count	370,000/µL (370 × 10⁹/L)
Alanine aminotransferase	55 U/L
Aspartate aminotransferase	30 U/L
Bile acids	Elevated
Total bilirubin	2.5 mg/dL (42.8 µmol/L)

Testing for hepatitis C and hepatis B viral infections is negative.

An ultrasound shows a normal liver with no dilated bile ducts.

Which of the following is the most appropriate next step in management?

(A) Liver biopsy

(B) Peripheral blood smear

(C) Topical glucocorticoids

(D) Ursodeoxycholic acid

Item 61

A 60-year-old woman is admitted to the hospital with sudden-onset, cramping abdominal pain of moderate severity in the right lower quadrant, followed several hours later by a bloody bowel movement. She has coronary artery disease; medications are atorvastatin, metoprolol, sublingual nitroglycerin, and low-dose aspirin.

On physical examination, the patient appears comfortable. Pulse rate is 110/min; BMI is 35. Other vital signs are normal. The abdomen is nondistended with normal bowel sounds. Deep palpation elicits tenderness in the right lower quadrant with no rebound or guarding.

A CT scan without contrast shows thickening of the ascending colon. Colonoscopy results show a segment of subepithelial hemorrhage, edema, and erythema from the cecum to the hepatic flexure.

Which of the following is the most appropriate test to perform next?

(A) CT angiography
(B) Doppler ultrasonography of mesenteric vessels
(C) MR angiography
(D) Selective catheter angiography

Item 62

A 73-year-old man is evaluated in the hospital for light-headedness. He also reports nonbloody, watery diarrhea of 4 months' duration and an unintentional 4.5-kg (9.9-lb) weight loss over the same time period. He has hypertension and hyperlipidemia. His medications are olmesartan and atorvastatin.

On physical examination, blood pressure is 100/50 mm Hg and pulse rate is 108/min; other vital signs are normal. Physical examination findings are unremarkable.

Results of laboratory studies, including serum creatinine, total IgA, and tissue transglutaminase IgA, are within normal limits.

The patient responds to fluid resuscitation with normalization of his pulse and blood pressure. Colonoscopy is grossly normal, and biopsy samples show no evidence of microscopic colitis. Upper endoscopy with duodenal biopsies shows villous flattening and increased intraepithelial lymphocytes.

Which of the following is the most appropriate next step in management?

(A) Discontinue atorvastatin
(B) Discontinue olmesartan
(C) Start a gluten-free diet
(D) Start prednisone

Item 63

A 65-year-old man is evaluated with upper endoscopy in follow-up for Barrett esophagus. He has had heartburn for more than 15 years, but his symptoms have been well controlled with daily omeprazole. He reports no weight loss or pain with swallowing and has no history of anemia. He stopped smoking 5 years earlier, but has a 40-pack-year history.

Vital signs and the remainder of the physical examination are normal.

On upper endoscopy, an area of salmon-colored mucosa is seen in the esophagus. Biopsies confirm evidence of Barrett esophagus with low-grade dysplasia. The pathology slides were reviewed by a second pathologist, confirming the presence of low-grade dysplasia.

Which of the following is the most appropriate next step in management?

(A) Endoscopic ablation
(B) Esophagectomy

(C) Fundoplication
(D) Repeat endoscopy in 6 months

Item 64

A 45-year-old man is evaluated for watery diarrhea accompanied by nausea and bloating. Symptoms began 4 weeks earlier with abdominal cramping and explosive watery stools. Now, he reports up to five loose bowel movements per day, with no blood and no nocturnal symptoms. He also describes generalized abdominal discomfort that is not relieved after a bowel movement. He works at a child care center. He is otherwise healthy and takes no medication.

On physical examination, vital signs are normal. Abdominal examination shows periumbilical tenderness with no rebound or guarding. The remainder of the examination is unremarkable.

Results of laboratory studies, including hemoglobin level and a comprehensive metabolic panel, are within normal limits.

Which of the following is the most appropriate next step in management?

(A) Colonoscopy
(B) CT scan of the abdomen and pelvis
(C) 24-Hour urine 5-hydroxyindoleacetic acid measurement
(D) Stool testing for *Giardia lamblia*

Item 65

A 45-year-old woman is evaluated for episodic nausea, bloating, and epigastric pain of 5 years' duration. In the past 3 months, the nausea has been accompanied by occasional vomiting. She also reports near-daily heartburn symptoms that have not responded to daily omeprazole. She has a 10-year history of type 2 diabetes mellitus that is treated with metformin and glyburide.

On physical examination, vital signs are normal; BMI is 29. Abdominal examination shows diffuse tenderness to deep palpation with no guarding. Other findings are normal.

Laboratory studies show a blood hemoglobin A_{1c} level of 7.5%. The basic metabolic panel is normal. A complete blood count and liver chemistry tests are normal.

Upper endoscopy shows a moderate amount of retained food in the stomach and patchy erythema of the gastric mucosa. Biopsies of the stomach are normal.

Which of the following is the most appropriate next step in management?

(A) Gastric emptying scintigraphy
(B) 24-Hour pH probe
(C) Initiation of domperidone
(D) Initiation of metoclopramide

Item 66

A 55-year-old man is evaluated after emergent treatment for an episode of hematemesis. Emergency endoscopy was performed in the emergency department, and the bleeding was successfully treated with band ligation. The endoscopy

CONT. revealed esophageal varices, one of which had stigmata of recent hemorrhage. Treatment with octreotide and a proton pump inhibitor was initiated. The patient has a history of cirrhosis due to hepatitis C viral infection. He has no other medical problems and takes no medication.

On physical examination, vital signs and other findings are normal.

Laboratory studies show a hemoglobin level of 8.9 g/dL (89 g/L), leukocyte count of 3600/μL (3.6 × 10⁹/L), and platelet count of 80,000/μL (80 × 10⁹/L).

Which of the following is the most appropriate next treatment?

(A) Blood transfusion
(B) Ciprofloxacin
(C) Platelet transfusion
(D) Transjugular intrahepatic portosystemic shunt placement

Item 67

A 56-year-old man is evaluated in the emergency department for altered mental status of 18 hours' duration. He has a history of cirrhosis due to hepatitis C viral infection and also has anxiety. He has not changed his diet recently, and he has no symptoms suggestive of gastrointestinal bleeding. His bowel movements have been regular and unchanged. His only medication is alprazolam started 2 weeks earlier, after a visit to an urgent care center.

On physical examination, vital signs are normal. Oxygen saturation is 96% breathing ambient air. Abdominal examination is unremarkable; there is no evidence of ascites. Psychomotor slowing and asterixis are noted. There are no focal neurologic findings. The remainder of the examination is unremarkable.

Complete blood count, serum electrolytes and creatinine, and blood glucose are normal.

In addition to starting lactulose, which of the following is the most appropriate next step in management?

(A) CT of the head
(B) Initiate a protein-restricted diet
(C) Initiate rifaximin
(D) Withdraw alprazolam

Item 68

A 38-year-old man is evaluated during a new-patient appointment. The patient reports no rectal bleeding or other gastrointestinal symptoms. His family history includes colon cancer diagnosed in his father at age 52 years. His personal medical history is unremarkable and he takes no medication.

All physical examination findings, including vital signs, are normal.

When should this patient undergo his first screening colonoscopy?

(A) Now
(B) Age 40 years
(C) Age 42 years
(D) Age 50 years

Item 69

A 64-year-old man is evaluated for hepatitis C virus–related cirrhosis with decompensation, including previous variceal hemorrhage, and ascites. His medications are furosemide, spironolactone, and nadolol.

On physical examination, vital signs are normal; BMI is 25. Spider angiomata are seen over the chest, and palmar erythema is noted. The abdomen is distended with flank dullness to percussion. The left liver lobe is palpable 5 cm below the xiphoid process. The spleen is palpable. Bilateral lower-extremity edema is noted. The remainder of the examination is normal.

A screening ultrasound examination shows a 3-cm mass with poorly defined margins and coarse, irregular internal echoes in the right hepatic lobe. A CT scan of the abdomen with contrast shows a 3-cm arterial enhancing lesion with portal venous phase washout in the periphery of the right lobe. The chest is normal on CT.

Which of the following is the most appropriate next step in management?

(A) Biopsy of the lesion
(B) Liver transplantation
(C) Sorafenib
(D) Surgical resection

Item 70

A 25-year-old man is evaluated for a sensation of solid food "sticking" several times per week. He reports that he sometimes forces himself to vomit when he feels food "stuck" in the esophagus, but he has never gone to the emergency department. He takes a multivitamin and is generally healthy.

On physical examination, vital signs and other findings, including those of an abdominal examination, are unremarkable.

Upper endoscopy findings are shown.

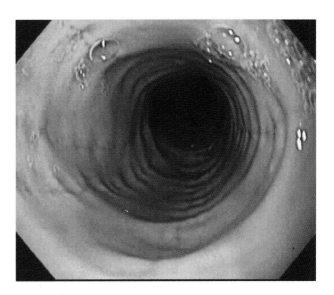

Biopsies of the esophagus show more than 18 eosinophils/hpf.

Which of the following is the most likely diagnosis?

(A) Achalasia

(B) *Candida* esophagitis

(C) Eosinophilic esophagitis

(D) Pill-induced esophagitis

Item 71

A 65-year-old man undergoes screening with ultrasonography for abdominal aortic aneurysm. He has no symptoms, his medical history is unremarkable, and he takes no medication.

Vital signs and other findings of the physical examination are normal.

On the abdominal ultrasound, the abdominal aorta appears normal. Multiple gallstones smaller than 1 cm in size are seen in the gallbladder. The liver has normal echogenicity, and there are no dilated bile ducts. No abnormalities are seen in the gallbladder wall.

Which of the following is the most appropriate management of this patient's gallstone disease?

(A) Cholecystectomy

(B) Endoscopic retrograde cholangiopancreatography

(C) Repeat ultrasonography in 6 months

(D) Clinical observation

Item 72

An 80-year-old man is evaluated in the emergency department after a bowel movement with initial passage of brown soft stool followed by a large volume of red blood. He reports intermittent chills and fevers over the past week. He also has peripheral vascular disease, hypertension, and hypercholesterolemia. His history includes an aortoiliac aneurysm treated with an aortic bifurcation graft 3 years earlier. His medications are atorvastatin, hydrochlorothiazide, losartan, and low-dose aspirin.

On physical examination, the patient is comfortable. His temperature is 38 °C (100.4 °F), blood pressure is 108/60 mm Hg, pulse rate is 112/min, and respiration rate is 18/min. Cardiopulmonary examination is unremarkable. There is midabdominal tenderness to palpation. Rectal examination reveals bright red blood mixed with brown stool.

Laboratory studies show a hemoglobin level of 9 g/dL (90 g/L). Leukocyte count is 14,000/µL (14 × 10⁹/L) with neutrophilia.

Which of the following is the most appropriate test to perform next?

(A) CT scan with contrast

(B) Mesenteric angiogram

(C) Tagged red blood cell scintigraphy

(D) Upper endoscopy

Item 73

A 72-year-old woman is evaluated after being hospitalized for gastrointestinal bleeding. She went to the emergency department after passing a large amount of bright red blood per rectum at home and became lightheaded. She had a second bloody bowel movement in the emergency department. She is otherwise healthy and takes no medication.

Findings on physical examination, including vital signs, are normal.

Laboratory studies show a hemoglobin level of 9 g/dL (90 g/L).

Which of the following is the most appropriate next step in management?

(A) Angiography and arterial embolization

(B) Colonoscopy within 8 hours with cleansing enemas

(C) Colonoscopy within 24 hours with oral bowel preparation

(D) Tagged red blood cell scintigraphy

(E) Transfusion of packed red blood cells

Item 74

A 58-year-old woman is evaluated in the emergency department for sharp, nonradiating pain in the left lower quadrant that has persisted for 2 days. She reports no fever, diarrhea, or blood in stools, and has not traveled recently. Her last colonoscopy, performed 1 year earlier, showed pandiverticulosis.

On physical examination, her temperature is 37.2 °C (99.0 °F), blood pressure is 130/85 mm Hg, pulse rate is 88/min, and respiratory rate is 18/min; BMI is 26. Abdominal examination is positive for left-lower-quadrant tenderness on palpation with no rebound or guarding.

Results of laboratory studies show an elevated leukocyte count; other findings are normal.

Abdominal CT shows focal diverticulitis in the sigmoid colon, without abscess.

Which of the following is the most appropriate next step in management?

(A) Colonoscopy

(B) Intravenous antibiotics

(C) Oral antibiotics

(D) Surgery

Item 75

A 66-year-old man is evaluated for breakthrough symptoms of gastroesophageal reflux disease (GERD) despite once-daily pantoprazole. He has a 5-year history of GERD.

On physical examination, his blood pressure is 118/70 mm Hg, pulse rate is 76/min, and respiratory rate is 18/min; BMI is 30. The abdomen is soft, nontender, and nondistended. Bowel sounds are hyperactive. The remainder of the examination is unremarkable.

Upper endoscopy shows Barrett esophagus. Biopsy results are indefinite for dysplasia.

Which of the following is the most appropriate next step in management?

(A) Endoscopic ablation therapy

(B) Esophagectomy

(C) Optimization of medical therapy followed by repeat upper endoscopy

(D) Repeat upper endoscopy in 1 year

Item 76

A 78-year-old woman is evaluated for frequent rectal urgency with the passage of explosive, loose to watery stool. She says she is often unable to get to the bathroom in time. Episodes have occurred after meals and in the early morning over the past 3 months. She has Alzheimer dementia and lives with her daughter. She also has hypertension and chronic back pain. Her history includes occasional constipation that resolves when treated with docusate. Her last screening colonoscopy at age 70 years showed diffuse diverticulosis. Her medications are lisinopril, acetaminophen, memantine, docusate as needed, and a calcium supplement with vitamin D.

On physical examination, vital signs are normal. Fecal soiling is noted. Rectal examination shows normal anal tone and brown stool in the rectal vault.

A complete blood count and thyroid-stimulating hormone level are normal.

Which of the following is the most appropriate next step in management?

(A) Abdominal radiograph
(B) Anorectal manometry
(C) Loperamide
(D) Psyllium

Item 77

A 68-year-old man is evaluated in the ICU for cramping abdominal pain in the left lower quadrant, which began approximately 3 hours before the evaluation. Twenty minutes before the evaluation, he had a loose stool with hematochezia. The patient has been in the ICU for 24 hours, after being admitted with fever and hypotension secondary to urosepsis. He was treated with intravenous fluids, vasopressors, and piperacillin-tazobactam. His medical history includes hypertension, benign prostatic hypertrophy, and hyperlipidemia. His daily medications are chlorthalidone, atorvastatin, and low-dose aspirin.

On physical examination, the patient is alert. Temperature is 38.7 °C (101.7 °F), blood pressure is 106/60 mm Hg, pulse rate is 90/min, respiration rate is 18/min, and oxygen saturation is 96% breathing ambient air. There is tenderness to palpation over the left side of the abdomen without guarding. The remainder of the examination is unremarkable.

Colonoscopy findings are shown.

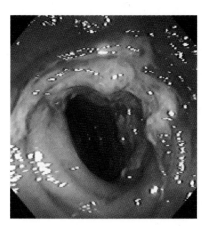

Which of the following is the most likely diagnosis?

(A) Acute mesenteric ischemia
(B) Diverticular bleeding
(C) Enterohemorrhagic *Escherichia coli*
(D) Ischemic colitis

Item 78

A 26-year-old woman with Crohn disease is evaluated for a 2-week history of worsening abdominal pain in the right lower quadrant. She reports passage of one to two formed and nonbloody stools per day with no changes in bowel habits. The patient has required three courses of prednisone for disease flares over the past year. Her only medication is azathioprine.

On physical examination, temperature is 37.7 °C (99.9 °F) and pulse rate is 115/min; other vital signs are normal. Abdominal examination shows fullness and tenderness in the right lower quadrant with no distinct mass. The remainder of the examination is unremarkable.

Laboratory studies show a hemoglobin level of 10.5 g/dL (105 g/L) and a C-reactive protein level of 32 mg/dL (320 mg/L). Leukocyte count and liver chemistry tests are normal.

CT enterography shows asymmetric mural thickening and mucosal inflammation of a long segment of distal ileum without luminal narrowing.

Which of the following is the most appropriate treatment?

(A) Budesonide
(B) Infliximab
(C) Mesalamine
(D) Prednisone

Item 79

A 30-year-old woman is evaluated during a new-patient appointment. Her personal medical history is unremarkable and she takes no medication. Her family history includes colon cancer diagnosed in her mother at age 48 years, endometrial cancer diagnosed in a maternal aunt at age 51 years, and colon cancer diagnosed in her maternal grandfather at age 55 years.

All physical examination findings, including vital signs, are normal.

Genetic testing for *MSH2* mutation is positive, consistent with Lynch syndrome.

Which of the following is the most appropriate next step?

(A) Colectomy
(B) Colonoscopy at age 38
(C) Colonoscopy at age 40
(D) Colonoscopy now

Item 80

A 38-year-old man is evaluated for epigastric discomfort and early satiety associated with an unintentional 4.5-kg (9.9-lb) weight loss over the preceding 5 months. His family history includes lobular breast cancer diagnosed in his mother at age 45 years, stomach cancer diagnosed in his maternal grandfather at age 48 years, and stomach cancer diagnosed in his maternal uncle at age 52 years. The patient's medical history is unremarkable, and he takes no medication.

On physical examination, vital signs are normal. Abdominal examination shows epigastric tenderness to palpation and normal bowel sounds.

Which of the following is the most appropriate diagnostic test to perform next?

(A) Colonoscopy
(B) Gastric emptying study
(C) *Helicobacter pylori* serology
(D) Upper endoscopy
(E) Upper gastrointestinal radiograph series

Item 81

A 32-year-old man is evaluated for a 1-week history of jaundice and pruritus. One month earlier, he completed treatment for sinusitis with amoxicillin-clavulanate. His sinusitis symptoms resolved with therapy.

On physical examination, vital signs are normal. BMI is 26. Jaundice is noted. Excoriations are seen on the extremities. The abdominal examination is normal.

Laboratory studies:

INR	1.0
Albumin	3.8 g/dL (38 g/L)
Alkaline phosphatase	580 U/L
Alanine aminotransferase	42 U/L
Aspartate aminotransferase	38 U/L
Total bilirubin	8.6 mg/dL (147.1 µmol/L)

Hepatitis A, B, and C virus and Epstein-Barr virus studies show no evidence of current or previous infection. Testing for antinuclear antibody and anti–smooth muscle antibody is negative. The ceruloplasmin level is normal.

Results of abdominal ultrasonography are normal, with no evidence of biliary dilation, gallstones, or hepatic parenchymal abnormalities.

Which of the following is the most appropriate next step in management?

(A) Endoscopic retrograde cholangiopancreatography
(B) Liver biopsy
(C) Prednisone administration
(D) Continued observation

Item 82

A 54-year-old woman is evaluated for a 1-year history of generalized abdominal pain that is constant throughout the day, every day. The pain is not triggered by eating and is not relieved by bowel movements. She reports no weight loss and no change in bowel habits. She also has depression. A screening colonoscopy done 8 months earlier was normal. Her only medication is escitalopram.

On physical examination, vital signs are normal; BMI is 28. The abdomen is tender to palpation in all quadrants

without guarding. The remainder of the examination is normal.

Results of laboratory studies, including a complete blood count and liver chemistry tests, are normal.

Which of the following is the most appropriate treatment?

(A) Alosetron
(B) Budesonide
(C) Cognitive-behavioral therapy
(D) Linaclotide

Item 83

A 55-year-old man is evaluated after being hospitalized for epigastric pain of 1 month's duration and melenic stools over the past 3 days associated with fatigue. He reports no hematochezia, hematemesis, chest pain, or shortness of breath. He has osteoarthritis treated with ibuprofen. He received an intravenous fluid bolus in the emergency department.

On physical examination, blood pressure is 135/75 mm Hg and other vital signs are normal, with no orthostatic changes. Abdominal examination reveals epigastric tenderness but is otherwise unremarkable. No stigmata of chronic liver disease are seen.

Laboratory studies show a hemoglobin level of 7.3 g/dL (73 g/L).

Upper endoscopy shows a 1.5-cm duodenal bulb ulcer with a clean base.

Which of the following is the most appropriate resuscitation measure?

(A) Transfuse red blood cells to a goal hemoglobin level of 8 g/dL (80 g/L)
(B) Transfuse red blood cells to a goal hemoglobin level of 9 g/dL (90 g/L)
(C) Transfuse red blood cells to a goal hemoglobin level of 10 g/dL (100 g/L)
(D) No transfusion

Item 84

A 28-year-old man is evaluated after hospitalization for lower gastrointestinal bleeding 6 weeks earlier. At that time, he was found to have innumerable adenomatous colon polyps during colonoscopy. He underwent total colectomy, and pathology showed a 2-cm adenocarcinoma in the transverse colon. There was no evidence of metastatic disease. Genetic testing confirmed a germline mutation in the adenomatous polyposis coli (*APC*) gene consistent with familial adenomatous polyposis syndrome. Family medical history is unremarkable.

On physical examination, vital signs are normal. Abdominal examination shows a well-healed scar and no tenderness to palpation.

Which of the following is the most appropriate test to perform next?

(A) Barium upper gastrointestinal series
(B) Double-balloon enteroscopy

(C) Upper endoscopy

(D) No further testing

Item 85

A 52-year-old man is evaluated after screening colonoscopy revealed three polyps in the descending colon, measuring 5 mm, 8 mm, and 3 mm in size. Colonoscopy preparation was excellent, and the procedure was complete to the cecum. The polyps were completely excised, and pathology showed all three to be tubular adenomas. The patient has no personal or family history of colorectal cancer. He reports no symptoms and takes no medication.

All physical examination findings, including vital signs, are normal.

Based on his colonoscopy findings, when should this patient next undergo surveillance colonoscopy?

(A) 1 year

(B) 3 years

(C) 5 years

(D) 10 years

Item 86

A 55-year-old woman is evaluated for a 6-month history of throbbing and sometimes burning epigastric pain. The pain occurs 2 to 3 times per week and often subsides with eating. She reports no weight loss, nausea, or vomiting, and no bowel symptoms. She tested negative for *Helicobacter pylori* infection. Her pain did not respond to a 4-week trial of omeprazole. The patient also has anxiety, hypothyroidism, and type 2 diabetes mellitus controlled by diet. Her family medical history is unremarkable. Her medications are lorazepam and levothyroxine.

On physical examination, vital signs are normal. Epigastric tenderness to palpation is noted. Other findings are normal.

A complete blood count, liver chemistry tests, and thyroid-stimulating hormone level are normal. Hemoglobin A_{1C} level is 6.7%.

Upper endoscopy findings are normal. Gastric and small-bowel biopsies are normal.

Which of the following is the most appropriate next step in management?

(A) CT scan of the abdomen

(B) Gastric emptying test

(C) Initiation of a tricyclic antidepressant

(D) Twice-daily proton pump inhibitor therapy

(E) Ultrasonography of the right upper quadrant

Item 87

A 61-year-old woman is evaluated for joint pain, a rash on her legs, and weakness. She has chronic genotype 1 hepatitis C viral infection. She takes no medication.

On physical examination, vital signs are normal. The lower extremities are shown (see top of next column). No evidence of muscle weakness, joint swelling or warmth is

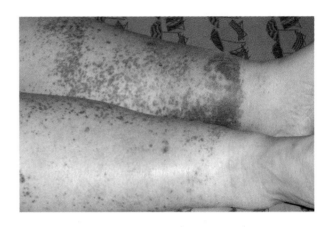

noted on musculoskeletal exam. The liver edge is palpable at the costal margin. The remainder of the physical examination is unremarkable.

Laboratory studies:

Complete blood count	Normal
Alanine aminotransferase	112 U/L
Aspartate aminotransferase	84 U/L
Total bilirubin	1 mg/dL (17.1 µmol/L)
Creatinine	Normal
Urinalysis	Normal

Which of the following is the most appropriate treatment?

(A) Cyclophosphamide

(B) Glucocorticoids

(C) Ledipasvir and sofosbuvir

(D) Pegylated interferon and ribavirin

(E) Rituximab

Item 88

A 63-year-old woman is evaluated for diarrhea characterized by three to four large-volume, watery stools per day over a period of 14 months with gradually increasing severity and frequency. She now reports occasional urge fecal incontinence and nocturnal diarrhea but no abdominal pain, bloody stools, or weight loss. She has been taking loperamide up to five times daily, but symptoms have persisted.

On physical examination, vital signs are normal; BMI is 26. Abdominal examination is normal with no tenderness or distention. Rectal examination reveals no blood or masses.

Results of routine laboratory studies are normal. Polymerase chain reaction testing of the stool for *Clostridium difficile* is negative.

Colonoscopy results are normal. Random colon biopsy specimens show lymphocytic infiltration of the mucosa with a subepithelial collagen band.

Which of the following is the most appropriate treatment?

(A) Bismuth subsalicylate

(B) Budesonide

(C) Mesalamine

(D) Prednisone

(E) Probiotics

Item 89

A 33-year-old woman is evaluated following an incidentally discovered hepatic adenoma. One week earlier, she was evaluated for nephrolithiasis with CT urogram. A 4-cm right-lobe liver lesion was also seen. Follow-up MRI identified findings consistent with hepatic adenoma. She is experiencing no symptoms now but has noted a sense of right-upper-quadrant abdominal discomfort in the past. Her only medication is an oral contraceptive agent.

All physical examination findings are normal.

Which of the following is the most appropriate management?

(A) Discontinue the oral contraceptive agent
(B) Radiofrequency ablation
(C) Surgical resection
(D) Observation

Item 90

A 75-year-old man is evaluated during a follow-up appointment for newly diagnosed iron deficiency anemia and stool testing positive for occult blood. He has undergone upper endoscopy and colonoscopy twice with no cause found for his gastrointestinal bleeding.

On physical examination, vital signs and other findings are unremarkable.

Laboratory studies show a serum ferritin level of 6 ng/mL (6 µg/L), a hemoglobin level of 9.9 g/dL (99 g/L), and a mean corpuscular volume of 78 fL.

Which of the following is the most appropriate next step in management?

(A) Capsule endoscopy
(B) CT enterography
(C) Push enteroscopy
(D) Small-bowel follow-through radiography

Item 91

A 40-year-old woman is evaluated at a follow-up appointment for hepatitis B virus (HBV) infection, which was diagnosed at age 23 years. The patient also has psoriasis. She is married and is sexually active. Medications are topical clobetasol and an oral contraceptive agent.

On physical examination, vital signs are normal. Psoriatic lesions are present on the elbows and knees. No hepatosplenomegaly is noted.

Laboratory studies:

Alanine aminotransferase	125 U/L
Aspartate aminotransferase	112 U/L
Hepatitis B surface antigen	Positive
Hepatitis B e antigen	Positive
HBV DNA	41,326 IU/mL

Which of the following is the most appropriate treatment?

(A) Adefovir
(B) Lamivudine
(C) Pegylated interferon

(D) Tenofovir
(E) No treatment

Item 92

A 40-year-old woman is evaluated for intermittent lower abdominal pain, daily bloating, and constipation. Her lower abdominal pain initially worsens then subsides after a bowel movement; it occurs nearly daily. She has bowel movements every 2 to 3 days and reports that most bowel movements are hard. The patient reports that adherence to a gluten-free diet has helped the bloating, but other symptoms have not responded. A twice-daily soluble fiber supplement has not affected symptoms. Her last thyroid-stimulating hormone measurement and complete blood count 6 months earlier were normal. Family history includes colon cancer diagnosed in her grandfather at age 60 years and a first cousin with celiac disease.

On physical examination, BMI is 29; all other findings are unremarkable.

Which of the following is the most appropriate next step in management?

(A) Colonoscopy
(B) Glucose breath test
(C) Polyethylene glycol 3350
(D) Serum tissue transglutaminase antibody measurement

Item 93

A 65-year-old man is evaluated after a positive stool antigen test for *Helicobacter pylori* infection obtained to confirm eradication after therapy. *H. pylori* gastritis was diagnosed in the setting of a duodenal ulcer. Four weeks ago, he completed a 10-day course of eradication therapy consisting of amoxicillin, clarithromycin, and omeprazole. He reports taking all medications as prescribed during treatment and reports no upper gastrointestinal symptoms or melena. The patient does not smoke cigarettes or drink alcohol. He has no known drug allergies.

Which of the following is the most appropriate 14-day treatment regimen?

(A) Amoxicillin, clarithromycin, and omeprazole
(B) Amoxicillin, metronidazole, and omeprazole
(C) Bismuth, metronidazole, omeprazole, and tetracycline
(D) Clarithromycin, metronidazole, and omeprazole

Item 94

A 61-year-old woman is evaluated in the hospital for abdominal discomfort and worsening ascites. She reports a significant decrease in urine output over the preceding 3 days. She has a history of cirrhosis due to primary biliary cholangitis. Her medications are furosemide and spironolactone.

On physical examination, blood pressure is 90/58 mm Hg; other vital signs are normal. The abdomen is distended with a positive fluid wave.

Laboratory studies show a serum creatinine level of 2.8 mg/dL (247.5 µmol/L) (3 weeks ago, 1.2 mg/dL [106.1 µmol/L]) and a serum sodium level of 133 mEq/L (133 mmol/L).

Urine studies show a sodium level of less than 10 mEq/L (10 mmol/L) and no protein, leukocytes, erythrocytes, or casts.

Analysis of ascitic fluid shows a leukocyte count of 180/µL with 30% neutrophils. Cultures of ascitic fluid are negative.

A kidney ultrasound shows no evidence of obstruction or kidney parenchymal disease.

Which of the following is the most likely diagnosis?

(A) Acute interstitial nephritis
(B) Acute tubular necrosis
(C) Hepatorenal syndrome
(D) Membranous glomerulonephritis

Item 95

A 48-year-old man is evaluated in the emergency department for left flank pain and dysuria. Six months earlier, the patient was hospitalized for severe acute gallstone pancreatitis. Contrast-enhanced CT of the pancreas showed lack of perfusion in the body of the pancreas. He recovered with supportive care and was discharged 2 weeks later. He had an uncomplicated laparoscopic cholecystectomy 4 weeks after discharge. He reports that he has felt well until the sudden onset of left flank pain today.

On physical examination, blood pressure is 130/80 mm Hg and pulse rate is 90/min; other vital signs are normal. Abdominal examination is notable for pain in the left lower quadrant on palpation. The remainder of the examination is normal.

Urinalysis shows hematuria.

A CT scan identifies nephrolithiasis and a small stone in the left ureter. The CT scan also shows a 6-cm fluid collection with solid debris in the body of the pancreas with a well-defined wall.

Which of the following is the most appropriate management of the fluid collection?

(A) Antibiotic therapy
(B) CT-guided fine-needle aspiration
(C) Drainage procedure
(D) Observation

Item 96

A 62-year-old woman is evaluated during a follow-up appointment 12 weeks after she completed treatment for genotype 1a hepatitis C virus (HCV) infection. She has Child-Turcotte-Pugh Class A cirrhosis (well-compensated cirrhosis). Small esophageal varices were noted on upper endoscopy 1 year earlier.

On physical examination, vital signs are normal; BMI is 26. Palmar erythema, spider angiomata over the chest, a firm liver edge 3 cm below the costal margin, and a palpable spleen tip are noted. The examination is otherwise normal.

Her HCV RNA is undetectable and her calculated Model for End-Stage Liver Disease score is 8.

Which of the following is the most appropriate management for this patient?

(A) Liver transplantation evaluation
(B) Measurement of HCV RNA in 12 weeks
(C) Ultrasonography of the liver every 6 months
(D) Upper endoscopy

Answers and Critiques

Item 1   Answer: D

Educational Objective: Treat opioid-induced constipation.

Switching to naloxegol is the most appropriate treatment for this patient. The clinical definition of constipation (as defined by the Rome 4 international working group) is a symptom complex that includes at least two of the following: straining during defecation, passage of lumpy or hard stool, sensation of incomplete defecation, use of manual maneuvers to facilitate a bowel movement, and/or frequency of fewer than three bowel movements per week. Oral naloxegol is a peripherally acting μ-opioid receptor antagonist that is FDA-approved for the treatment of opioid-induced constipation in adults with chronic noncancer pain. This patient's constipation can be classified as opioid-induced because her constipation symptoms developed after the initiation of chronic opioid analgesic therapy for reflex sympathetic dystrophy syndrome. First-line laxative therapies, including over-the-counter stool softeners, bulk laxatives (fiber supplements), a stimulant laxative (bisacodyl), and an osmotic laxative (polyethylene glycol [PEG]), have all been ineffective. Current maintenance laxative therapy should be stopped before the initiation of naloxegol and can be added to the naloxegol after 3 days of monotherapy as symptoms dictate.

Surfactants such as docusate sodium or docusate calcium are weak laxatives with an excellent safety profile. As such, they are most appropriate for very mild, intermittent constipation and will not be effective in this patient.

Adding a second osmotic agent such as lactulose is unlikely to improve the patient's reduced stool frequency, which is the result of slowed colonic motility caused by her chronic opioid analgesic use. Also, lactulose use is likely to lead to bloating.

Increasing the dose of PEG will not provide any additional benefit because the patient reports soft stool with the current dose. The patient's altered colonic motility will not improve with additional PEG. Furthermore, an increased dose of PEG is likely to cause bloating.

KEY POINT

- Oral naloxegol is a peripherally acting μ-opioid receptor antagonist that is FDA-approved for the treatment of opioid-induced constipation in adults with chronic noncancer pain.

Bibliography

Chey WD, Webster L, Sostek M, Lappalainen J, Barker PN, Tack J. Naloxegol for opioid-induced constipation in patients with noncancer pain. N Engl J Med. 2014;370:2387-96. [PMID: 24896818] doi:10.1056/NEJMoa1310246

Item 2   Answer: D

Educational Objective: Manage the immune-tolerant phase of hepatitis B viral infection.

Repeat liver chemistry testing in 6 months is the most appropriate next step in the management of this patient. The patient has hepatitis B virus (HBV) infection in the immune-tolerant phase, which can be determined by the likely vertical transmission and the patient's young age, positive hepatitis B e antigen (HBeAg), high viral load, and normal aminotransferase levels. Therefore, the patient only requires serial monitoring of aminotransferase levels. There are four typical phases of HBV infection: (1) immune tolerant; (2) immune active, HBeAg positive; (3) immune control (inactive); and (4) reactivation, HBeAg negative. Not all patients go through each phase. Patients with infection in the immune-tolerant phase do not have significant hepatic inflammation and have no fibrosis, and, therefore, do not require treatment. However, infection can progress to the immune-active, HBeAg-positive phase, in which hepatic inflammation, elevated aminotransferase levels, and fibrosis develop, underscoring the need for surveillance of aminotransferase levels.

Patients with HBV infection in the immune-active, HBeAg-positive and reactivation, HBeAg-negative phases require treatment if the alanine aminotransferase level is elevated. Antiviral therapy is also required for patients who present with acute liver failure, all patients with cirrhosis, and patients undergoing treatment with certain immunosuppressive or chemotherapy regimens. None of these scenarios apply to this patient, so she does not require antiviral treatment such as tenofovir, entecavir, or pegylated interferon.

Patients with HBV infection are at increased risk for hepatocellular carcinoma, even in the absence of cirrhosis. Patients from Southeast Asia should undergo hepatocellular carcinoma surveillance with ultrasonography starting at age 40 years for men and at age 50 years for women, and patients from sub-Saharan Africa should begin at age 20 years. Other indications include persistent inflammatory activity (defined as an elevated alanine aminotransferase level and HBV DNA levels greater than 10,000 IU/mL for at least a few years) and a family history of hepatocellular carcinoma. The preferred surveillance strategy is liver ultrasonography with or without α-fetoprotein measurement. This patient is not yet old enough to warrant hepatocellular carcinoma surveillance, so hepatic ultrasonography is not indicated.

KEY POINT

- Patients with hepatitis B infection in the immune-tolerant phase require serial monitoring of aminotransferase levels.

Bibliography

Terrault NA, Bzowej NH, Chang KM, Hwang JP, Jonas MM, Murad MH; American Association for the Study of Liver Diseases. AASLD guidelines for treatment of chronic hepatitis B. Hepatology. 2016;63:261-83. [PMID: 26566064] doi:10.1002/hep.28156

Item 3   Answer: D

Educational Objective: Manage aspirin use before and after polypectomy.

This patient should not discontinue aspirin use. Aspirin does not need to be discontinued before colonoscopy in any scenario, and data from studies of patients who have undergone polypectomy show no difference in the risk for postprocedure bleeding with discontinuation or continuation of aspirin use. The American College of Gastroenterology's 2016 guidelines for management of lower gastrointestinal bleeding (LGIB) recommend the continuation of aspirin for secondary cardiovascular prophylaxis after polypectomy. Discontinuing aspirin is recommended after polypectomy in patients without established cardiovascular disease who are using aspirin as primary prophylaxis. In patients with established cardiovascular disease, such as this patient, the risks of a potential cardiovascular event outweigh those of potential gastrointestinal bleeding.

Holding aspirin for a period of time after a polypectomy, such as 48 hours, has not been shown to reduce postprocedure LGIB and may increase risk for a thromboembolic event in a patient with established cardiovascular disease.

KEY POINT

- Aspirin for secondary prophylaxis in patients with established cardiovascular disease should be continued after colonoscopy with polypectomy.

Bibliography

Strate LL, Gralnek IM. ACG clinical guideline: management of patients with acute lower gastrointestinal bleeding. Am J Gastroenterol. 2016;111:459-74. [PMID: 26925883] doi:10.1038/ajg.2016.41

Item 4   Answer: C

Educational Objective: Diagnose nonalcoholic fatty liver disease.

The most likely diagnosis is nonalcoholic fatty liver disease (NAFLD). Up to 108 million Americans have NAFLD, which far exceeds the prevalence of any other form of chronic liver disease. Risk factors include obesity, diabetes mellitus, insulin resistance, hypertension, and hyperlipidemia. This patient has three risk factors for NAFLD, as well as an enlarged liver on physical examination. Her elevated alanine aminotransferase and aspartate aminotransferase levels are within the typical range for patients with NAFLD. Alkaline phosphatase (ALP) levels may be slightly elevated as well, typically less than 2 to 2.5 times the upper limit of normal. The finding of a hyperechoic liver on ultrasonography is also consistent with NAFLD. Because other liver diseases may also result in hepatic steatosis, patients with elevated liver chemistries and suspected nonalcoholic steatohepatitis should be evaluated to exclude other causes of chronic liver disease.

The diagnosis of primary biliary cholangitis (PBC) is generally made on the basis of a cholestatic liver enzyme profile in the setting of a positive antimitochondrial antibody test. The predominant liver enzyme abnormality is an increase in serum ALP levels, but a mild to moderate increase in aminotransferase levels is also seen. Antimitochondrial antibody–negative PBC accounts for about 10% of cases of PBC. This patient's liver chemistry profile is hepatocellular (elevations primarily of aminotransaminase levels), not cholestatic, making PBC unlikely.

Although this patient has a positive anti–smooth muscle antibody test, the low titer alone is not diagnostic of autoimmune hepatitis. Autoimmune hepatitis is typically accompanied by higher autoantibody titers and elevated γ-globulin levels. It requires a liver biopsy to establish the diagnosis. Between 20% and 30% of patients with NAFLD exhibit low-titer autoantibodies.

This patient has a minimally elevated ALP level, which helps to exclude primary sclerosing cholangitis (PSC) or PBC. In addition, the patient's risk factors and ultrasound findings make these diagnoses unlikely. MR cholangiopancreatography is required to diagnose PSC.

KEY POINT

- Nonalcoholic fatty liver disease is the most common cause of abnormal liver test results in the United States.

Bibliography

Chalasani N, Younossi Z, Lavine JE, Diehl AM, Brunt EM, Cusi K, et al. The diagnosis and management of non-alcoholic fatty liver disease: practice guideline by the American Association for the Study of Liver Diseases, American College of Gastroenterology, and the American Gastroenterological Association. Hepatology. 2012;55:2005-23. [PMID: 22488764] doi:10.1002/hep.25762

Item 5   Answer: D

Educational Objective: Diagnose pseudoachalasia.

This patient likely has pseudoachalasia, and endoscopic ultrasound should be used to diagnose a possible tumor of the distal esophagus or gastric cardia. The other causes of pseudoachalasia are benign disease, such as amyloidosis and sarcoidosis, and postsurgical status (for example, after Nissen fundoplication or bariatric surgery). The clinical presentation of achalasia consists of dysphagia to both solids and liquids along with regurgitation of undigested food and saliva. Other conditions can mimic achalasia and can have identical clinical, barium-imaging, and manometric findings, as well as identical endoscopic appearance. These include pseudoachalasia, secondary achalasia, and Chagas disease. Pseudoachalasia is caused by a tumor at the gastroesophageal junction infiltrating the myenteric plexus causing esophageal motor abnormalities. Tumors capable of infiltrating the myenteric plexus include those of the distal esophageus, gastric cardia, pancreatic, breast, lung, and hepatocellular. Patients with pseudoachalasia are often in their sixth decade of life or older, have a short duration of symptoms, and experience sudden and profound weight loss. Endoscopic ultrasonography can exclude an infiltrating tumor, and guidelines recommend its use in patients with a strong suspicion for malignancy.

Achalasia affects men and women equally, with an annual incidence of 1 in 100,000 individuals. It tends to occur between the ages of 30 and 60 years. Typical achalasia has an insidious onset and long duration of symptoms, often measured in years, before patients seek medical attention. This patient's age, short duration of symptoms, and rapid weight loss argue against the diagnosis of achalasia.

Chagas disease is caused by infection with the vector-borne parasite *Trypanosoma cruzi* in rural areas of Latin America. The major manifestations of Chagas disease include enteric myenteric destruction, resulting in achalasia, megacolon, heart disease, and other neurologic disorders. The lack of travel and absence of other manifestations of Chagas disease make this diagnosis unlikely.

Eosinophilic esophagitis is inconsistent with this patient's symptoms and endoscopic examination. Its typical presentation is in younger patients with food bolus obstruction. Endoscopy findings in eosinophilic esophagitis include rings and furrows.

KEY POINT

- Pseudoachalasia is caused by a tumor at the gastroesophageal junction infiltrating the myenteric plexus causing esophageal motor abnormalities; symptoms, barium-imaging and manometric findings, and endoscopic appearance are similar to achalasia.

Bibliography
Vaezi MF, Pandolfino JE, Vela MF. ACG clinical guideline: diagnosis and management of achalasia. Am J Gastroenterol. 2013;108:1238-49; quiz 1250. [PMID: 23877351] doi:10.1038/ajg.2013.196

Item 6   **Answer:**   **C**

Educational Objective: Treat diarrhea-predominant irritable bowel syndrome.

A low-FODMAP (Fermentable Oligosaccharides, Disaccharides, Monosaccharides, And Polyols) diet is the most appropriate treatment for this patient. FODMAPs consist of short-chain carbohydrates that are poorly absorbed and rapidly fermented by gut bacteria, resulting in the production of gas and an increased osmotic fluid load within the gut lumen. The patient has diarrhea-predominant irritable bowel syndrome (IBS-D). IBS is a heterogeneous symptom complex characterized by abdominal pain and altered bowel habits. The diagnosis of IBS requires symptoms of recurrent abdominal pain or discomfort at least 1 day a week for a period of 3 months, along with two of the following three additional criteria: pain relieved by defecation, change in stool frequency,

or change in bowel consistency. IBS can then be further subtyped into IBS with predominant constipation (IBS-C), predominant diarrhea, mixed bowel habits, or unclassified.

The effects of dietary FODMAPs may contribute to the symptoms of IBS-D. A randomized controlled trial involving 84 adults with IBS-D compared a low-FODMAP diet to a diet based on modified National Institute for Health and Care Excellence (mNICE) guidelines. In this study, more patients on the low-FODMAP diet reported adequate relief of their IBS-D symptoms (52% versus 41%) and response in abdominal pain (51% versus 23%) than those on the mNICE diet.

Alosetron is a peripherally acting serotonin type 3–receptor antagonist approved by the FDA for the treatment of IBS-D in women aged 18 years or older after failure of conventional therapy. Due to the risk for adverse events with the use of alosetron, including serious complications of constipation and ischemic colitis, a prescriber must first complete an FDA-mandated Risk Evaluation and Mitigation Strategy training program that is available online (www.alosetronrems.com). Alosetron is not FDA-approved for the treatment of men with IBS-D due to the small number of men involved in the pivotal clinical trials, and it would not be appropriate as an initial treatment for IBS in this male patient.

Linaclotide is a peripherally acting guanylate cyclase-C activator approved by the FDA for the treatment of IBS-C. Lubiprostone is a peripherally acting chloride channel activator that is approved by the FDA for the treatment of IBS-C in women aged 18 years or older. In this patient whose predominant bowel symptom is diarrhea, use of either of these agents will worsen his diarrhea and is therefore not indicated.

KEY POINT

- A low-FODMAP (Fermentable Oligosaccharides, Disaccharides, Monosaccharides, And Polyols) diet can reduce abdominal pain and bloating and improve stool consistency, frequency, and urgency in patients with diarrhea-predominant irritable bowel syndrome.

Bibliography
Eswaran SL, Chey WD, Han-Markey T, Ball S, Jackson K. A randomized controlled trial comparing the low FODMAP diet vs. modified NICE guidelines in US adults with IBS-D. Am J Gastroenterol. 2016;111:1824-1832. [PMID: 27725652] doi:10.1038/ajg.2016.434

Item 7   **Answer:**   **A**

Educational Objective: Diagnose a Zenker diverticulum.

Barium esophagram is the most appropriate next diagnostic test for this patient. The patient's primary symptom of dysphagia associated with regurgitation of undigested food is the classic presentation of a Zenker diverticulum. Other commonly reported symptoms include halitosis, aspiration, and gurgling in the chest, but esophageal dysphagia is the most common symptom, reported by the majority of patients with a Zenker diverticulum. This type of diverticulum is located in the cervical esophagus and may lead to complications such as aspiration and pneumonia. The best initial test is a barium esophagram, which will identify the diverticulum. Treatment is reserved for symptomatic patients and endoscopic diverticulectomy is favored where surgical expertise is available. In medical centers without such expertise, surgery by external neck incision is used.

Esophageal manometry is used when there is concern for a motility disorder, such as achalasia. Patients with motility disorders commonly report dysphagia to liquids or both solids and liquids; this patient's dysphagia to solid food does not suggest a motility disorder.

Ambulatory pH testing and impedance-pH testing can be valuable tools in identifying acid exposure within the esophagus. Impedance-pH testing can identify both acid and nonacid reflux. Testing can be done with a 48-hour wireless capsule or 24-hour transnasal catheter to detect active acid reflux. The wireless capsule has been shown to have better patient tolerability. A 24-hour pH manometry test is often used to further evaluate a patient with symptoms of gastroesophageal reflux disease that have not responded to medical therapy (usually a trial of an acid-reducing agent such as a proton pump inhibitor). A peptic stricture causing solid-food dysphagia may result from untreated reflux, but this patient reports dysphagia and regurgitation of undigested food, symptoms strongly suggestive of Zenker diverticulum.

Endoscopy is used to inspect the mucosal surface of the esophagus, stomach, and duodenum to identify conditions within the upper gastrointestinal tract. Because this patient's symptoms are consistent with the presentation of a Zenker diverticulum, a barium esophagram is a more appropriate choice than upper endoscopy. Although endoscopy may identify the diverticulum, there is risk for perforation if the endoscope enters the diverticulum.

KEY POINT

- Patients with dysphagia associated with regurgitation of undigested food should be evaluated with a barium esophagram for the presence of a Zenker diverticulum.

Bibliography

Smith CD. Esophageal strictures and diverticula. Surg Clin North Am. 2015;95:669-81. [PMID: 25965138] doi:10.1016/j.suc.2015.02.017

Item 8   Answer: C

Educational Objective: Diagnose hepatopulmonary syndrome.

Echocardiography with agitated saline is the most appropriate next test for this patient. Hepatopulmonary syndrome is a complication of cirrhosis caused by dilation of the pulmonary vasculature in the setting of advanced liver disease and portal hypertension. A high alveolar-arterial oxygen gradient results from functional shunting. Patients with hepatopulmonary syndrome usually have a preexisting diagnosis of liver disease and present with shortness of breath. Dilation of pulmonary vasculature occurs at the base of the lungs, so hypoxemia is most noted when patients are upright or sitting, when shunting is maximal. Classic features are platypnea (worsening shortness of breath in the upright position) and orthodeoxia (worsening arterial oxygen saturation in the upright position). Pulse oximetry is often used to screen for changes in the arterial oxygen saturation level with changes of position. The diagnosis is made by demonstrating an arterial oxygen tension less than 80 mm Hg (10.7 kPa) breathing ambient air, or an alveolar-arterial gradient of 15 mm Hg (2 kPa) or greater, along with evidence of intrapulmonary shunting on echocardiography with agitated saline or macroaggregated albumin study. The detection of intrapulmonary shunting of blood is best confirmed by echocardiography with agitated saline (also known as a bubble study), during which bubbles are identified in the left side of the heart after 5 beats, demonstrating that the shunting of blood is not intracardiac. Clinically significant hepatopulmonary syndrome is treated with supplemental oxygen and liver transplantation. Hepatopulmonary syndrome is a progressive condition that is ultimately fatal without liver transplantation.

Bronchoscopy is of no value in the diagnosis of platypnea or shunting disorders. It is potentially useful in the diagnosis of a pulmonary infiltrate or relief of an airway obstruction.

CT angiography can demonstrate the presence of large vascular shunts in the lungs but is rarely required to establish the diagnosis of hepatopulmonary syndrome. An additional benefit of CT angiography is its ability to show pulmonary emboli. In this patient, the presence of orthopnea is not consistent with pulmonary embolism. Transthoracic echocardiography with agitated saline is the gold standard for detecting pulmonary vascular dilatation and diagnosing hepatopulmonary syndrome.

Pulmonary function testing is useful for evaluating the presence of obstructive lung disease as well as restrictive lung disease. The normal pulmonary examination and normal chest radiography suggest that neither restrictive nor obstructive lung disease is contributing to this patient's presentation.

KEY POINT

- The diagnosis of hepatopulmonary syndrome is made by demonstrating an arterial oxygen tension less than 80 mm Hg (10.7 kPa) breathing ambient air, or an alveolar-arterial gradient of 15 mm Hg (2 kPa) or greater, along with evidence of intrapulmonary shunting on echocardiography with agitated saline or macroaggregated albumin study.

Bibliography

Krowka MJ, Fallon MB, Kawut SM, Fuhrmann V, Heimbach JK, Ramsay MA, et al. International Liver Transplant Society practice guidelines: diagnosis and management of hepatopulmonary syndrome and portopulmonary hypertension. Transplantation. 2016;100:1440-52. [PMID: 27326810] doi:10.1097/TP.0000000000001229

Item 9   Answer: A

Educational Objective: Treat acalculous cholecystitis.

Cholecystostomy tube placement is the most appropriate next step in management for this patient. She has risk factors as well as clinical and radiologic findings that are consistent with acalculous cholecystitis. Cholecystectomy is the definitive treatment for acalculous cholecystitis in stable patients. However, this patient is now hemodynamically unstable and, therefore, requires a temporizing cholecystostomy tube to allow time for her to stabilize and for gallbladder inflammation to improve before cholecystectomy. Risk factors for acalculous cholecystitis include diabetes mellitus, sepsis, trauma, burns, vasculitis, cardiovascular disease, mechanical ventilation, and total parenteral nutrition. Acalculous cholecystitis can present with biliary colic symptoms in the alert patient or with unexplained leukocytosis, sepsis, and jaundice in the critically ill patient. On physical examination, a mass may be palpated in the right upper quadrant. Ultrasound may show some of the features seen in this patient (distended gallbladder with wall thickening and pericholecystic fluid), gas bubbles in the fundus ("champagne sign"), or nonvisualization of the gallbladder altogether. No stones or sludge are present in the gallbladder. Management includes bacterial cultures, intravenous antibiotics to cover gram-negative organisms, and cholecystostomy tube placement in the unstable patient or cholecystectomy in the stable patient.

The role of endoscopic retrograde cholangiopancreatography with stenting is evolving. It has been used in case series to decompress the gallbladder in patients with acalculous cholecystitis, but it is not yet considered a first- or second-line treatment option due to less robust evidence to support this practice and the need for experienced endoscopists to perform the procedure.

A hepatobiliary iminodiacetic acid scan may be used when ultrasonography is equivocal, and it would show nonopacification of the gallbladder in cases of cholecystitis. It is unnecessary in this patient who has clinical and radiologic features consistent with acalculous cholecystitis.

This patient's ultrasonographic findings of a distended and thick-walled gallbladder with associated pericholecystic fluid and a lack of gallstones, in addition to her risk factors for acalculous cholecystitis, make further imaging, such as MR cholangiopancreatography, unnecessary and possibly dangerous due to the need for urgent gallbladder decompression.

KEY POINT

- Acalculous cholecystitis can present with biliary colic symptoms in the alert patient or with unexplained leukocytosis, sepsis, and jaundice in the critically ill patient.

Bibliography

Huffman JL, Schenker S. Acute acalculous cholecystitis: a review. Clin Gastroenterol Hepatol. 2010;8:15-22. [PMID: 19747982] doi:10.1016/j.cgh.2009.08.034

Item 10   Answer: B

Educational Objective: Prevent recurrent NSAID-related peptic ulcer disease.

Celecoxib plus omeprazole is the most appropriate treatment regimen for this patient. Patients who have bleeding ulcers while taking NSAIDs should discontinue NSAIDs permanently if possible. In cases where this is not possible, strategies to reduce the risk for recurrent bleeding should be instituted. Selective cyclooxygenase-2 (COX-2) inhibitors, such as celecoxib, preferentially inhibit the COX-2 isoenzyme, which primarily modulates pain and inflammation, and minimally inhibit the COX-1 isoenzyme, which promotes generation of the gastric mucosal protective barrier, decreases gastric acid secretion, and helps to maintain good mucosal blood flow. The risk for gastroduodenal ulcers and ulcer complications is significantly lower in patients taking COX-2 inhibitors compared with nonselective NSAIDs such as naproxen; however, in high-risk patients, such as those with previous peptic ulcer disease, a COX-2 inhibitor alone is no better than a nonselective NSAID coadministered with a proton pump inhibitor in preventing ulcer complications, with rebleeding rates of approximately 4% to 6% within 6 months.

A single 12-month randomized study showed an ulcer rebleeding rate of 0% in patients treated with celecoxib plus omeprazole compared with 9% in patients treated with a celecoxib alone. A direct comparison of naproxen plus omeprazole to celecoxib plus omeprazole in the prevention of NSAID bleeding in high-risk patients has not been performed. There is also evidence that COX-2 inhibitors and nonselective NSAIDs, with the possible exception of naproxen, increase the risk for cardiovascular complications; therefore, the decision to use a COX-2 inhibitor requires a harm-benefit analysis that weighs the gastrointestinal risks of an NSAID with the potential cardiovascular risks of a COX-2 inhibitor.

The use of ibuprofen, a nonselective NSAID, is no safer than the use of naproxen for lessening the likelihood of development of peptic ulcers.

Other gastroprotective agents, such as H_2 blockers (including ranitidine) and misoprostol, have been ineffective in preventing NSAID-related peptic ulcers in patients at low or moderate risk; however, their efficacy in high-risk patients (such as this patient with a previous NSAID-induced gastric ulcer) has not been demonstrated. Misoprostol is associated with adverse effects, including diarrhea and abdominal pain. Also, the required twice-daily dosing for ranitidine and four-times-daily dosing for misoprostol may lead to patient nonadherence, which further reduces the efficacy of such therapy.

KEY POINT

- In patients requiring NSAIDs, an evidence-based treatment strategy to prevent recurrent NSAID-induced peptic ulcers is the use of a cyclooxygenase-2 selective NSAID plus a proton pump inhibitor.

Bibliography

Laine L. CLINICAL PRACTICE. Upper gastrointestinal bleeding due to a peptic ulcer. N Engl J Med. 2016;374:2367-76. [PMID: 27305194] doi:10.1056/NEJMcp1514257

Item 11   Answer: D

Educational Objective: Manage follow-up colonoscopy for hyperplastic polyps.

This patient should undergo colonoscopy in 10 years. Serrated polyps are classified into three histologic types: hyperplastic polyps, sessile serrated polyps, and traditional serrated adenomas. Hyperplastic polyps are the most common type of serrated polyp. They are non-neoplastic and are composed of normal mucosal elements; small hyperplastic polyps, often found in the rectosigmoid colon, are believed to have no clinical significance. As a result, the interval until the next screening examination is 10 years, the same as for patients who do not have polyps found on baseline examination. Sessile serrated polyps (also known as sessile serrated adenomas) and traditional serrated adenomas are both neoplastic and are precursors to colorectal cancer; they should be completely excised. Substantial variability has been demonstrated in the ability of a pathologist to differentiate a hyperplastic polyp from a sessile serrated polyp; therefore, guidelines recommend managing large (>10 mm) hyperplastic polyps as if they are sessile serrated polyps.

The patient's family history of a second-degree relative with colon cancer diagnosed at age 80 years does not increase her risk for colon cancer or indicate the need for more frequent or early colonoscopy.

A 1-year surveillance interval is not appropriate for this patient. It is indicated in patients with more than 10 adenomas found on colonoscopy, those with a diagnosed polyposis syndrome, or those with Lynch syndrome. *Lynch syndrome* is the term used to describe patients who meet the Amsterdam II criteria for hereditary nonpolyposis colorectal cancer and have an identified germline mutation in one of the four mismatch repair genes (*MLH1*, *MSH2*, *MSH6*, *PMS2*) or the epithelial cell adhesion molecule gene (*EPCAM*).

A 3-year surveillance interval is recommended for patients who have three or more adenomas (or sessile serrated polyps) found on baseline colonoscopy, one adenoma larger than 10 mm in size, or an adenoma with any degree of villous or high-grade dysplasia.

A surveillance interval of 5 years is recommended for patients with two or fewer adenomas (or sessile serrated polyps) found on baseline colonoscopy and for patients with a first-degree relative with colon cancer diagnosed at an age younger than 60 years. Sessile serrated polyps are more frequently found in the proximal colon and may be difficult to detect on colonoscopy due to their flat appearance. Like tubular adenomas, surveillance colonoscopy is based on size and presence of dysplasia.

KEY POINT

- Patients with small (<10 mm) hyperplastic polyps on baseline colonoscopic examination should undergo surveillance colonoscopy in 10 years.

Bibliography

Lieberman DA, Rex DK, Winawer SJ, Giardiello FM, Johnson DA, Levin TR; United States Multi-Society Task Force on Colorectal Cancer. Guidelines for colonoscopy surveillance after screening and polypectomy: a consensus update by the US Multi-Society Task Force on Colorectal Cancer. Gastroenterology. 2012;143:844-57. [PMID: 22763141] doi:10.1053/j.gastro.2012.06.001

Item 12   Answer: B

Educational Objective: Treat acute cholangitis with biliary obstruction.

Endoscopic retrograde cholangiopancreatography (ERCP) is the most appropriate next step in the management of this patient. The patient presents with the Charcot triad of symptoms—fever, abdominal pain in the right upper quadrant, and jaundice—which is consistent with a diagnosis of cholangitis. In patients with evidence of biliary obstruction (as seen in this patient's findings on ultrasonography) and more than mild disease, biliary decompression with ERCP is an essential component of therapy. Obstruction is typically indicated by a dilated bile duct and persistently elevated liver enzyme levels. Indications for urgent ERCP include ongoing septic physiology (persistently elevated leukocyte count and temperature greater than 38.9 °C [102 °F]) despite resuscitative measures and antibiotics, hyperbilirubinemia (>5 mg/dL [85.5 µmol/L]), and altered mental status, which may also herald a worsened prognosis.

When duct decompression with ERCP is not possible, percutaneous cholangiography with biliary tube placement can be performed. Most patients with cholangitis also have cholelithiasis, elevated aminotransferase levels, and hyperbilirubinemia. Acute cholangitis is usually caused by *Escherichia coli*, *Klebsiella* species, *Pseudomonas* species, and enterococci and can progress to septic shock with or without liver abscess formation. The mainstay of therapy for cholangitis is the initiation of antibiotic therapy targeting enteric organisms; for mild to moderate community-acquired disease, options include cefazolin, cefuroxime, or ceftriaxone.

Patients who have complicated gallstone disease with evidence of choledocholithiasis should be considered for cholecystectomy; however, in the acute setting, this intervention should be deferred until after antibiotic therapy and biliary decompression with ERCP. Cholecystectomy will remove the source of future gallstones, but it will not decompress this patient's obstructed common bile duct or reduce the risk for sepsis.

MR cholangiopancreatography is a diagnostic test that is unlikely to yield additional information other than what this patient's ultrasound has already shown. In this patient with a very high likelihood of finding a common bile duct stone, a therapeutic procedure such as ERCP is more appropriate.

CONT.

A percutaneous cholecystostomy can be used to treat cholecystitis, but in the setting of cholangitis, as in this patient, percutaneous cholecystostomy would not necessarily provide decompression of the biliary obstruction if the bile duct is obstructed above the insertion point of the cystic duct. Due to their higher rates of morbidity, percutaneous approaches to decompression of the biliary system should only be considered if endoscopic approaches are unavailable or contraindicated.

KEY POINT

- Patients who have cholangitis with evidence of biliary obstruction should be treated with antibiotic therapy and biliary decompression with endoscopic retrograde cholangiopancreatography.

Bibliography

Demehri FR, Alam HB. Evidence-based management of common gallstone-related emergencies. J Intensive Care Med. 2016;31:3-13. [PMID: 25320159] doi:10.1177/0885066614554192

Item 13 Answer: B

Educational Objective: Treat an esophageal stricture.

Endoscopy with dilation is the most appropriate treatment for this patient, who has eosinophilic esophagitis, refractory symptoms of dysphagia despite fluticasone therapy, and the finding of an esophageal stricture on endoscopy. Eosinophilic esophagitis can cause patients to develop a fibrostenotic esophageal stricture, which can be treated using endoscopy with dilation. Endoscopic dilation relieves the dysphagia but has no effect on underlying inflammation; therefore, medical therapy must be maintained. For unclear reasons, patients with eosinophilic esophagitis are more prone to mucosal tears with dilation than are patients with other stricturing diseases. It is imperative that the extent of dilation be limited in amount to avoid these complications; multiple dilations may be required to adequately treat the dysphagia.

Most patients respond quickly after initiation of the fluticasone; therefore, continued or increased fluticasone alone will not alleviate the patient's dysphagia symptoms. Continued fluticasone may be necessary as maintenance therapy for this patient. Eosinophilic esophagitis is a chronic disease that often recurs after treatment is stopped; therefore, repeat or maintenance therapy may be needed.

Omeprazole and other proton pump inhibitors (PPIs) are not effective in relieving dysphagia due to stricture. PPIs can reduce inflammation and eosinophil count and are often used before initiating fluticasone therapy to determine if the patient has PPI-responsive eosinophilic esophagitis.

Limited data suggest that prednisone may be useful in patients with eosinophilic esophagitis who do not experience relief of symptoms with fluticasone therapy. However, like the swallowed aerosolized glucocorticoids, relapse is common when the medication is stopped, and relatively high doses are typically required, which carry associated risks of immunosuppression and other side effects. Additionally, this patient's esophageal stricture is fibrotic rather than inflammatory, so oral prednisone would not be effective for his dysphagia symptoms.

KEY POINT

- Esophageal stricture in patients with eosinophilic esophagitis requires treatment with endoscopic dilation when symptoms do not respond to medical therapy.

Bibliography

Dellon ES, Gonsalves N, Hirano I, Furuta GT, Liacouras CA, Katzka DA; American College of Gastroenterology. ACG clinical guideline: evidenced based approach to the diagnosis and management of esophageal eosinophilia and eosinophilic esophagitis (EoE). Am J Gastroenterol. 2013; 108:679-92; quiz 693. [PMID: 23567357] doi:10.1038/ajg.2013.71

Item 14 Answer: A

Educational Objective: Treat toxic megacolon.

This patient requires colectomy. He has a history of ulcerative colitis and presents with fever, tachycardia, hypotension, and a dilated colon on abdominal radiography; the diagnosis is toxic megacolon, a life-threatening condition that complicates approximately 5% of acute, severe cases of ulcerative colitis. Toxic megacolon is defined by the presence of toxicity (fever, tachycardia, hypotension, and leukocytosis) along with evidence of colonic dilation. Patients with this condition have an increased risk for complications such as colonic perforation. Intravenous fluid resuscitation, intravenous high-dose corticosteroids, and broad-spectrum antibiotics (for example, a third-generation cephalosporin with metronidazole) should be initiated in patients with toxic megacolon. Management requires close collaboration with a surgeon; therefore, emergent surgical consultation for consideration of subtotal colectomy is required because of the impending risk for perforation and peritonitis in patients with toxic megacolon. Some patients may respond to medical therapy with high-dose glucocorticoids (in addition to intravenous fluids and broad-spectrum antibiotics), but there should be a low threshold for surgical intervention due to the potential harms associated with toxic megacolon.

Colonoscopy is contraindicated because it would increase the risk for perforation and complications related to toxic megacolon.

CT of the abdomen and pelvis is the optimal imaging modality to evaluate suspected toxic megacolon and may better assess for the presence of colonic necrosis; however, in this case, the diagnosis of toxic megacolon can be confidently made based on the patient's presentation and abdominal radiography, and urgent surgical evaluation is necessary.

Stool studies for enteric pathogens may identify a precipitant of toxic megacolon but require a minimum of 24 hours before test results are received. Surgical consultation should not be delayed to wait for results of stool testing.

KEY POINT

- Toxic megacolon is defined by the presence of toxicity and evidence of colonic dilation; it requires prompt surgical treatment.

Answers and Critiques

Bibliography
Seah D, De Cruz P. Review article: the practical management of acute severe ulcerative colitis. Aliment Pharmacol Ther. 2016;43:482-513. [PMID: 26725569] doi:10.1111/apt.13491

Item 15   Answer: B

Educational Objective: Diagnose microscopic colitis.

Based on the patient's age, sex, and clinical presentation, microscopic colitis is the most likely diagnosis. Microscopic colitis is the underlying cause in 10% to 15% of patients with chronic, watery diarrhea. In contrast to inflammatory bowel disease, microscopic colitis is more common in older persons and does not cause endoscopically visible inflammation. The symptoms of microscopic colitis are similar to other chronic causes of nonbloody diarrhea, such as celiac disease and irritable bowel syndrome; therefore, colonic mucosal biopsies are required for diagnosis. Lymphocytic and collagenous colitis are the two subtypes of microscopic colitis, and they are distinguishable only by histology. Random biopsies from multiple colonic segments are recommended to establish the diagnosis because the disease can be patchy. In some patients, certain medications (such as NSAIDs and proton pump inhibitors) have been implicated as causative agents. Microscopic colitis is associated with other autoimmune diseases such as diabetes mellitus and psoriasis. The association with celiac disease is of particular clinical importance because the symptoms of these conditions are similar. Therefore, in patients with celiac disease or microscopic colitis whose symptoms do not respond to appropriate therapy, the other condition must be ruled out.

Giardia lamblia is a common infectious cause of persistent diarrhea in immunocompetent patients in developed countries and should be considered in patients with exposure to young children or potentially contaminated water, such as lakes and streams. This patient has no risk factors for *Giardia* infection.

Small intestinal bacterial overgrowth (SIBO) causes diarrhea, often with bloating, flatulence, and weight loss. Several conditions can predispose patients to SIBO due to effects on stomach acid, intestinal transit, or disruption of normal antibacterial defense mechanisms. Gastric bypass surgery is an increasingly common cause of SIBO. The absence of malabsorption symptoms and weight loss make this diagnosis unlikely.

Ulcerative colitis typically presents with bloody diarrhea and abdominal discomfort, the severity of which is related to the extent and severity of inflammation. Because ulcerative colitis typically involves the rectum, patients with this condition commonly present with tenesmus, urgency, rectal pain, and fecal incontinence. Some patients with distal inflammation can present with constipation owing to rectal spasm and stasis of stool. Fever and weight loss suggest severe disease. The patient's symptoms are not typical for ulcerative colitis.

KEY POINT

- Microscopic colitis is a cause of nonbloody, watery diarrhea in older adults and is diagnosed by colonoscopy with random biopsies from multiple colonic segments.

Bibliography
Pardi DS. Diagnosis and management of microscopic colitis. Am J Gastroenterol. 2017;112:78-85. [PMID: 27897155] doi:10.1038/ajg.2016.477

Item 16   Answer: D

Educational Objective: Treat autoimmune pancreatitis.

Prednisone is the most appropriate treatment for this patient. Based on his typical symptom of painless jaundice and the characteristic "sausage-shaped" pancreas on imaging, the patient has type 1 autoimmune pancreatitis, a frequent manifestation of IgG4 disease. He also has associated IgG4-related conditions, sialadenitis, and probable retroperitoneal fibrosis. Autoimmune pancreatitis is rare and has an unclear pathogenesis. Type 1 autoimmune pancreatitis is a systemic fibroinflammatory disease, defined as an inflammatory condition causing tissue damage and scarring. Pancreatic involvement is only one manifestation of IgG4 disease, which is characterized by abundant IgG4-producing plasma cells seen on tissue biopsy. Most IgG4-related conditions are characterized by plasma-cell infiltration of the affected tissue and the clinical consequences that infiltration entails. Almost any organ can be involved; lymph nodes are frequently affected. The initial treatment is oral prednisone with a taper over 2 to 3 months, and symptoms usually resolve within 2 to 4 weeks with treatment. Almost all patients (>90%) enter clinical remission in response to glucocorticoids. Treatment response may be limited by the amount of fibrosis present before initiation of therapy. The relapse rate is approximately 30% in type 1 autoimmune pancreatitis.

Azathioprine is an immunosuppressive drug that has been used to treat relapsing IgG4-related disease and can be used as a glucocorticoid-sparing agent. It may take 6 to 8 weeks to reach a therapeutic drug level and provoke a clinical response. Therefore, it is not considered initial first-line therapy for symptomatic IgG4-related disease.

Endoscopic retrograde cholangiopancreatography with bile-duct stenting is usually not required in patients with autoimmune pancreatitis because most patients' symptoms respond quickly to oral prednisone. Glucocorticoid therapy also treats the underlying immunologic disorder, making it the preferred first-line treatment.

Pancreaticoduodenectomy (Whipple surgery) is not indicated in patients with autoimmune pancreatitis. It may be considered to treat pancreatic adenocarcinoma occurring in the head of the pancreas, which can be mistaken for autoimmune pancreatitis. Because this patient's histology findings confirm IgG4-related disease, a trial of immunosuppressive therapy is the most appropriate treatment.

Answers and Critiques

KEY POINT

- Almost all patients (>90%) with autoimmune pancreatitis enter clinical remission in response to glucocorticoids.

Bibliography

Okazaki K, Uchida K. Autoimmune pancreatitis: the past, present, and future. Pancreas. 2015;44:1006-16. [PMID: 26355544] doi:10.1097/MPA.0000000000000382

Item 17   Answer: B

Educational Objective: Treat acute fatty liver of pregnancy with immediate delivery of the fetus.

Immediate delivery of the fetus is the most appropriate next step in management. This patient has findings of acute fatty liver of pregnancy, which is a rare but serious condition occurring most commonly in the third trimester. Women with this condition typically present with a 1- to 2-week history of nausea and vomiting, right-upper-quadrant or epigastric pain, headache, jaundice, anorexia, and/or polyuria and polydipsia (due to associated transient diabetes insipidus). Maternal and neonatal mortality rates are high in this setting. This patient's presentation with coagulopathy, hypoglycemia, and somnolence consistent with hepatic encephalopathy are indications of acute liver failure, which can result from acute fatty liver of pregnancy. Immediate delivery of the fetus is indicated to prevent fetal mortality and to reverse the mother's liver failure and improve her condition. Prompt delivery typically results in improvement of the mother's medical condition within 48 to 72 hours. Acute fatty liver of pregnancy can reoccur in subsequent pregnancies. It is also associated with long-chain 3-hydroxyacyl CoA dehydrogenase deficiency, and affected women and their children should be screened for this deficiency. HELLP (Hemolysis, Elevated Liver enzymes, and Low Platelets) syndrome can also occur in the third trimester of pregnancy. It has similarly life-threatening consequences and also requires emergent delivery of the fetus to resolve the condition. HELLP syndrome can present similarly to acute fatty liver of pregnancy in that manifestations of liver failure are present.

This patient's ultrasound showed no dilation of bile ducts, and no stones were seen in the common bile duct; therefore, endoscopic retrograde cholangiopancreatography is not indicated.

This patient's drowsiness is due to impending liver failure. Lactulose, which is used for treatment of hepatic encephalopathy in patients with chronic liver disease, is not indicated for patients with acute liver failure because it may exacerbate symptoms of ileus, and there is no evidence of benefit in the acute setting. Any symptoms referable to hepatic encephalopathy will resolve with delivery of the fetus, which resolves acute fatty liver of pregnancy.

Intrahepatic cholestasis of pregnancy occurs during the second or third trimester and resolves after delivery. The most common laboratory findings are elevated bilirubin and alkaline phosphatase levels. The condition is believed to result from sex hormone–induced inhibition of bile salt export from hepatocytes. It is treated with ursodeoxycholic acid, which can result in alleviation of symptoms. Although the maternal effects of intrahepatic cholestasis of pregnancy are mild, it can cause fetal distress and premature labor. Because this patient's clinical profile is not compatible with intrahepatic cholestasis of pregnancy, ursodeoxycholic acid therapy is not indicated.

KEY POINT

- The fetus should be delivered immediately upon recognition of acute fatty liver of pregnancy.

Bibliography

Bacak SJ, Thornburg LL. Liver failure in pregnancy. Crit Care Clin. 2016;32:61-72. [PMID: 26600444] doi:10.1016/j.ccc.2015.08.005

Item 18   Answer: A

Educational Objective: Treat a gallbladder polyp.

Cholecystectomy is indicated for this patient with a gallbladder polyp and gallstones because of the increased risk for gallbladder cancer when the two conditions coexist. The finding of a gallbladder polyp larger than 1 cm in size is an indication for cholecystectomy, even if the patient is asymptomatic. An additional indication for prophylactic cholecystectomy is the presence of a gallbladder polyp larger than 8 mm in size in the setting of primary sclerosing cholangitis. Gallbladder polyps are found on approximately 5% of ultrasounds. Although only a small percentage of gallbladder polyps are neoplastic (adenoma or adenocarcinoma), the risk for neoplasia increases as polyp size increases.

Further evaluation of the polyp with abdominal CT, endoscopic retrograde cholangiopancreatography, or MR cholangiopancreatography is not indicated because gallbladder ultrasonography is adequately sensitive for the detection of gallbladder lesions. These tests could be considered if this patient had symptoms or elevated liver chemistry tests suggesting bile-duct obstruction or malignancy.

In a patient with an 8-mm gallbladder polyp in the absence of gallstones or primary sclerosing cholangitis, repeat ultrasonography in 6 months would be indicated. However, follow-up ultrasonography is not appropriate for this patient with a gallbladder polyp and gallstones, which increase the risk for gallbladder cancer.

Bile acids, such as ursodeoxycholic acid, work by reducing biliary cholesterol secretion, thereby increasing biliary bile-acid concentrations and, as a result, reducing the cholesterol saturation index and gallstone size. Bile-acid therapy works best for small, primarily cholesterol gallstones and is indicated in patients who cannot or will not undergo laparoscopic cholecystectomy. More importantly, ursodeoxycholic acid therapy would not address this patient's gallbladder polyp.

Answers and Critiques

KEY POINT

- The finding of a gallbladder polyp larger than 1 cm in size, or a polyp of any size associated with gallstones, is an indication for cholecystectomy even if the patient is asymptomatic.

Bibliography

Gallahan WC, Conway JD. Diagnosis and management of gallbladder polyps. Gastroenterol Clin North Am. 2010;39:359-67, x. [PMID: 20478491] doi:10.1016/j.gtc.2010.02.001

Item 19   Answer: C

Educational Objective: Evaluate for *Helicobacter pylori* eradication following treatment.

A urea breath test is the most appropriate next test for this patient. Testing to confirm eradication should be pursued in all cases of identified and treated *Helicobacter pylori* infection because of the established risks for peptic ulcer disease and gastric malignancy in patients with chronic *H. pylori* infection. To maximize the accuracy of testing to confirm eradication, testing should be performed a minimum of 4 weeks after completion of *H. pylori* eradication therapy and after proton pump inhibitor therapy has been discontinued for 1 to 2 weeks and H_2-blockers for 1 to 2 days. The test chosen should be highly accurate in identifying active infection; appropriate tests include the urea breath test, fecal antigen test, or biopsy-based testing. The urea breath test is limited by need for specialized equipment and personnel and by its cost. The fecal antigen test is limited by the collection of stool but is less expensive than the urea breath test. Biopsy-based testing is expensive and invasive. Unless upper endoscopy is indicated for other reasons, noninvasive testing modalities (the urea breath test or the fecal antigen test) are more appropriate for confirmation of eradication or assessment for reinfection. Both testing modalities are equivalent with regard to accuracy; therefore, the specific test chosen should be based on patient preference and/or test availability.

Serologic antibody testing is an inaccurate means of testing to confirm eradication because antibodies can remain present despite successful eradication of active infection; therefore, serologic testing cannot distinguish between past and current *H. pylori* infection.

Invasive (endoscopic) tests for *H. pylori* include the rapid urease test, histology, and culture; all invasive testing modalities identify active infection. Due to its expense and invasive nature, biopsy-based testing should be reserved for patients requiring a repeat upper endoscopy for other reasons (for example, follow-up endoscopy for high-risk gastric ulcer). In this patient with no indications for repeat upper endoscopy, one of the two noninvasive tests, either the urea breath test or fecal antigen test, is preferable.

KEY POINT

- After eradication therapy for *Helicobacter pylori* infection, eradication should be confirmed using the urea breath test or fecal antigen test.

Bibliography

Lopes AI, Vale FF, Oleastro M. *Helicobacter pylori* infection–recent developments in diagnosis. World J Gastroenterol. 2014;20:9299-313. [PMID: 25071324] doi:10.3748/wjg.v20.i28.9299

Item 20   Answer: B

Educational Objective: Treat gallstone pancreatitis with prompt cholecystectomy.

Laparoscopic cholecystectomy before discharge from the hospital is the most appropriate treatment. Gallstone acute pancreatitis can be diagnosed based on elevated liver transaminases on presentation, a lipase level elevated to more than three times the upper limit of normal, characteristic severe abdominal pain, and ultrasonographic evidence of cholelithiasis. This patient showed clinical improvement within 3 days of hospitalization. Her laboratory values have normalized, suggesting spontaneous passage of a gallstone through the common bile duct, which occurs in most patients with gallstone pancreatitis. In a multicenter randomized controlled trial, same-admission cholecystectomy reduced rates of gallstone-related complications compared with interval cholecystectomy 25 to 30 days after hospital discharge for patients with mild gallstone pancreatitis.

Endoscopic retrograde cholangiopancreatography (ERCP) is indicated within the first 24 hours for patients with acute pancreatitis and ascending cholangitis (fever, abdominal pain, and jaundice) due to choledocholithiasis. If there is evidence of ongoing biliary obstruction in patients hospitalized with acute pancreatitis, ERCP may be indicated to remove a retained gallstone from the common bile duct. This patient's symptoms and laboratory abnormalities resolved quickly, which supports the spontaneous passage of a gallstone without evidence of ongoing biliary obstruction.

MR cholangiopancreatography (MRCP) can be used to identify causes of biliary obstruction. MRCP is not needed in this patient because she has normal-caliber bile ducts on abdominal ultrasonography and normal liver chemistry test results, indicating that a biliary obstruction is unlikely.

Ursodeoxycholic acid has been used to medically dissolve small cholesterol gallstones in patients who are not candidates for surgery. The medication works slowly and may take longer than 1 year to dissolve small stones, leaving patients at risk for recurrent attacks of gallstone pancreatitis or other gallstone-related complications. This patient is young and without comorbidities, making surgery a more appropriate treatment.

KEY POINT

- Same-admission cholecystectomy reduces rates of gallstone-related complications compared with cholecystectomy after hospital discharge for patients with mild gallstone pancreatitis.

Bibliography

da Costa DW, Bouwense SA, Schepers NJ, Besselink MG, van Santvoort HC, van Brunschot S, et al; Dutch Pancreatitis Study Group. Same-admission versus interval cholecystectomy for mild gallstone pancreatitis (PONCHO): a multicentre randomised controlled trial. Lancet. 2015;386:1261-8. [PMID: 26460661] doi:10.1016/S0140-6736(15)00274-3

Item 21   Answer: B

Educational Objective: Treat cholangitis using endoscopic retrograde cholangiopancreatography.

Endoscopic retrograde cholangiopancreatography (ERCP) is the most appropriate next test for this patient. This patient with primary sclerosing cholangitis (PSC) presents with fever, rigors, right-upper-quadrant pain, and leukocytosis, all of which are consistent with bacterial cholangitis. Indications for ERCP in patients with PSC are bacterial cholangitis (as in this patient), increasing jaundice, increasing pruritus, or a dominant stricture seen on imaging. Symptoms of bacterial cholangitis, increasing jaundice, and pruritus can signify strictures that may improve with dilation or stenting, or, alternatively, removing sludge or stone debris in the bile ducts via ERCP. A dominant stricture in a patient with PSC must be evaluated for cholangiocarcinoma by obtaining biliary brushings for cytologic examination, and, if available, fluorescent in situ hybridization to evaluate chromosomal abnormalities.

The CA 19-9 level will be elevated in the setting of bacterial cholangitis. The risk for false-positive results makes CA 19-9 measurement inappropriate in this context. CA 19-9 levels can be used as an adjunctive tool in the diagnosis of cholangiocarcinoma, but the diagnosis cannot be made based only on this marker.

IgG4 levels should be checked in patients with a new diagnosis of presumed PSC because IgG4 cholangitis is a steroid-responsive condition, whereas PSC is not. Testing for IgG4 does not assist in the management of this patient's cholangitis.

A percutaneous transhepatic biliary tube can be employed when ERCP is unsuccessful at traversing a biliary stricture, but because of its invasiveness and inconvenience, it would not be a first-line tool for assessing and treating a patient with bacterial cholangitis.

The role of PET in the evaluation and management of cholangiocarcinoma is evolving. However, this is not the test of choice in a patient with bacterial cholangitis because it does not allow for biliary intervention. Furthermore, PET scans can be associated with false-positive results for malignancy in the setting of bacterial cholangitis, and also with false-negative results due to the desmoplastic reaction of cholangiocarcinoma tumors.

KEY POINT

- Indications for endoscopic retrograde cholangiopancreatography in patients with primary sclerosing cholangitis are bacterial cholangitis, increasing jaundice, increasing pruritus, or a dominant stricture on imaging.

Bibliography

Lindor KD, Kowdley KV, Harrison ME; American College of Gastroenterology. ACG clinical guideline: primary sclerosing cholangitis. Am J Gastroenterol. 2015;110:646-59; quiz 660. [PMID: 25869391] doi:10.1038/ajg.2015.112

Item 22   Answer: B

Educational Objective: Evaluate rectal bleeding in a young patient.

Colonoscopy is the most appropriate next step in management for this patient. Her symptoms of weight loss, abdominal pain, and rectal bleeding with iron deficiency anemia warrant further evaluation with colonoscopy. Inflammatory bowel disease is a possibility in this patient; however, colon cancer also needs to be excluded. In the United States, the overall incidence of colon cancer has decreased by 3% to 4% since the early 2000s; however, in adults younger than age 50 years, the incidence of colorectal cancer is increasing at a rate of 2.1% per year.

Anoscopy enables a limited examination and would not assist in evaluating the patient's iron deficiency anemia and weight loss.

Flexible sigmoidoscopy allows examination of only the lower third of the colon, and if negative, a full colonoscopy would still be required. There has been a gradual shift from left-sided to right-sided colon cancers. A number of factors have been suggested to explain this, including inadequate colon preparation, incomplete colonoscopy, and difficulty recognizing serrated polyps that are typically flat and occur more often on the right side. However, there also appears to be a true increase in tumors of the proximal and right colon that may be missed if only a sigmoidoscopy is performed.

Hemorrhoids are arteriovenous communications covered by cushions of connective tissue in the anal canal. Internal hemorrhoids cause most hemorrhoidal symptoms (bright red blood dripping in the toilet bowl or seen on toilet paper, with no accompanying pain; a protrusion of tissue; itching; and pain). Patients with alarm features (such as unexplained weight loss, change in bowel movements, iron deficiency anemia, age older than 50 years, or personal or family history of colorectal cancer or inflammatory bowel disease) warrant colonoscopy. Initial treatment of internal and external hemorrhoids consists of dietary and lifestyle modifications to soften bowel movements and avoid constipation, straining, and prolonged time on the toilet. Increased fiber intake has been shown to reduce symptomatic prolapse and bleeding. Local therapy such as topical anesthetics and glucocorticoids may relieve pain and itching, but data to support their use are scant.

KEY POINT

- Red-flag symptoms such as rectal bleeding with iron deficiency anemia, abdominal pain, and weight loss should prompt evaluation by colonoscopy for colorectal cancer regardless of the patient's age or the presence of bleeding hemorrhoids.

Bibliography

Inra JA, Syngal S. Colorectal cancer in young adults. Dig Dis Sci. 2015;60:722-33. [PMID: 25480403] doi:10.1007/s10620-014-3464-0

Item 23   Answer: D

Educational Objective: Diagnose narcotic bowel syndrome.

Narcotic bowel syndrome is the most likely diagnosis in this patient. Narcotic bowel syndrome, also known as opiate-induced gastrointestinal hyperalgesia, is a centrally mediated disorder of gastrointestinal pain characterized by a paradoxical increase in abdominal pain with increasing doses of narcotics. Many patients are prescribed opioid pain medication for an unrelated medical condition but have increasing pain over time despite clinical evidence of improvement or resolution of the initial condition. Patients often fear tapering off opioids and believe the opioids are the only treatment that alleviates their pain.

Chronic pancreatitis may result from a severe episode of acute pancreatitis or recurrent episodes of acute pancreatitis. It may require opioid pain medication for flares of pain or for constant, daily pain, but the pain is usually relieved with opioids. This patient only had one episode of uncomplicated pancreatitis and has no other risk factors for chronic pancreatitis and no evidence of chronic pancreatitis (pancreatic calcifications) on abdominal imaging.

Distal intestinal obstruction syndrome is caused by thickened intestinal contents that completely or partially block the small intestinal lumen in patients with cystic fibrosis. It is characterized by progressive, crampy abdominal pain in the right lower quadrant, sometimes progressing to vomiting. This patient has no history of cystic fibrosis and no symptoms of a small-bowel obstruction making this an unlikely diagnosis.

The diagnosis of irritable bowel syndrome is typically made in the presence of recurrent abdominal pain or discomfort at least 3 days per month in the last 3 months that is associated with two or more of the following: relief with defecation, onset associated with a change in frequency of stool, or onset associated with a change in form (appearance) of stool. While this patient has abdominal pain and constipation, her symptoms are worsened with eating, not relieved with defecation, and the onset of pain is clearly tied to an acute abdominal diagnosis and treatment with an opioid, making IBS an unlikely diagnosis.

KEY POINT

- Narcotic bowel syndrome, also known as opiate-induced gastrointestinal hyperalgesia, is a centrally mediated disorder of gastrointestinal pain characterized by a paradoxical increase in abdominal pain with increasing doses of opioids.

Bibliography

Keefer L, Drossman DA, Guthrie E, Simrén M, Tillisch K, Olden K, et al. Centrally mediated disorders of gastrointestinal pain. Gastroenterology. 2016. [PMID: 27144628] doi:10.1053/j.gastro.2016.02.034

Item 24   Answer: B

Educational Objective: Treat pain in chronic pancreatitis.

The most appropriate initial treatment is the use of NSAIDs, a low-fat diet, and smoking cessation. The hallmark symptom of chronic pancreatitis is abdominal pain that often radiates to the back; however, pain can be absent. Pain is typically intermittent, with attacks interrupted by varying pain-free intervals. Constant pain may occur from local anatomic causes (compressing pseudocyst, biliary or pancreatic duct stricture) or from visceral hyperalgesia (increased sensation in response to stimuli) from chronic narcotic use and centralization of pain. Management focuses on reducing pain and detecting and treating complications. Unfortunately, the treatment of persistent pain is difficult, and the evidence supporting most treatment modalities is of low quality and often contradictory. Most authorities recommend that persistent pain be treated in a stepwise approach beginning with lifestyle modification (discontinue alcohol and cigarettes), use of simple analgesics, adding low-dose tricyclic antidepressants, and gabapentinoids (gabapentin and pregabalin). Smoking has been identified as an important and independent risk factor for chronic pancreatitis, and cessation of smoking and alcohol use is recommended to prevent recurrent attacks of pancreatitis. An important goal is to control pain with opioid-sparing adjunctive agents to minimize chronic opioid use, owing to concerns for opioid dependence and gastrointestinal side effects. This would especially be true in a patient with a history of opioid or other substance abuse, such as this patient.

Nerve blocks, such as celiac plexus blocks, and neurolysis procedures are not recommended for the management of pain related to chronic pancreatitis because the response rate is low (15%), and pain relief, if achieved at all, is short-lived.

Opioid pain medications, such as oxycodone, are used in acute pancreatitis and during acute flares of chronic pancreatitis, but they should be avoided in the long-term management of ongoing pain due to the risk for hyperesthesia and the development of tolerance and/or addiction.

Pancreatic enzyme replacement therapy is often recommended for the treatment of persistent pain associated with chronic pancreatitis. A large systematic review found conflicting evidence for the efficacy of pancreatic enzymes in relieving pain in patients with chronic pancreatitis but found that they may improve fat absorption. If used, acid suppression therapy with a proton pump inhibitor should be given as an adjunct to uncoated pancreatic enzymes in order to reduce the inactivation of enzymes by gastric acid. Simple analgesics and lifestyle modifications can be effective for some patients and should be initiated first.

KEY POINT

- Treatment of chronic pancreatitis-related persistent pain should proceed in a stepwise approach beginning with lifestyle modifications (discontinue alcohol and cigarettes) and the use of simple analgesics (acetaminophen, NSAIDs).

Bibliography

Majumder S, Chari ST. Chronic pancreatitis. Lancet. 2016;387:1957-66. [PMID: 26948434] doi:10.1016/S0140-6736(16)00097-0

Item 25   Answer: A

Educational Objective: Treat hepatitis B virus–related polyarteritis nodosa.

The most appropriate treatment is entecavir. Hepatitis B virus (HBV)–related polyarteritis nodosa (PAN) is the most likely diagnosis in this patient. The patient has fever, arthralgia, and evidence of cutaneous vasculitis (rash). There is also evidence of hepatitis (elevated bilirubin and aminotransferase levels) likely related to his use of intravenous drugs. Testing for hepatitis B surface antigen and hepatitis B e antigen is positive, as is IgM antibody to hepatitis B core antigen, with a significant HBV DNA viral load; all of these results are consistent with a recent HBV infection. PAN and mixed cryoglobulinemia are rare HBV-associated vasculitides. This patient has undetectable serum cryoglobulins, excluding the diagnosis of mixed cryoglobulinemia. There are no data from randomized trials to guide therapy in patients with HBV-related PAN. Patients with HBV infection and mild manifestations of PAN are usually treated with antiviral agents such as entecavir. Patients (such as this one) with mild PAN have constitutional symptoms, arthritis or arthralgia, anemia, and skin lesions. More severe disease is characterized by organ dysfunction (for example, myocarditis, kidney insufficiency and hypertension, mononeuritis multiplex) or life-threatening systemic manifestations. Patients with severe manifestations of PAN are often treated with an antiviral agent and a short course of prednisone and plasma exchange.

Prednisone and cyclophosphamide are agents typically used to treat mild and severe manifestations of idiopathic PAN, the most commonly recognized form of PAN. Because this patient has HBV-related PAN, treating the causative viral infection with an antiviral agent is the preferred management.

Sofosbuvir and ledipasvir are direct-acting antiviral agents used to treat hepatitis C virus (HCV) infection and would be an appropriate choice for mild HCV-related PAN. However, this patient's hepatitis C antibody is negative and these agents are not indicated.

Tenofovir, emtricitabine, and raltegravir are used to treat HIV infection. This drug combination would be an appropriate choice for HIV-related PAN, but the patient's HIV test is negative and these agents are not indicated. Tenofovir alone would be a reasonable treatment for this patient.

KEY POINT

- Mild hepatitis B virus–related polyarteritis nodosa is treated with antiviral agents.

Bibliography

Forbess L, Bannykh S. Polyarteritis nodosa. Rheum Dis Clin North Am. 2015;41:33-46, vii. [PMID: 25399938] doi:10.1016/j.rdc.2014.09.005

Item 26   Answer: A

Educational Objective: Treat acute necrotic pancreatitis with enteral feeding.

Placement of a nasoenteric tube for enteral feeding is the most appropriate next step in this patient's management. The patient has taken nothing by mouth (NPO) since hospitalization 4 days earlier and requires nutritional support. She continues to have abdominal pain requiring intravenous opioid pain medication, as well as nausea and no appetite. Enteral nutrition is preferred in patients with acute pancreatitis because of the benefit of maintaining a healthy mucosal barrier in the gut to prevent translocation of bacteria. Both nasogastric and nasojejunal enteral feeding are safe and have comparable effectiveness. Studies show nasogastric tube feeding is well tolerated in these patients, and placement of a nasogastric tube may be easier, more cost effective, and faster than placement of a nasojejunal tube.

Total parenteral nutrition (TPN) is discouraged in patients with acute pancreatitis because the mucosal barrier is not maintained when patients are NPO for prolonged periods, which may lead to higher rates of bacterial translocation into necrotic pancreatic tissue. TPN also increases the risk for bacterial and fungal bloodstream infections, as well as venous thrombosis associated with more proximal indwelling intravenous catheters required for TPN administration.

Cholecystectomy will not be an option for this patient in the near future (likely not during this hospitalization) because she has severe necrotic acute pancreatitis. Maintaining NPO status for a prolonged period of time before surgery is not appropriate clinical management of her nutritional needs.

There are no data to support withholding feeding in patients with acute pancreatitis based on enzyme levels. Lipase levels three to five times the upper level of normal are used as diagnostic criteria for acute pancreatitis but have no impact on clinical management decisions.

KEY POINT

- Enteral nutrition is preferred in patients with acute pancreatitis because of the benefit of maintaining a healthy gut mucosal barrier to prevent translocation of bacteria.

Bibliography

Forsmark CE, Vege SS, Wilcox CM. Acute pancreatitis. N Engl J Med. 2016;375:1972-1981. [PMID: 27959604]

Item 27   Answer: C

Educational Objective: Prevent spontaneous bacterial peritonitis.

Initiation of indefinite primary prophylaxis with ciprofloxacin is the most appropriate next step in the management of this patient with ascites. Patients with ascites are at risk for developing spontaneous bacterial peritonitis (SBP), a common infection in patients with cirrhosis. SBP has a mortality

CONT.

rate of 20%. Long-term primary antibiotic prophylaxis may reduce mortality in patients at high risk for SBP. Criteria for patients at high risk include an ascitic-fluid total protein level less than 1.5 g/dL (15 g/L) in conjunction with any of the following: serum sodium level less than or equal to 130 mEq/L (130 mmol/L), serum creatinine level greater than or equal to 1.2 mg/dL (106.1 µmol/L), blood urea nitrogen level greater than or equal to 25 mg/dL (8.9 mmol/L), serum bilirubin level greater than or equal to 3 mg/dL (51.3 µmol/L), or Child-Turcotte-Pugh class B or C cirrhosis. Patients who have had a bout of SBP should also receive lifelong antibiotic prophylaxis to reduce the risk for recurrence. In the setting of variceal hemorrhage, a limited 7-day course of antibiotics initiated at the time of bleeding is indicated to prevent infectious complications from intestinal bacterial translocation.

Increasing this patient's propranolol is not indicated because, although β-blocker therapy can reduce the risk for variceal bleeding, the patient already has a pulse rate of less than 60/min. Nonselective β-blockers such as propranolol may be associated with higher transplant-free survival in patients with cirrhosis overall but may decrease transplant-free survival in the first 6 months after SBP or in patients with refractory ascites, and discontinuation should be considered at that time.

Albumin infusion may decrease the frequency of hepatorenal syndrome and improves survival in patients with SBP, but its role in primary prevention of SBP is undefined and its use for primary prevention not recommended.

Systemic blood pressure decreases in patients with decompensated cirrhosis resulting in reductions in renal perfusion and glomerular filtration rate. This leads to elevated levels of vasopressin, angiotensin, and aldosterone. ACE inhibitors, such as lisinopril, and angiotensin receptor blockers impair these compensatory efforts to maintain blood pressure and can worsen kidney perfusion in the setting of ascites due to portal hypertension; therefore, initiating lisinopril is inappropriate in this patient.

KEY POINT

- Primary prophylactic antibiotic therapy is indicated for patients at high risk for the development of spontaneous bacterial peritonitis, including patients with very low ascitic-fluid protein levels and those with advanced liver failure.

Bibliography

Solà E, Solé C, Ginès P. Management of uninfected and infected ascites in cirrhosis. Liver Int. 2016;36 Suppl 1:109-15. [PMID: 26725907] doi:10.1111/liv.13015

Item 28   Answer: A

Educational Objective: Diagnose dumping syndrome after gastrojejunostomy.

Dumping syndrome is the most likely diagnosis in this patient. Rapid gastric emptying of hyperosmolar chyme

into the small intestine after partial gastric resection can lead to postprandial vasomotor symptoms known as dumping syndrome. This patient had a gastrojejunostomy 1 year earlier, and her symptoms started after the surgery. Common early symptoms of dumping symptoms are palpitations, tachycardia, diaphoresis, and lightheadedness with abdominal pain and diarrhea presenting within 30 minutes of eating. Late symptoms can occur 1 to 3 hours after eating in 25% of patients and include sweating, tremor, hunger, and difficulty with concentration and cognition (hypoglycemia). A minority of patients have both early and late symptoms. The diagnosis is usually made based on clinical findings. Initial treatment for dumping syndrome is dietary: eating small frequent meals and saving liquids until after a meal, which this patient has already found to help her symptoms.

Dumping syndrome is misdiagnosed as gastroparesis in up to 37% of patients. Gastroparesis involves delayed gastric emptying and is typically associated with nausea and vomiting after eating. The prominent vasomotor symptoms this patient describes are uncommon in gastroparesis.

Irritable bowel syndrome is more common in younger patients, and rarely causes weight loss. Symptoms that occur after a gastrointestinal surgery should suggest an alternative diagnosis.

Small intestinal bacterial overgrowth (SIBO) is an excess number and alteration in type of bacteria cultured from the small intestine. Digestive enzymes and intestinal motility normally limit the growth of excessive bacteria, but SIBO can occur in conditions in which these functions are disrupted, including gastrojejunostomy, which creates a blind loop of small intestine. Clinical features of SIBO are diarrhea, bloating, and weight loss. Patients may have a combination of fat, protein, or carbohydrate malabsorption. Unlike in dumping syndrome, symptoms are not immediately related to eating and are not associated with prominent vasomotor symptoms such as palpitations, tachycardia, diaphoresis, and lightheadedness.

KEY POINT

- Rapid gastric emptying of hyperosmolar chyme into the small intestine after partial gastric resection can lead to postprandial vasomotor symptoms, abdominal pain, and diarrhea, collectively known as dumping syndrome.

Bibliography

Berg P, McCallum R. Dumping syndrome: a review of the current concepts of pathophysiology, diagnosis, and treatment. Dig Dis Sci. 2016;61:11-8. [PMID: 26396002] doi:10.1007/s10620-015-3839-x

Item 29   Answer: B

Educational Objective: Treat chronic idiopathic constipation unresponsive to first-line treatment.

Linaclotide is the most appropriate treatment for this patient. Linaclotide is a peripherally acting guanylate

Answers and Critiques

cyclase-C receptor agonist that is FDA approved for the treatment of chronic idiopathic constipation in adults. Linaclotide increases intracellular and extracellular cyclic guanosine monophosphate, which results in chloride and bicarbonate secretion into intestinal lumen, increasing intestinal fluid content and accelerated transit time. Its superiority to placebo in the treatment of constipation was demonstrated in two 12-week, high-quality randomized controlled trials. Diarrhea occurred in 16% of patients receiving linaclotide (compared to 4.7% in those receiving placebo) in the 12-week clinical trials. The potential for diarrhea can be minimized by taking linaclotide on an empty stomach, ideally 30 minutes before the first meal of the day. Plecanatide is the second guanylate cyclase-C receptor agonist to receive FDA approval for the treatment of chronic idiopathic constipation. Diarrhea was also the most commonly reported side effect of plecanatide therapy in the 12-week clinical trials (5% versus 1% in the placebo group). Lubiprostone, a chloride channel agonist, is a third agent with FDA approval for the treatment of chronic idiopathic constipation. The most common side effects reported in clinical trials were nausea, reported by 29% of patients taking lubiprostone, and diarrhea, reported by 12%. The efficacy and safety of linaclotide, plecanatide, and lubiprostone have not been established in patients aged younger than 18 years nor in pregnant patients. Because of cost effectiveness, over-the-counter laxatives, such as fiber supplements, polyethylene glycol, and bisacodyl, should be pursued first in patients with constipation, but they were ineffective in this patient.

Osmotic laxatives include magnesium hydroxide, lactulose, sorbitol, and polyethylene glycol (PEG); clinical trials have demonstrated the superiority and safety of PEG. The patient tried over-the-counter PEG, and it was poorly tolerated due to bloating. Substituting another, less effective, osmotic agent (for example, lactulose) will lead to similar adverse effects without relieving constipation.

Methylnaltrexone, an injectable peripheral opioid antagonist that does not cross the blood-brain barrier, is very effective in treating opioid-induced constipation without adversely affecting analgesia. Bowel obstruction is an absolute contraindication to methylnaltrexone. Because this patient does not have opioid-induced constipation, methylnaltrexone is an inappropriate choice.

Rifaximin is a nonabsorbable antibiotic used in the treatment of irritable bowel syndrome predominated by diarrhea, hepatic encephalopathy, and travelers' diarrhea. It has no proven efficacy in chronic idiopathic constipation and is therefore not indicated in this patient.

KEY POINT

- Linaclotide is a peripherally acting guanylate cyclase-C receptor agonist that is FDA approved for the treatment of chronic idiopathic constipation in adults with symptoms refractory to first-line therapies.

Bibliography

Lembo AJ, Schneier HA, Shiff SJ, Kurtz CB, MacDougall JE, Jia XD, et al. Two randomized trials of linaclotide for chronic constipation. N Engl J Med. 2011;365:527-36. [PMID: 21830967] doi:10.1056/NEJMoa1010863

Item 30   Answer: D

Educational Objective: Prevent vertical transmission of hepatitis B viral infection.

Tenofovir is the most appropriate next step in management of this patient, with the goal of preventing vertical transmission of hepatitis B virus (HBV) infection from mother to child during the course of delivery. Guidelines recommend treatment with lamivudine, telbivudine, or tenofovir for the prevention of vertical transmission in pregnant women who have HBV DNA levels greater than 200,000 IU/mL at 24 to 28 weeks' gestation. There are no head-to-head data comparing these regimens, but tenofovir is preferred over telbivudine and lamivudine due to lower rates of resistance. Tenofovir and telbivudine are the only FDA pregnancy category B agents. Lamivudine and other oral drugs used to treat HBV are category C agents, though there are reasonable data on the safety of lamivudine use in pregnancy in the HIV population. Only a few patients will become hepatitis B surface antigen–negative with treatment; therefore, cure of HBV infection is an unrealistic goal for most chronically infected patients.

There are no data suggesting that cesarean delivery is effective at preventing vertical transmission of HBV. All babies born to mothers with chronic HBV infection should receive active HBV vaccination and passive immunization (HBV immune globulin). The risk for developing chronic HBV infection is high (90%) in newborns who acquire HBV.

Because the patient's HBV DNA level is high enough (>200,000 IU/mL) to warrant treatment to prevent vertical transmission of HBV, measuring her HBV DNA level again in 3 months would not be appropriate without first instituting treatment.

Pegylated interferon is not considered safe in pregnancy and, therefore, would be an inappropriate choice for this patient. Pegylated interferon can be used to treat HBV infection in patients with high alanine aminotransferase levels, low HBV DNA levels, and without cirrhosis. Candidates for interferon have a desire for finite therapy, do not have cirrhosis, are not pregnant, and do not have significant psychiatric disease, cardiac disease, seizure disorder, cytopenia, or autoimmune disease.

KEY POINT

- Pregnant women who have hepatitis B virus DNA levels greater than 200,000 IU/mL at 24 to 28 weeks' gestation should be treated with tenofovir to prevent vertical transmission during delivery.

Bibliography

Terrault NA, Bzowej NH, Chang KM, Hwang JP, Jonas MM, Murad MH; American Association for the Study of Liver Diseases. AASLD guidelines for treatment of chronic hepatitis B. Hepatology. 2016;63:261-83. [PMID: 26566064] doi:10.1002/hep.28156

Answers and Critiques

Item 31   Answer: A

Educational Objective: Diagnose pancreatic cancer.

Contrast-enhanced CT of the abdomen is the most appropriate next step in this patient's management. Pancreatic neoplasm must be considered as a cause of acute pancreatitis in patients older than age 40 years when no other cause has been identified and/or when worrisome features such as weight loss or new onset of diabetes mellitus are present. This patient had no identifiable cause and has worrisome features of decreased appetite, back pain, and weight loss. Contrast-enhanced multidetector CT has a 90% sensitivity for detecting malignancy in patients in whom pancreatic cancer is suspected. CT also provides staging information.

Endoscopic retrograde cholangiopancreatography (ERCP) is not appropriate for this patient because laboratory data, abdominal ultrasound, and physical examination show no evidence of biliary obstruction. ERCP may be indicated in patients with biliary obstruction for stenting of the bile duct. This may occur in the setting of a neoplasm in the head of the pancreas.

Endoscopic ultrasound (EUS) examination resembles standard endoscopy, but the endoscope has an ultrasound transducer at the tip that emits acoustic waves to the surrounding tissues, allowing for the acquisition of real-time views of the pancreas, bile ducts, and blood vessels. In the diagnosis of pancreatic lesions, EUS is useful for the detection of small tumors that may be below the resolution of the CT scan and allows tissue diagnosis by fine-needle aspiration when required. In patients in whom pancreatic cancer is suspected, contrast-enhanced multidetector CT is the preferred initial diagnostic study.

No further testing is indicated for patients younger than age 40 years who are asymptomatic after treatment for a first case of mild acute pancreatitis in the absence of worrisome features. This patient's age, lack of an identifiable cause, and worrisome clinical features warrant further evaluation rather than continuing current management.

KEY POINT

- Pancreatic neoplasm must be considered as a cause of acute pancreatitis in patients older than age 40 years when no other cause has been identified and/or when worrisome features, such as weight loss or new onset of diabetes mellitus, are present.

Bibliography

Tenner S, Baillie J, DeWitt J, Vege SS; American College of Gastroenterology. American College of Gastroenterology guideline: management of acute pancreatitis. Am J Gastroenterol. 2013;108:1400-15; 1416. [PMID: 23896955] doi:10.1038/ajg.2013.218

Item 32   Answer: A

Educational Objective: Manage antithrombotic therapy after gastrointestinal bleeding.

This patient's warfarin therapy should be restarted now. The risk for warfarin-associated bleeding is determined by the INR, patient comorbid conditions, and duration of therapy. For patients with an INR in or slightly above the therapeutic range (up to 2.7), normalization of the INR does not reduce rebleeding risk but delays endoscopy and decreases the sensitivity of endoscopy to identify important prognostic indicators related to risk for rebleeding. There are few data to guide the clinician's decision of when to resume antithrombotic therapy after gastrointestinal bleeding. In general, once endoscopic hemostasis has been achieved, anticoagulation should be reinitiated, and in most cases, this can be done on the same day as the procedure. After temporary discontinuation of warfarin, antithrombotic therapy should be reinitiated within 7 days of initial drug discontinuation to avoid an increased risk for a thromboembolic event. Hemostasis has been achieved in this patient, with no evidence of ongoing gastrointestinal bleeding seen for 24 hours after the procedure; therefore, it is appropriate to reinitiate warfarin therapy now.

Retrospective studies have shown that resumption of warfarin therapy is associated with a decreased risk for mortality and thrombosis without a significantly increased risk for recurrent hemorrhage in patients with gastrointestinal bleeding. Waiting 10 or 30 days to resume warfarin therapy increases the risk for a thromboembolic event with no reduction in risk for recurrent gastrointestinal bleeding.

This patient's CHA_2DS_2-VASc (Congestive heart failure, Hypertension, Age ≥75 years, Diabetes mellitus, Stroke or transient ischemic attack or thromboembolism, Vascular disease, Age 65-74 years, Sex category) score is 5, predicting a nearly 7% annual risk for stroke and thromboembolism event at 1-year follow-up evaluation. This is a moderately high annual risk for thromboembolism; therefore, holding warfarin therapy indefinitely is inappropriate.

KEY POINT

- Once endoscopic hemostasis has been achieved in a patient with gastrointestinal bleeding, anticoagulation should be reinitiated, and in most cases, this can be done on the same day as the procedure.

Bibliography

Abraham NS. Management of antiplatelet agents and anticoagulants in patients with gastrointestinal bleeding. Gastrointest Endosc Clin N Am. 2015;25:449-62. [PMID: 26142031] doi:10.1016/j.giec.2015.02.002

Item 33   Answer: D

Educational Objective: Diagnose celiac disease.

Testing for anti–tissue transglutaminase (tTG) IgA antibody is the most appropriate next test for this patient, who has symptoms of celiac disease, including diarrhea, bloating, and weight loss. She is underweight due to malabsorption related to immune destruction of small intestinal villi, and she has laboratory abnormalities associated with celiac disease, including iron deficiency anemia and elevated liver transaminases. Her family history of autoimmune diseases is also consistent with celiac disease due to common genetic predisposition (*HLA-DQ2* and *DQ8*). The best initial screening test for celiac disease is anti–tTg IgA antibody testing. Given increased prevalence of IgA deficiency in celiac disease, total IgA levels should be measured in patients with high suspicion for celiac disease. If patients are IgA deficient, IgG-based antibody testing (such as deamidated gliadin peptide [DGP] IgG) should be performed. Positive antibody screening for celiac disease should prompt upper endoscopy and biopsies of the duodenum for definitive diagnosis. Treatment is a lifelong, strict gluten-free diet.

Gliadin antibodies are neither sensitive nor specific for the diagnosis of celiac disease and are no longer recommended for the evaluation of celiac disease. Newer gliadin-based serology tests, anti-DGP IgA and anti-DGP IgG, have greater sensitivity and specificity than older antigliadin antibodies. Anti-DGP IgG is particularly useful in cases of total IgA deficiency for diagnosing celiac disease.

Anti-*Saccharomyces cerevisiae* antibodies have been proposed as a serologic method for differentiating Crohn disease from ulcerative colitis, but they are neither adequately sensitive nor specific and can lead to false-positive results if used as a screening test for gastrointestinal symptoms. In addition, the absence of fever, bloody diarrhea, or abdominal pain makes the diagnosis of inflammatory bowel disease unlikely in this patient.

Anti–smooth muscle antibody testing can be helpful in the diagnosis of autoimmune hepatitis. Autoimmune hepatitis is a chronic inflammatory liver disease that is usually seen in women and can be associated with other autoimmune diseases (most commonly autoimmune thyroiditis, synovitis, or ulcerative colitis). The disease presentation ranges from asymptomatic to acute liver failure. Serum aminotransferase levels are elevated and range from mild elevations to greater than 1000 U/L. Serum IgG levels are also elevated. Patients with autoimmune hepatitis do not present with loose stools, bloating, and weight loss.

KEY POINT

- Anti–tissue transglutaminase IgA antibody testing is the best screening test for celiac disease.

Bibliography
Rubio-Tapia A, Hill ID, Kelly CP, Calderwood AH, Murray JA; American College of Gastroenterology. ACG clinical guidelines: diagnosis and management of celiac disease. Am J Gastroenterol. 2013;108:656-76; quiz 677. [PMID: 23609613] doi:10.1038/ajg.2013.79

Item 34   Answer: A

Educational Objective: Monitor for colorectal neoplasia after colon cancer resection.

This patient's next surveillance colonoscopy should take place now (1 year after diagnosis) according to the American Gastroenterological Association (AGA) and American Society of Clinical Oncology (ASCO) guidelines. Patients who undergo a complete perioperative colonoscopy with clearing of synchronous neoplasia and curative surgical resection for colon cancer should have a subsequent surveillance colonoscopy within 1 year. If the colonoscopy is normal, the AGA recommends repeat examination in 3 years; ASCO recommends repeat examination in 5 years. If normal, colonoscopy should be repeated every 5 years thereafter until the benefit of continued surveillance is outweighed by risks and diminished life expectancy. If neoplasms are detected during any follow-up examination, then the surveillance interval should be adjusted based on polyp size, number, and histology.

Colonoscopy is the preferred modality for surveillance in patients with a personal history of colon cancer. There is insufficient evidence to support CT colonography, fecal immunochemical testing, or fecal DNA testing for surveillance after colon cancer.

Surveillance colonoscopy every 1 to 2 years is recommended in individuals with Lynch syndrome, regardless of whether the patient has a personal history of colon cancer. Lynch syndrome is unlikely because the patient's family history does not meet the Amsterdam II criteria, which require that three family members are affected by a Lynch syndrome–associated cancer, at least two successive generations are affected, one of the affected family members is a first-degree relative of the other two affected family members, and at least one cancer was diagnosed in a family member younger than age 50 years, with familial adenomatous polyposis excluded and tumors verified histologically.

A 5-year or 10-year interval is not appropriate for this patient because the risk for metachronous cancer (multiple primary tumors developing at different time intervals) is increased for about 2 to 3 years after colon cancer resection.

According the American Cancer Society's *Colorectal Cancer Survivorship Care Guidelines* published in 2015, a history and physical examination should be performed every 3 to 6 months for the first 2 years, then every 6 months for 5 years. After treatment for stages 1, 2, or 3 colorectal cancer, patients at high risk for recurrence (for example, with poorly differentiated histology, lymphatic or vascular invasions, or positive resection margins) should receive annual abdominal-pelvic and chest CT scans for 5 years after resection. A history and physical examination should also be performed every 3 to 6 months for 5 years. Carcinoembryonic antigen measurement is recommended every 3 to 6 months for the first 2 years, then every 6 months to 5 years if the patient is a potential candidate for further intervention. Follow-up evaluation recommendations from other expert organizations vary.

KEY POINT

- After treatment of colon cancer, patients should undergo surveillance colonoscopy 1 year after diagnosis.

Bibliography
American Gastroenterology Association. AGA institute guidelines for colonoscopy surveillance after cancer resection: clinical decision tool. Gastroenterology. 2014;146:1413-4. [PMID: 24742563] doi:10.1053/j.gastro.2014.03.029

Item 35   Answer: D

Educational Objective: Treat main-duct intraductal papillary mucinous neoplasm of the pancreas.

Pancreatic resection is the most appropriate next step in management. Pancreatic cysts are classified as pancreatic cystic neoplasms (the most common), nonneoplastic pancreatic cysts, and pseudocysts. The two most common pancreatic cystic neoplasms are mucinous cystic neoplasms (MCNs) and intraductal papillary mucinous neoplasms (IPMNs), which involve the main duct, branch ducts, or both. Most pancreatic cysts are branch-duct IPMNs. Main-duct IPMNs can be diagnosed based on diffuse dilation of the main pancreatic duct and the characteristic feature of mucin exuding from the ampulla during endoscopic visualization. Main-duct IPMNs carry a greater than 65% risk for malignant transformation. Surgical resection is the only option for treatment of these high-risk cystic lesions of the pancreas in patients who are appropriate surgical candidates.

Diagnosis of solitary cysts is challenging. It may require endoscopic ultrasonography and fine-needle aspiration to distinguish between cystic neoplasms (branch-duct IPMNs, MCNs, and serous tumors) and pseudocysts based on cytology. This patient has endoscopic ultrasonographic findings showing characteristic features of main-duct IPMN. The best course of action is pancreatic resection and not endoscopic ultrasound surveillance in 1 year.

MRI of the abdomen in 1 year is the standard surveillance recommendation for asymptomatic, low-risk cystic lesions of the pancreas. Main-duct IPMN is considered a high-risk cystic lesion and, therefore, MRI surveillance is not appropriate.

Oral prednisone is used to treat autoimmune pancreatitis, a frequent manifestation of IgG4-related disease. The characteristic finding of autoimmune pancreatitis on imaging is a narrowed main pancreatic duct with parenchymal swelling, known as the "sausage-shaped" pancreas, which is not consistent with this patient's findings.

KEY POINT

- Surgical resection is the best management option for high-risk cystic lesions of the pancreas, such as intraductal papillary mucinous neoplasms that involve the main duct.

Bibliography
Vege SS, Ziring B, Jain R, Moayyedi P; Clinical Guidelines Committee. American Gastroenterological Association Institute guideline on the diagnosis and management of asymptomatic neoplastic pancreatic cysts. Gastroenterology. 2015;148:819-22; quize12-3. [PMID: 25805375] doi:10.1053/j.gastro.2015.01.015

Item 36   Answer: D

Educational Objective: Diagnose the cause of hematochezia.

Upper endoscopy is the most appropriate test to perform next. The patient's presentation is consistent with rapid upper gastrointestinal bleeding (UGIB), likely from an NSAID-induced peptic ulcer. Fifteen percent of patients with presumed lower gastrointestinal bleeding are found to have an upper gastrointestinal source. Factors in this patient that favor a diagnosis of UGIB include young age, hemodynamic instability on presentation, and NSAID use. Approximately 80% of UGIB is due to four causes: peptic ulcer disease, esophagogastric varices, esophagitis, and Mallory-Weiss tear. Bleeding typically stops spontaneously; however, 20% of patients have persistent or recurrent bleeding, which increases mortality. Guidelines recommend upper endoscopy within 24 hours of presentation in patients with features of UGIB.

Angiography is used to diagnose the cause of obscure gastrointestinal bleeding when more common sources are not found on routine upper and lower endoscopy. It is also used for treatment, such as embolization, when a bleeding source has been identified.

Capsule endoscopy employs a wireless capsule camera that is swallowed by the patient to take images of the small bowel. These images are transmitted to a radiofrequency receiver worn by the patient. Capsule endoscopy allows visualization of the entire small bowel. This patient's bleeding is very likely to be accessible by upper endoscopy, the preferred diagnostic test.

Colonoscopy requires bowel preparation for adequate visualization of bleeding sources, and in the setting of acute bleeding with hemodynamic instability, a more urgent diagnostic and therapeutic test is indicated. Colonoscopy would be indicated if the source of bleeding were not identified on upper endoscopy.

KEY POINT

- Hematochezia associated with hemodynamic instability in a young patient is likely due to an upper gastrointestinal source.

Bibliography
Strate LL, Gralnek IM. ACG clinical guideline: management of patients with acute lower gastrointestinal bleeding. Am J Gastroenterol. 2016;111:459-74. [PMID: 26925883] doi:10.1038/ajg.2016.41

Item 37   Answer: D

Educational Objective: Diagnose secretory diarrhea.

Secretory diarrhea is the diagnosis most compatible with the patient's presentation. In the evaluation of chronic diarrhea, it is often useful to categorize the condition as secretory or osmotic, as well as to determine whether the cause is due to chronic infection or an inflammatory condition, which will guide further evaluation and treatment. Secretory and osmotic diarrhea can often be distinguished by clinical history. Patients with secretory diarrhea may pass liters of stool daily, causing severe dehydration and electrolyte disturbances, with persistent stooling despite fasting. Patients with osmotic diarrhea often have stool volumes of less than 1 L/d and have cessation of stooling when they are fasting. This patient's large-volume, watery diarrhea that persists despite fasting is compatible with secretory diarrhea. Another clue to this patient's diagnosis is hypokalemia. Hypokalemia from lower-gastrointestinal losses is most common when the losses occur over a prolonged period. Fecal electrolytes can be used to calculate the fecal osmotic gap:

$$290 - (2 \times [\text{stool sodium} + \text{stool potassium}])$$

An osmotic gap of less than 50 mOsm/kg suggests secretory diarrhea, and a gap greater than 75 mOsm/kg suggests osmotic diarrhea.

Examples of conditions that can cause a chronic secretory diarrhea include medications (colchicine, NSAIDs), hormone-producing tumors (carcinoid, gastrinoma, VIPoma), small intestinal bacterial overgrowth, bile acid malabsorption (short-bowel syndrome), and villous adenoma. Additional testing may be warranted in patients with secretory diarrhea. Patients found to have a small-bowel tumor in the setting of diarrhea as well as symptoms such as flushing should be considered for additional testing, including radioimmunoassays for peptides and/or 24-hour urine 5-hydroxyindoleacetic acid measurement for carcinoid tumors. Colonoscopy can be used to evaluate for villous adenomas and is also indicated if the patient is not up-to-date for colon cancer screening.

Infections leading to chronic diarrhea can be caused by parasites such as *Giardia*. *Giardia* leads to a malabsorptive condition; it would not present with large-volume diarrhea that persists despite fasting.

Inflammatory causes of chronic diarrhea include inflammatory bowel diseases (ulcerative colitis and Crohn disease) and microscopic colitis. Patients with inflammatory causes of chronic diarrhea present with bloody stools, nocturnal symptoms, and sometimes anemia. This patient is less likely to have an inflammatory cause for her chronic diarrhea given the absence of these signs and symptoms. Blood or leukocytes in the stool suggest an inflammatory cause.

Causes of chronic osmotic diarrhea include medications (laxatives), undigested sugars (lactose), celiac disease, and fat maldigestion or absorption leading to steatorrhea (chronic pancreatitis). When laxative abuse is suspected, a stool or urine laxative screen can aid in the diagnosis. Celiac disease can be evaluated with serology testing and small intestinal biopsy. A positive 72-hour stool collection for fecal fat confirms steatorrhea; a random fecal fat assessment may be helpful if a timed collection is not possible.

KEY POINT

- Patients with secretory diarrhea may pass liters of stool daily, causing severe dehydration and electrolyte disturbances, with persistent stooling despite fasting.

Bibliography
Schiller LR, Pardi DS, Spiller R, Semrad CE, Surawicz CM, Giannella RA, et al. Gastro 2013 APDW/WCOG Shanghai working party report: chronic diarrhea: definition, classification, diagnosis. J Gastroenterol Hepatol. 2014;29:6-25. [PMID: 24117999] doi:10.1111/jgh.12392

Item 38   Answer: A

Educational Objective: Diagnose Crohn disease.

The patient has Crohn colitis presenting as a chronic inflammatory diarrhea. Common symptoms are abdominal pain, diarrhea, and weight loss; overt gastrointestinal bleeding is a less common manifestation. Crohn disease has varied presentations that can make diagnosis difficult. The pattern of inflammation and histologic features in this case allow distinction of Crohn disease from other inflammatory conditions. Colonoscopy findings are consistent with Crohn colitis based on patchy distribution of mucosal inflammatory changes with normal intervening mucosa, called "skip areas." The biopsy results show distorted and branching colonic crypts, which are indicative of chronic colitis. The skip areas of normal intervening mucosa and biopsy results for involved mucosa showing features of chronicity (distorted and branching colonic crypts) make Crohn disease the most likely diagnosis.

The patient is at risk for *Giardia lamblia* infection because she works in a child care center. However, *Giardia* is a small-bowel protozoal pathogen and does not cause the symptoms of colonic inflammation with bloody diarrhea. Although most patients with giardiasis are asymptomatic, those with symptoms note abdominal pain and cramping with diarrhea, often consisting of large-volume, watery, and foul-smelling stools. Symptoms may be acute or chronic.

Microscopic colitis does not cause bloody diarrhea but rather is a cause of chronic watery diarrhea predominantly in women, with a peak onset between ages 60 and 70 years. Also, colonoscopy results are normal in patients with this condition, with inflammation only seen on biopsy.

Ulcerative colitis typically presents with bloody diarrhea and abdominal discomfort, the severity of which is related to the extent and severity of inflammation. Because ulcerative colitis typically involves the rectum, tenesmus, urgency, rectal pain, and fecal incontinence are common. Patients with ulcerative colitis have distorted and branching colonic crypts on biopsy, but the distribution of inflammation begins in the rectum and progresses up the colon in a continuous and symmetric pattern, without skip areas.

KEY POINT

- Colonoscopy results in Crohn disease show patchy distribution of mucosal inflammatory changes with "skip areas" of normal intervening mucosa, and biopsy results for involved mucosa show features of chronicity (distorted and branching colonic crypts).

Bibliography
Lee JM, Lee KM. Endoscopic diagnosis and differentiation of inflammatory bowel disease. Clin Endosc. 2016;49:370-5. [PMID: 27484813] doi:10.5946/ce.2016.090

Item 39   Answer: B

Educational Objective: Manage follow-up colonoscopy after uncomplicated diverticulitis.

This patient should undergo colonoscopy in 1 to 2 months following treatment of uncomplicated diverticulitis. According to the American Gastroenterological Association Institute Technical Review on the Management of Acute Diverticulitis, patients with a recent episode of acute diverticulitis should undergo colonoscopy 4 to 8 weeks after an episode of acute diverticulitis. Follow-up colonoscopy may identify a few cases of colorectal carcinoma. The risk for perforation after a case of diverticulitis is uncertain. The technical review estimated that 1 in 67 patients with confirmed acute diverticulitis would have a misdiagnosed colorectal cancer found on follow-up colonoscopy. Almost all of the misdiagnosed colorectal cancers included in the technical review were located in the area of diverticulitis. Assessing the patient for underlying inflammatory bowel disease is another reason for performing follow-up colonoscopy.

Colonoscopy during the acute phase of illness is contraindicated because acute diverticulitis causes acute colonic inflammation, which may increase the risk for perforation. The risk for perforation has been reported to be as high as 0.3%, but it is generally thought to be less than 0.1%, based on data from large populations undergoing screening colonoscopy. If the results of colonoscopy performed within the past 12 to 24 months are negative, then repeat colonoscopy is not needed.

Delaying colonoscopy beyond 1 to 2 months places the patient at risk for a missed diagnosis that could be important and time sensitive, such as a diagnosis of colon cancer.

KEY POINT

- Patients with uncomplicated diverticulitis should undergo colonoscopy 1 to 2 months after the episode of acute diverticulitis, when colonic inflammation has resolved.

Bibliography

Strate LL, Peery AF, Neumann I. American Gastroenterological Association Institute technical review on the management of acute diverticulitis. Gastroenterology. 2015;149:1950-1976.e12. [PMID: 26453776] doi: 10.1053/j.gastro.2015.10.001

Item 40   Answer: D

Educational Objective: Diagnose atrophic gastritis.

Upper endoscopy with gastric biopsy is the most appropriate next diagnostic study. The two forms of atrophic gastritis are *Helicobacter pylori*–associated and autoimmune. *H. pylori*–associated atrophic gastritis typically resolves with *H. pylori* eradication, whereas autoimmune atrophic gastritis has no cure. This patient's hematologic findings and positive testing for serum antiparietal antibodies confirm the diagnosis of pernicious anemia and suggest the presence of autoimmune atrophic gastritis. Iron deficiency anemia is a common comorbidity of autoimmune gastritis, as is

autoimmune thyroid disease. Autoimmune gastritis is associated with parietal cell loss, reduced gastric acid production, and secondary hypergastrinemia. Hypergastrinemia is associated with an increased risk for the development of gastric carcinoid and adenocarcinoma. It is prudent to perform upper endoscopy and gastric biopsy at the time of pernicious anemia diagnosis to evaluate for these cancers; however, the benefit on ongoing surveillance endoscopy is unclear. Autoimmune-related pernicious anemia and associated iron deficiency anemia are likely to require lifelong vitamin B_{12} and iron replacement, respectively.

Capsule endoscopy is typically used to evaluate obscure causes of gastrointestinal bleeding. This patient had a normal colonoscopy 4 years earlier, and stool evaluation is negative for blood. Finally, this patient's iron deficiency anemia is most likely due to atrophic gastritis–related achlorhydria, which decreases iron absorption by impairing the conversion of ferric iron to absorbable ferrous iron; in many patients, iron deficiency precedes vitamin B_{12} deficiency. Additional testing for iron deficiency beyond upper endoscopy is likely unnecessary.

Although small intestinal bacterial overgrowth (SIBO) can be associated with anemia, the diagnosis is unlikely in this patient with no risk factors or typical symptoms of SIBO; therefore, a glucose breath test to assess for SIBO is likely to be of low yield.

The serum gastrin level is elevated in patients with any form of atrophic gastritis and has no diagnostic or prognostic value in this setting.

KEY POINT

- Patients with newly diagnosed pernicious anemia should be evaluated for gastric adenocarcinoma and gastric carcinoid with upper endoscopy and gastric biopsy.

Bibliography

Minalyan A, Benhammou JN, Artashesyan A, Lewis MS, Pisegna JR. Autoimmune atrophic gastritis: current perspectives. Clin Exp Gastroenterol. 2017;10:19-27. [PMID: 28223833] doi:10.2147/CEG.S109123

Item 41   Answer: D

Educational Objective: Treat acute anal fissure.

Sitz baths and psyllium are the most appropriate next step in the management of this patient, who has an acute anal fissure that is most likely the result of worsening constipation induced by the recent use of opioid analgesic therapy. Anal fissures are tears in the anoderm below the dentate line that can be seen on inspection of the perianal area, often unaided by the use of an anoscope. They are usually in the posterior position and are less often in the anterior midline. The classic symptom is pain with and after defecation, which may be associated with bright red blood on the toilet tissue. Most acute fissures heal spontaneously. The most effective treatment approach is daily warm-water sitz baths and the use of the bulk laxative psyllium. This combination therapy was superior to topical lidocaine or hydrocortisone in a randomized clinical trial.

Anal botulinum toxin injection is reserved for chronic anal fissures that do not respond to more conservative treatment measures, including sitz baths, fiber supplementation, and topical therapy (nitroglycerin or calcium channel blocker) applied to the anal canal. This initial acute presentation of anal fissure is best managed by more conservative, less invasive treatment measures first.

A flexible sigmoidoscopy is not indicated because the diagnosis of anal fissure can be accurately made by history and examination. Furthermore, the patient's family history is not significant enough to warrant endoscopic evaluation.

Although topical anti-inflammatory therapy can alleviate the pain associated with anal fissure, the placement of a suppository may be uncomfortable. In addition, the patient has already tried over-the-counter topical hemorrhoid therapy with no relief of symptoms, so a glucocorticoid suppository is unlikely to help.

Topical glucocorticoid therapy is less effective in the treatment of anal fissure than sitz baths and fiber. Lubiprostone is a peripherally acting chloride channel activator with FDA approval for the treatment of opioid-induced constipation. This patient's opioid analgesic use is temporary after shoulder surgery, and lubiprostone use is more appropriate in the setting of more chronic opioid use.

KEY POINT

- The most effective treatment approach for anal fissure is daily warm-water sitz baths and the use of the bulk laxative psyllium.

Bibliography

Beaty JS, Shashidharan M. Anal fissure. Clin Colon Rectal Surg. 2016;29:30-7. [PMID: 26929749] doi:10.1055/s-0035-1570390

Item 42   Answer: A

Educational Objective: Diagnose familial adenomatous polyposis.

Colonoscopy is the best next step in the evaluation of this patient. The patient has multiple fundic gland polyps, which can be associated with familial adenomatous polyposis (FAP). Fundic gland polyps related to FAP are usually numerous (>30 polyps) and frequently harbor low-grade dysplasia, but they rarely progress to gastric cancer. Colonoscopy to rule out FAP is recommended in patients younger than age 40 years with dysplastic or numerous fundic gland polyps. Classic FAP results in the development of hundreds to thousands of colorectal adenomas that often manifest by the second decade of life. Without treatment, colorectal cancer typically develops in all patients by age 40 years. Therefore, a colonoscopy is indicated in this patient to evaluate for colonic polyposis. If colonic polyposis identified, the patient should undergo genetic testing to make the definitive diagnosis of FAP. FAP is caused by mutations in the *APC* gene. Mutations can be inherited in an autosomal dominant

pattern with multiple generations affected, but de novo mutations account for up to 25% of cases. If FAP is confirmed in this patient, it is likely due to a de novo mutation because of his unremarkable family history.

There is no role for surgical management of fundic gland polyps because they rarely progress to gastric cancer, so gastrectomy is not indicated for this patient.

An upper endoscopy in 3 months is not indicated for diagnosis of FAP. If FAP is confirmed, the patient should have regular surveillance of the upper gastrointestinal tract with a forward and side-viewing scope to assess for duodenal polyps. Duodenal polyps occur commonly in FAP, and risk for duodenal cancer is elevated. The interval for surveillance upper endoscopy in FAP depends on the number, size, and pathology of the duodenal polyps. This upper endoscopy also includes surveillance for gastric adenomas and cancer.

For sporadic fundic gland polyps, no further evaluation would be needed. Sporadic fundic gland polyps can arise in the setting of proton pump inhibitor (PPI) therapy; however, this usually occurs with prolonged therapy. Because this patient has only been taking a PPI for 4 months, his fundic gland polyposis is unlikely to be caused by PPI therapy. The patient's young age and the number of gastric polyps should prompt evaluation by colonoscopy.

KEY POINT

- Patients with multiple fundic gland polyps found at a young age should be evaluated for familial adenomatous polyposis.

Bibliography

Syngal S, Brand RE, Church JM, Giardiello FM, Hampel HL, Burt RW; American College of Gastroenterology. ACG clinical guideline: genetic testing and management of hereditary gastrointestinal cancer syndromes. Am J Gastroenterol. 2015;110:223-62; quiz 263. [PMID: 25645574] doi:10.1038/ajg.2014.435

Item 43   Answer: D

Educational Objective: Diagnose primary sclerosing cholangitis.

Primary sclerosing cholangitis (PSC) is the most likely diagnosis in this patient. The patient has elevated liver chemistry test results in a predominantly cholestatic pattern and concomitant inflammatory bowel disease (IBD). Disorders are considered cholestatic when the most prominent abnormality of liver chemistry testing is an elevation of the serum alkaline phosphatase level. Approximately 5% of patients with IBD will develop PSC during the course of their disease. In most patients, PSC presents as a stricturing process in the medium to large bile ducts, readily identifiable by MR cholangiopancreatography (alternating strictures and dilations resulting in a "string of beads" pattern). However, a minority of patients may present with involvement of only the small bile ducts, called small-duct PSC. The cholangiogram is normal in these patients; the diagnosis of small-duct PSC can only be made by liver biopsy. Small-duct PSC is associated with a better prognosis than typical PSC, although 10% to

Answers and Critiques

20% of patients with small-duct PSC eventually develop changes in the medium and large ducts.

The diagnosis of primary biliary cholangitis (PBC) is generally made on the basis of a cholestatic liver enzyme profile in the setting of a positive antimitochondrial antibody test. Case reports have described PBC associated with IBD, but the association between the two conditions is not well accepted, making the diagnosis of PBC unlikely. Although 10% of patients with PBC may test negative for antimitochondrial antibody, the absence of antibody makes this diagnosis less likely. A liver biopsy is required to establish the diagnosis of antimitochondrial antibody–negative PBC.

Drug-induced liver injury can occur in patients taking medications used to treat IBD, such as azathioprine and tumor necrosis factor-α inhibitors. Drug-induced liver injury is not a common adverse effect of mesalamine; therefore, this diagnosis is unlikely in this patient.

Nonalcoholic fatty liver disease is the most common liver disease in the United States. It is unlikely in this patient because it usually does not present with alkaline phosphatase levels greater than 2 to 2.5 times the upper limit of normal. Furthermore, MRI has a reasonable sensitivity (>80%) for the detection of fatty liver, which was not seen in this patient.

KEY POINT

- Approximately 5% of patients with inflammatory bowel disease will develop primary sclerosing cholangitis during the course of their disease, typically presenting as cholestatic liver injury with a characteristic imaging study showing bile duct strictures and dilations ("string of beads").

Bibliography

Lindor KD, Kowdley KV, Harrison ME; American College of Gastroenterology. ACG clinical guideline: primary sclerosing cholangitis. Am J Gastroenterol. 2015;110:646-59; quiz 660. [PMID: 25869391] doi:10.1038/ajg.2015.112

Item 44   Answer: C

Educational Objective: Treat gastroesophageal reflux disease.

The most appropriate next step in the management of this patient is the initiation of a proton pump inhibitor (PPI) in conjunction with lifestyle and dietary changes. The diagnosis of gastroesophageal reflux disease (GERD) is made clinically. This patient's symptoms of burning pain in his abdomen and chest and a sour taste in his mouth occurring more than a few times a week are consistent with GERD. Due to the frequency of his symptoms, the best initial treatment is a once-daily PPI for a period of up to 8 weeks. Weight reduction is suggested for patients with recent weight gain or who are overweight. Interventions such as raising the head of the bed and eliminating meals within 2 to 3 hours of bedtime are helpful for nocturnal GERD. Cessation of alcohol and tobacco use is universally supported. Treatment for less

frequent symptoms could include famotidine or other H_2 blockers. Symptom relief with the use of a PPI confirms the diagnosis of GERD.

Ambulatory pH testing is used to determine acid exposure in the esophagus in patients considering antireflux surgery. Indications for surgery include patient preference to stop taking medication, medication side effects, and refractory symptoms despite optimized medical therapy. Laparoscopic fundoplication and bariatric surgery (in obese patients) are surgical methods used to treat GERD. This patient has no surgical indications.

A barium esophagram is the initial test for evaluation of achalasia. The main symptom of achalasia is dysphagia to both solids and liquids along with regurgitation of undigested food and saliva. Patients may also report unintentional weight loss, chest pain, and heartburn. A barium esophagram is not indicated because this patient's symptoms are more consistent with GERD than with achalasia.

Upper endoscopy is indicated in patients with alarm symptoms, such as dysphagia or weight loss, and in patients whose symptoms do not respond to a PPI. Upper endoscopy is not indicated in this patient with typical GERD symptoms because most patients with typical symptoms have normal upper-endoscopy findings. Upper endoscopy is useful for the evaluation of the esophagus to identify damage in the form of erosive esophagitis, stricture, or Barrett esophagus.

KEY POINT

- Patients with a clinical diagnosis of gastroesophageal reflux disease should start an empiric trial of a proton pump inhibitor in conjunction with lifestyle and dietary changes, with no further testing.

Bibliography

Katz PO, Gerson LB, Vela MF. Guidelines for the diagnosis and management of gastroesophageal reflux disease. Am J Gastroenterol. 2013 Mar;108(3):308-28; quiz 329. Erratum in: Am J Gastroenterol. 2013 Oct;108(10):1672. [PMID: 23419381]

Item 45   Answer: A

Educational Objective: Screen for osteoporosis in a patient with cirrhosis.

Bone densitometry to screen for osteoporosis is the most appropriate next intervention for this patient with cirrhosis. Patients with cirrhosis are at twice the risk for the development of osteoporosis as demographically similar patients without cirrhosis, and women (especially those who are postmenopausal) are at higher risk than men. Initial studies of metabolic bone disease in patients with cirrhosis focused on those with primary biliary cholangitis (PBC) or alcoholic liver disease. Subsequently, it has been recognized that all patients with cirrhosis are at increased risk for bone fractures due to osteoporosis. Standard evaluation should include measurement of serum calcium, phosphate, and vitamin D levels. Up to two thirds of patients with cirrhosis are deficient in vitamin D. Dual-energy x-ray absorptiometry is recommended for patients with cirrhosis or PBC (even if noncirrhotic).

Patients with primary sclerosing cholangitis (PSC) have a high likelihood of ulcerative colitis with associated risk for colonic dysplasia and colon cancer. Eighty percent of patients with PSC have inflammatory bowel disease, usually ulcerative colitis. This association with ulcerative colitis is not seen in patients with PBC. This patient is at average risk for colorectal cancer, and colonoscopy is not indicated until age 50 years.

Contrast-enhanced abdominal CT with arterial and portal venous phase imaging can be helpful in evaluating for hepatocellular cancer; however, in this patient whose ultrasound showed no hepatic mass, a CT scan is not necessary.

Patients with cirrhosis who develop an infection have a 30% mortality rate at 1 month, and another 30% die within 12 months; this underscores the importance of preventing infection. However, the herpes zoster vaccine is not indicated in patients younger than age 60 years. It is recommended for individuals aged 60 years and older, regardless of whether they have had a previous zoster episode, but vaccination should be avoided in immunocompromised patients. Patients with decompensated cirrhosis are considered immunocompromised due to impaired reticuloendothelial cell function, impaired neutrophil function, and possible concomitant malnutrition.

KEY POINT

- Patients with cirrhosis are at increased risk for the development of osteoporosis and should be screened using bone densitometry.

Bibliography

Santos LA, Romeiro FG. Diagnosis and management of cirrhosis-related osteoporosis. Biomed Res Int. 2016;2016:1423462. [PMID: 27840821]

Item 46 Answer: C

Educational Objective: Prevent venous thromboembolism in a hospitalized patient with inflammatory bowel disease.

Subcutaneous heparin is the most appropriate venous thromboembolism (VTE) prophylaxis for this patient. VTE is a common clinical problem and is associated with substantial morbidity and mortality among hospitalized patients. Most medical patients have one or more risk factors for VTE. More than a quarter of patients with undiagnosed and untreated pulmonary embolism (PE) will have a subsequent fatal PE, and between 5% and 10% of all in-hospital deaths are a direct result of PE. VTE is one of the most common extraintestinal manifestations of inflammatory bowel disease (IBD); patients with IBD have a three-fold risk for VTE compared to patients without IBD. VTE represents a significant cause of morbidity and mortality in patients with IBD, and risk for VTE is highest at the time of disease flare. Although the incidence of VTE increases with age, the highest relative risk for VTE in IBD is observed in patients younger than 40 years

old. Patients with IBD who develop VTE have an increased mortality rate, and the most important risk factor for development of VTE is active IBD. For these reasons, prevention of VTE in patients with IBD is essential. All hospitalized patients with IBD should be given pharmacologic VTE prophylaxis with subcutaneous heparin. Systematic reviews of trials comparing prophylactic low-molecular-weight heparin with unfractionated heparin have not shown a statistically significant difference for mortality or major bleeding events, although there was a nonsignificant trend favoring low-molecular-weight heparin in the prevention of PE.

Mechanical VTE prophylaxis with graduated compression stockings or intermittent pneumatic compression devices is not recommended either with or in place of pharmacologic prophylaxis, although intermittent pneumatic compression has shown some efficacy in surgical patients and may be an option for nonsurgical patients with a contraindication to pharmacologic therapy, such as severe gastrointestinal bleeding. Compression stocking are no more effective than placebo in preventing VTE and are associated with harm in the form of increased incidence of skin breakdown.

Aspirin and low-dose warfarin have no role in VTE prophylaxis for hospitalized medical patients or patients with IBD.

KEY POINT

- All hospitalized patients with inflammatory bowel disease should be given pharmacologic venous thromboembolism prophylaxis with subcutaneous heparin.

Bibliography

Seah D, De Cruz P. Review article: the practical management of acute severe ulcerative colitis. Aliment Pharmacol Ther. 2016;43:482-513. [PMID: 26725569] doi:10.1111/apt.13491

Item 47 Answer: C

Educational Objective: Diagnose Lynch syndrome.

This patient should be referred to a genetic counselor for genetic testing. The patient could have Lynch syndrome based on his personal history of colon cancer diagnosed before age 50 years and his family history of colon cancers. His family history meets the Amsterdam II criteria for Lynch syndrome because three individuals in the family are affected with a Lynch syndrome–associated cancer, at least two successive generations are affected, one of the affected family members is a first-degree relative of the other two affected family members, and at least one cancer was diagnosed in a family member younger than age 50 years (the "3-2-1-1" pattern). Additional criteria are that familial adenomatous polyposis has been excluded and tumors have been verified histologically. Guidelines recommend tumor testing (microsatellite instability testing or immunohistochemistry) to screen for Lynch syndrome in all colon cancers. The results of tumor testing can help determine if Lynch syndrome is likely and inform genetic testing. Lynch syndrome is only diagnosed in individuals who meet the Amsterdam criteria and have an identified constitutional mutation in a mismatch repair gene (*MLH1*, *MSH2*, *MSH6*, or *PMS2*) or the epithelial cell adhesion molecule (*EPCAM*) gene. Diagnosis of Lynch syndrome will inform colonoscopy surveillance recommendations for this patient. Identification of a Lynch syndrome mutation will also affect the recommendation for screening of other cancers (gastric, skin, urinary tract, and, in women, ovarian and endometrial cancers). In addition, if he has an identifiable mutation associated with Lynch syndrome, genetic testing should be offered to his first-degree relatives.

A 3-year interval for colonoscopy cannot be recommended until the results of the genetic evaluation are available. If Lynch syndrome is confirmed, the screening interval is every 1 to 2 years, not every 3 years.

Colonoscopy is preferred for screening high-risk patients such as those with a previous colorectal cancer; therefore, screening using fecal immunochemical testing, other fecal-based testing, or colonic imaging is not appropriate.

In patients with Lynch syndrome, upper endoscopy is recommended to screen for upper gastrointestinal cancers and to sample for *Helicobacter pylori*. However, this cannot be recommended until results from genetic testing are available. Patients with Lynch syndrome have an increased risk for small-intestinal cancer. However, routine cancer screening with capsule endoscopy is controversial and not routinely recommended even in patients with confirmed Lynch syndrome.

KEY POINT

- Patients with a family history suggesting Lynch syndrome (three family members are affected with a Lynch syndrome–associated cancer, at least two successive generations are affected, one of the affected family members is a first-degree relative of the other two affected family members, and at least one cancer was diagnosed in a family member younger than age 50 years) should be referred for genetic counseling.

Bibliography

Syngal S, Brand RE, Church JM, Giardiello FM, Hampel HL, Burt RW; American College of Gastroenterology. ACG clinical guideline: genetic testing and management of hereditary gastrointestinal cancer syndromes. Am J Gastroenterol. 2015;110:223-62; quiz 263. [PMID: 25645574] doi:10.1038/ajg.2014.435

Item 48   Answer: A

Educational Objective: Evaluate persistent gastroesophageal reflux disease.

Ambulatory pH testing is the most appropriate next diagnostic test for this patient. The patient has persistent cough, which may be an extraesophageal symptom of gastroesophageal reflux disease (GERD) resulting from laryngopharyngeal reflux. Additional extraesophageal symptoms of GERD include asthma, globus sensation, hoarseness, throat clearing, and chronic laryngitis. It appears that the laryngopharynx is more sensitive to the erosive effects of acid, and small

amounts of reflux may produce symptoms. The selection of a diagnostic test to confirm or exclude laryngopharyngeal reflux is controversial. Ambulatory pH testing, if positive, can help to confirm the diagnosis of GERD and supports the diagnosis of laryngopharyngeal reflux. Negative ambulatory pH testing suggests that the patient does not have GERD and that proton pump inhibitor therapy should be discontinued and another cause of the persistent hoarseness sought. Other experts propose laryngoscopy as the gold standard to diagnose laryngopharyngeal reflux. Common findings during laryngoscopy include edema and erythema, but these findings are also seen in 80% of healthy controls. While laryngoscopy should not be used as the sole test to diagnose extraesophageal GERD, abnormal findings in patients with an appropriate clinical history suggest that cough is related to GERD. Other causes of cough may include allergy, smoking, and voice abuse, and these should be ruled out with an ear, nose, and throat evaluation.

Barium esophagography should not be used as the initial diagnostic test for GERD and is not useful for evaluating this patient's symptoms, which primarily involve the laryngopharynx.

Esophageal manometry is used for patients suspected of having an underlying motility disorder involving peristalsis or lower esophageal sphincter dysfunction. This patient reports no dysphagia, a common presenting symptom of motility disorders, and his heartburn symptoms are controlled, so esophageal manometry is not indicated.

Upper endoscopy is the primary tool used to evaluate patients with GERD for complications such as erosive esophagitis, stricture, Barrett esophagus, and esophageal cancer. Because this patient does not have esophageal symptoms and had a normal endoscopy 1 year ago, upper endoscopy is not indicated.

KEY POINT

- Ambulatory pH testing can be a helpful diagnostic test in patients with suspected extraesophageal manifestations of gastroesophageal reflux disease.

Bibliography

Katz PO, Gerson LB, Vela MF. Guidelines for the diagnosis and management of gastroesophageal reflux disease. Am J Gastroenterol. 2013;108:308-28; quiz 329. [PMID: 23419381] doi:10.1038/ajg.2012.444

Item 49   Answer: A

Educational Objective: Treat ascites caused by portal hypertension.

Discontinuing lisinopril is the most appropriate next step in the management of this patient with ascites. Blood pressure falls with worsening cirrhosis, resulting in reduced renal blood flow and glomerular filtration. A compensatory upregulation of the renin-angiotensin system results in increased levels of vasoconstrictors, including vasopressin, angiotensin, and aldosterone, which support systemic blood pressure and kidney function. ACE inhibitors and angiotensin receptor blockers impair the compensatory response to cirrhosis-related hypotension and thereby impair the ability to excrete excess sodium and water and may also affect survival. Medications that decrease kidney perfusion, including NSAIDs, ACE inhibitors such as lisinopril, and angiotensin receptor blockers, should be discontinued because their use often worsens ascites due to portal hypertension. The mainstay of therapy of ascites is to initiate dietary changes, restricting sodium intake to less than 2000 mg (87 mEq) daily. If sodium restriction does not result in significant improvement of ascites, the initiation of diuretic therapy with spironolactone with or without furosemide can be effective in increasing urinary sodium excretion.

Free-water restriction can be useful for the management of dilutional hyponatremia that is sometimes seen in patients with advanced liver dysfunction. This patient has a normal serum sodium concentration, so free-water restriction is not indicated.

Propranolol and other nonselective β-blockers are often used prophylactically for the prevention of variceal hemorrhage, but they do not have a role in the management of ascites. Furthermore, in some patients with ascites that is refractory to medical management, β-blockers may worsen clinical outcomes, including survival.

Indwelling drains for ascites have been used for patients with malignant ascites, but in the setting of portal hypertensive ascites, such as seen in this patient, indwelling drains are associated with a high risk for infection and their use is contraindicated.

KEY POINT

- Medications that decrease kidney perfusion, including NSAIDs, ACE inhibitors, and angiotensin receptor blockers, should be discontinued in patients with ascites.

Bibliography
Runyon BA; AASLD. Introduction to the revised American Association for the Study of Liver Diseases Practice Guideline management of adult patients with ascites due to cirrhosis 2012. Hepatology. 2013;57:1651-3. [PMID: 23463403] doi:10.1002/hep.26359

Item 50 Answer: D
Educational Objective: Treat acute liver failure.

Referral for liver transplantation is the most appropriate choice for this patient with acute liver failure. Acute liver failure is defined by the manifestation of hepatic encephalopathy within 26 weeks of developing symptoms of liver disease. The development of jaundice was this patient's first symptom of liver disease. Within 6 weeks, he developed coagulopathy, with an INR of 2.6, as well as symptoms of hepatic encephalopathy (confusion and asterixis). Liver injury is distinct from acute liver failure and presents with elevated liver test results and/or jaundice in the absence of evidence of liver function failure. The most common causes

of acute liver failure are medications, especially acetaminophen, and viral infections, although many cases are due to indeterminate causes. The prompt recognition of acute liver failure is essential due to high rates of mortality. Patients require frequent monitoring for hypoglycemia, hypophosphatemia, acute kidney injury, infections, and progressive hepatic encephalopathy, which can be accompanied by cerebral edema and intracranial hypertension. Liver transplantation improves the survival rate; therefore, referral to a liver transplantation center is essential upon recognition of acute liver failure.

The presence of an elevated INR reflects decreased synthesis of liver-derived clotting factors, and the administration of fresh frozen plasma is not indicated in the absence of demonstrable bleeding or the need for invasive procedures.

Kidney failure is common in the setting of acute liver failure, and many patients require renal replacement therapy, which should be performed in a liver transplant center. Most patients requiring hemodialysis in this setting tolerate continuous renal replacement therapy better than intermittent hemodialysis.

There are several appropriate indications for endoscopic retrograde cholangiopancreatography (ERCP), and one of the most common is the evaluation of biliary obstruction. In these cases, ERCP can both be diagnostic and therapeutic if the obstruction can be removed or bypassed. In this patient, ERCP is not indicated because the ultrasound shows no signs of biliary obstruction.

KEY POINT

- Acute liver failure is an indication for immediate referral to a liver transplantation center.

Bibliography
Lee WM, Stravitz RT, Larson AM. Introduction to the revised American Association for the Study of Liver Diseases position paper on acute liver failure 2011. Hepatology. 2012;55:965-7. [PMID: 22213561] doi:10.1002/hep.25551

Item 51 Answer: D
Educational Objective: Treat left-sided ulcerative colitis.

Oral mesalamine with mesalamine enema is the most appropriate treatment. Ulcerative colitis typically presents with bloody diarrhea and abdominal discomfort, the severity of which is related to the extent and severity of inflammation. The distribution of ulcerative colitis is generally divided into proctitis (involving the rectum only), left-sided colitis (inflammation does not extend beyond the splenic flexure), and pancolitis (inflammation extends above the splenic flexure). The choice of treatment depends on the extent and severity of inflammation. This patient's stool passage frequency (three per day), intermittent hematochezia, normal blood count and C-reactive protein level, and normal vital signs categorize her disease as mild. Results of colonoscopy with biopsy show moderate inflammation of the rectum and a sigmoid colon consistent with chronic idiopathic left-sided ulcerative colitis.

Mesalamine preparations are the mainstay of treatment in patients with mild to moderate disease. Mesalamine given orally or topically is effective in inducing and maintaining remission in ulcerative colitis. Evidence suggests that combined mesalamine therapy (oral and topical) is superior for induction of remission in mild to moderately active disease compared with oral or topical therapies alone; however, patient adherence to this dual treatment regimen can be difficult.

A mesalamine enema has topical effects up to the splenic flexure of the colon and would be a more effective topical agent when combined with oral mesalamine in this patient.

A mesalamine suppository is appropriate for treatment of ulcerative proctitis but is not effective for topical treatment of inflammation above the rectum.

KEY POINT

- Combined mesalamine therapy (oral and topical) is superior for induction of remission in mild to moderately active ulcerative colitis compared with oral or topical therapies alone.

Bibliography

Bressler B, Marshall JK, Bernstein CN, Bitton A, Jones J, Leontiadis GI, et al; Toronto Ulcerative Colitis Consensus Group. Clinical practice guidelines for the medical management of nonhospitalized ulcerative colitis: the Toronto consensus. Gastroenterology. 2015;148:1035-1058.e3. [PMID: 25747596] doi:10.1053/j.gastro.2015.03.001

Item 52   Answer: B

Educational Objective: Evaluate dyspepsia.

Stool antigen testing for *Helicobacter pylori* is the most appropriate next step in the management of this patient. The American College of Gastroenterology and Canadian Association of Gastroenterology have issued a joint recommendation that patients younger than age 60 years presenting with dyspepsia should first undergo a noninvasive test for *H. pylori* followed by eradication therapy if testing is positive. The committee gave a strong recommendation based on high-quality evidence for the "test and treat" strategy.

The pooled data from four trials including a total of 1608 patients with dyspepsia found no difference in the prevalence of dyspepsia at the end of 1 year of follow-up between patients undergoing the "test and treat" strategy versus those receiving a course of empirical proton pump inhibitor (PPI) therapy. Furthermore, there was a trend toward a reduction in cost for the "test and treat" strategy compared to empirical PPI therapy. For these reasons, testing for *H. pylori* is a more appropriate initial strategy for this patient than a course of omeprazole. In patients whose testing is negative for *H. pylori*, an empiric trial of PPI therapy (for example, omeprazole) can be considered before proceeding to any other testing.

Upper endoscopy should be performed in patients older than 60 years with persistent dyspeptic symptoms despite eradication of *H. pylori* and/or a trial of PPI therapy. Upper endoscopy could also be considered, regardless of age, in patients with a combination of alarm features, including a family history of gastric cancer, immigration from a region with increased risk for gastric cancer (Asia, Russia, and South America), and severe symptoms. Upper endoscopy is considered the gold standard for the exclusion of upper gastrointestinal structural causes of dyspepsia.

No other biochemical, structural (including right upper quadrant ultrasonography), or physiologic studies should be performed routinely for the evaluation of dyspepsia.

KEY POINT

- Patients younger than age 60 years presenting with dyspepsia should first undergo a noninvasive test for *Helicobacter pylori* followed by eradication therapy if testing is positive.

Bibliography

Moayyedi PM, Lacy BE, Andrews CN, Enns RA, Howden CW, Vakil N. ACG and CAG clinical guideline: management of dyspepsia. Am J Gastroenterol. 2017;112:988-1013. [PMID: 28631728] doi:10.1038/ajg.2017.154

Item 53   Answer: B

Educational Objective: Treat amebic liver abscess.

Metronidazole plus paromomycin is the most appropriate treatment for this patient with an amebic liver abscess. The two most common types of hepatic abscess are pyogenic and amebic. Pyogenic liver abscesses are the most common hepatic abscesses in the United States, whereas amebic abscesses are seen more frequently in the developing world. Pyogenic abscesses are typically polymicrobial, originating from gastrointestinal flora in the setting of intra-abdominal infections, malignancies, or procedures. Amebic abscesses are usually caused by the organism *Entamoeba histolytica*, and the mechanism of formation involves enteric infection with the invasion of amoeba through the intestinal mucosa and via the portal vein. With amebic abscesses, infection of the liver is asymptomatic until hepatic necrosis results in abscess development, at which time abdominal pain, fever, and leukocytosis develop. Amebic liver abscesses are seen in patients from endemic areas, such as India, Africa, or Central or South America, or in patients who have traveled to endemic areas. The typical presentation in travelers occurs 3 to 5 months after infection. Nearly all patients with an amebic abscess have positive serological studies for *E. histolytica*. The diagnosis is usually established with compatible imaging and serologic testing. Ultrasonography is less sensitive for the detection of pyogenic liver abscesses (CT is preferred) but may be equally sensitive for the detection of amebic abscesses. The mainstay of therapy for an amebic liver abscess is antibiotic therapy, such as metronidazole, plus a luminal agent, such as paromomycin, to eradicate the coexisting intestinal infection.

Meropenem is an effective broad-spectrum antibiotic that is often used to treat pyogenic liver abscesses. It has no role in the treatment of an amebic abscess.

Percutaneous drainage and surgical resection of an abscess are treatment options indicated for pyogenic liver abscesses. Surgical intervention is usually necessary for abscesses 5 cm or larger in size, complex abscesses, presence of gas-forming organisms, hemodynamic instability, biliary fistulization, or presence of a foreign body. These procedures are typically not needed in the treatment of amebic liver abscesses, which usually resolve with anti-microbial therapy.

KEY POINT

- The mainstay of therapy for amebic liver abscesses is antibiotic therapy, such as metronidazole, plus a luminal agent, such as paromomycin, to eradicate the coexisting intestinal infection.

Bibliography

Bonder A, Afdhal N. Evaluation of liver lesions. Clin Liver Dis. 2012;16:271-83. [PMID: 22541698] doi:10.1016/j.cld.2012.03.001

Item 54   Answer: D

Educational Objective: Diagnose ulcerative colitis.

Ulcerative colitis is the most likely diagnosis in this patient. The differential diagnosis of chronic bloody diarrhea includes inflammatory bowel disease (ulcerative colitis or Crohn colitis) and chronic ulcerating infections such as cytomegalovirus or *Entamoeba histolytica*. This patient's stool studies for enteric pathogens are negative, making Crohn colitis or ulcerative colitis the most likely cause of her symptoms. The mucosal biopsy results showing crypt architectural distortion confirm a chronic colitis such as ulcerative colitis or Crohn disease. The endoscopic description of inflammation beginning at the anorectal verge and extending proximally in a continuous fashion with transition to normal mucosa at splenic flexure is consistent with left-sided ulcerative colitis. Crohn disease characteristically has a patchy progression pattern resulting in "skip lesions" and may spare the rectum, making Crohn colitis less likely in this case.

Entamoeba histolytica causes amoebic dysentery. In the United States, amebiasis is usually diagnosed in immigrants or travelers returning from endemic areas, or in institutional settings. Although most infected persons are asymptomatic, others may develop bloody or watery diarrhea, abdominal pain, and fever. Rarely, a chronic syndrome of diarrhea, weight loss, and abdominal pain can mimic inflammatory bowel disease. Stool microscopy for ova and parasites can aid in the diagnosis by detecting the protozoa, but stool antigen testing is more sensitive. This patient's negative travel history and findings on colonoscopy and biopsy are not consistent with amebiasis.

Cytomegalovirus infection is an uncommon infection in immunocompetent patients but can occur and cause significant symptoms. The most common presenting symptoms are diarrhea, fever, and abdominal pain; half of patients have grossly bloody stools. The most common finding on endoscopy is well-demarcated ulcerations. On biopsy, histological findings include multinucleated giants cells with eosinophilic inclusions. The rarity of this condition coupled with the patient's colonoscopy and biopsy findings make cytomegalovirus infection an unlikely diagnosis.

KEY POINT

- Chronic bloody diarrhea and abdominal discomfort are typical presenting symptoms of inflammatory bowel disease; endoscopic findings help distinguish ulcerative colitis from Crohn disease.

Bibliography

Danese S, Fiocchi C. Ulcerative colitis. N Engl J Med. 2011;365:1713-25. [PMID: 22047562] doi:10.1056/NEJMra1102942

Item 55   Answer: C

Educational Objective: Test for Wilson disease.

Serum ceruloplasmin measurement is the most appropriate test for this patient. Wilson disease is an autosomal recessive disorder of copper excretion with subsequent accumulation of copper in the liver and central nervous system, cornea, kidney, joints, and cardiac muscle resulting in organ dysfunction. Children aged 10 years or younger with Wilson disease tend to present with acute liver failure; older patients (aged 30 years or younger) present with chronic liver disease and/or neurologic manifestations. Wilson disease should be considered in all patients younger than age 40 years who have unexplained liver disease. When Wilson disease causes acute hepatitis, usually in young patients, the sudden release of copper from liver cells can also induce hemolytic anemia. In this patient with evidence of hepatic encephalopathy, hemolytic anemia, low alkaline phosphatase level, and unconjugated bilirubinemia, the diagnosis of Wilson disease should be considered. The serum ceruloplasmin level is used to test for Wilson disease. Slit-lamp examination of the cornea can be performed to evaluate for Kayser-Fleischer rings, which most commonly occur in patients with neurologic manifestations of Wilson disease. A 24-hour urine copper assessment can be performed to confirm an excessive amount of copper excretion.

The diagnosis of primary biliary cholangitis is generally made on the basis of a cholestatic liver enzyme profile in the setting of a positive antimitochondrial antibody test. The predominant liver enzyme abnormality is an increase in serum alkaline phosphatase level. This patient's biochemical profile reflects hepatocellular injury, not cholestasis, and an antimitochondrial antibody test is not indicated.

With a negative test for hepatitis B virus surface antigen, this patient is very unlikely to have a hepatitis B viral infection and measurement of a hepatitis B virus DNA level is not indicated.

Symptomatic hereditary hemochromatosis is usually diagnosed after age 40 years and is often diagnosed later in women than in men, due to iron losses associated with menstruation, pregnancy, and lactation. The most sensitive initial diagnostic study is measurement of the serum transferrin saturation. The patient's sex, young age, and presence of a hemolytic anemia make the diagnosis of hereditary hemochromatosis unlikely and the measurement of a transferrin level unnecessary.

KEY POINT

- Wilson disease should be considered in all patients younger than age 40 years who have unexplained liver disease.

Bibliography

Eapen CE, Kumar S, Fleming JJ, Ramakrishna B, Abraham L, Ramachandran J. Copper and liver disease. Gut. 2012;61:63. [PMID: 22139599] doi:10.1136/gutjnl-2011-301743

Item 56   Answer: A

Educational Objective: Treat achalasia with botulinum toxin injection.

Endoscopic botulinum toxin injection is the best treatment option for this patient because his cardiac status places him at an unacceptable surgical risk. Achalasia is a motility disorder of the esophagus that results in aperistalsis and inadequate relaxation of the lower esophageal sphincter (LES). The cause of achalasia is unknown, but the pathophysiologic process involves ganglion cell and myenteric plexus degeneration in the esophageal body and LES. This nerve imbalance leads to uncontested action by cholinergic nerves and incomplete LES relaxation. The clinical presentation of achalasia consists of dysphagia to both solids and liquids. Additional symptoms may include regurgitation, chest pain, and heartburn. Standard treatments for achalasia include surgical myotomy and endoscopic pneumatic dilation. Botulinum toxin injection inhibits acetylcholine release, resulting in relaxation of the LES and relief of achalasia symptoms in up to 85% of patients. However, approximately 50% of patients will experience recurrent symptoms within 6 to 24 months after injection.

Medical therapy with calcium channel blockers or long-acting nitrates is considered third-line therapy because its effectiveness is limited. Medications may be used early in treatment, in patients who decline other interventions, before definitive treatment, and in patients who have a recurrence in symptoms after botulinum toxin injection for achalasia.

Studies have shown that endoscopic pneumatic dilation and surgical myotomy result in similar clinical outcomes in patients with achalasia, with choice of therapy depending on local expertise. Pneumatic dilation is the most effective nonsurgical treatment and is more cost-effective than surgical myotomy, but it is associated with serious complications,

such as esophageal perforation. Therefore, patients who are not surgical candidates should not undergo endoscopic dilation treatment of achalasia.

KEY POINT

- Patients with achalasia who are at high surgical risk should be treated with endoscopic botulinum toxin injection.

Bibliography

Vaezi MF, Pandolfino JE, Vela MF. ACG clinical guideline: diagnosis and management of achalasia. Am J Gastroenterol. 2013;108:1238-49; quiz 1250. [PMID: 23877351] doi:10.1038/ajg.2013.196

Item 57   Answer: B

Educational Objective: Recognize atypical chest pain and evaluate before starting treatment for gastroesophageal reflux disease.

The most appropriate next step in management of this patient is electrocardiography followed by evaluation for cardiac disease. Although gastroesophageal reflux disease (GERD) can present with symptoms of chest pain, this patient's pain is also exertional (occurs while walking up stairs), which is not typical in GERD. Failure to identify underlying cardiac disease in the setting of atypical chest pain can be catastrophic. Although this patient may have GERD, it is essential to evaluate her for heart disease before beginning empiric treatment for GERD. GERD is the most common cause of noncardiac chest pain, and chest pain caused by esophageal disorders can be difficult to distinguish from cardiac chest pain because of the anatomic proximity and common innervation of the esophagus and the heart.

Barium esophagography is recommended as the initial test for evaluation of dysphagia but is not recommended for the evaluation of typical GERD symptoms.

In patients with typical GERD symptoms, no additional testing is required and an empiric trial of a proton pump inhibitor (PPI) can be initiated. Failure to improve after 8 weeks of standard therapy should prompt further evaluation. In patients with atypical chest pain, treatment with a PPI is appropriate after ruling out cardiac disease as a cause of the chest pain.

An upper endoscopy is indicated in patients with gastrointestinal alarm symptoms such as anemia, dysphagia, or unintentional weight loss. Upper endoscopy is the primary tool to evaluate mucosal inflammation in the upper gastrointestinal tract.

KEY POINT

- In patients with atypical chest pain, a cardiac cause must be ruled out before starting treatment for gastroesophageal reflux disease.

Bibliography

Katz PO, Gerson LB, Vela MF. Guidelines for the diagnosis and management of gastroesophageal reflux disease. Am J Gastroenterol. 2013;108:308-28; quiz 329. [PMID: 23419381] doi:10.1038/ajg.2012.444

Answers and Critiques

Item 58 Answer: D

Educational Objective: Diagnose the relapsing, remitting variant of hepatitis A viral infection.

Relapsing, remitting hepatitis A virus (HAV) infection is the most likely diagnosis. This patient returned from Mexico with an icteric illness and tested positive for HAV IgM, consistent with acute HAV infection. Her HAV-infection symptoms resolved and liver chemistry tests normalized, but she developed an icteric illness 3 months later. This presentation is most consistent with an atypical course of HAV infection known as relapsing, remitting HAV infection. It is rare but was reported to occur in up to 10% of patients with HAV infection in one series. Patients may have multiple clinical or biochemical relapses but will spontaneously improve within months to 1 year without intervention. The relapses tend to be milder, are more likely to be associated with cholestasis, and may be associated with extrahepatic manifestations including nephritis, arthralgia, vasculitis, and cryoglobulinemia.

In rare cases, HAV infection has been observed to trigger autoimmune hepatitis. However, testing does not show the typical antibodies (anti–smooth muscle or antinuclear antibodies) or elevated IgG levels commonly seen in patients with autoimmune hepatitis.

Acute leptospirosis is manifested by high fever, headache, severe myalgia, conjunctival injection, abdominal pain, diarrhea, pharyngitis, and occasionally a pretibial rash. The patient's clinical course is not compatible with leptospirosis.

Malarial infection can result in jaundice due to hemolysis or, less commonly, cholestasis. However, Mexico is considered to be a very low-risk travel destination for acquisition of malaria.

KEY POINT

- The relapsing, remitting variant of hepatitis A viral infection is characterized by multiple clinical or biochemical relapses with spontaneous improvement within months to 1 year without intervention.

Bibliography

Matheny SC, Kingery JE. Hepatitis A. Am Fam Physician. 2012;86:1027-34; quiz 1010-2. [PMID: 23198670]

Item 59 Answer: A

Educational Objective: Manage chronic proton pump inhibitor therapy.

The most appropriate next step in management is an attempt to discontinue or reduce pantoprazole. Guidelines recommend that patients with symptomatic gastroesophageal reflux disease (GERD) syndromes without esophagitis be treated with a short course of a proton pump inhibitor (PPI) to achieve symptom control. Maintenance PPI therapy is recommended for patients with GERD who continue to have symptoms after the initial course of a PPI is discontinued, and for those who have erosive esophagitis or Barrett esophagus.

In 2010, the FDA revised the prescription and nonprescription labels for PPIs to include possible increased risk for hip, wrist, and spine fractures. The FDA concluded that fracture risk was greatest with higher doses of PPIs or PPI exposure for 1 year or longer. The evidence associating PPI therapy with hip fracture was inconsistent, and guidelines recommend not stopping PPI therapy when it is otherwise indicated in patients at risk for osteoporosis. Other possible PPI-related adverse reactions include vitamin B_{12} and mineral (calcium and magnesium) malabsorption, as well as increased risk for community-acquired pneumonia, *Clostridium difficile* infection, and cardiovascular events. Many guidelines recommend that long-term PPI therapy be given at the lowest effective dose, which may include as-needed therapy. Other recommendations encourage an attempt to either reduce or stop chronic PPI therapy for uncomplicated GERD at least once per year.

Upper endoscopy is not indicated in patients whose GERD symptoms are controlled in the absence of alarm symptoms, such as dysphagia, weight loss, or anemia.

Prokinetic agents such as metoclopramide should not be used in the treatment of GERD unless gastroparesis is also present. Prokinetic drugs are no more effective than placebo, and these drugs can be associated with acute dystonic reaction and tardive dyskinesia. H_2 blockers, such as ranitidine, can be used alone in patients without erosive esophagitis whose symptoms respond to H_2-blocker therapy.

Sucralfate is sulfated sucrose complexed with aluminum hydroxide and can bind to damaged mucosa. It has been shown to prevent acute mucosal damage and heals chronic ulcers without altering gastric acid concentration or pepsin secretion. Sucralfate has no role in the treatment of GERD because, as with metoclopramide, studies have shown that it is no more effective than placebo.

KEY POINT

- Long-term proton pump inhibitor (PPI) therapy for uncomplicated gastroesophageal reflux disease should be given at the lowest effective dose possible, and consideration should be given to reducing or stopping PPI therapy at least once a year.

Bibliography

Katz PO, Gerson LB, Vela MF. Guidelines for the diagnosis and management of gastroesophageal reflux disease. Am J Gastroenterol. 2013;108:308-28; quiz 329. [PMID: 23419381] doi:10.1038/ajg.2012.444

Item 60 Answer: D

Educational Objective: Treat intrahepatic cholestasis of pregnancy with ursodeoxycholic acid.

Ursodeoxycholic acid therapy is the most appropriate management for this patient. Intrahepatic cholestasis of pregnancy is a liver condition that affects pregnant women in the second or third trimester. This condition spontaneously improves within 48 hours of delivery. Typical symptoms include diffuse pruritus, and there is typically a mild increase

Answers and Critiques

in serum transaminase concentrations. Associated risks include premature delivery as well as higher rates of fetal death. Mutations in bile salt transporters have been implicated in the pathophysiology. The mainstay of therapy for intrahepatic cholestasis of pregnancy is ursodeoxycholic acid, which is associated with alleviated symptoms, improved fetal outcomes, and improved liver test abnormalities.

Cholestasis of pregnancy can be diagnosed in pregnant women with otherwise unexplained pruritus and abnormal liver chemistry tests. Elevated levels of total serum bile acid in a pregnant woman with pruritus are considered diagnostic for cholestasis of pregnancy in the absence of an alternative diagnosis. In this patient with findings compatible with intrahepatic cholestasis of pregnancy and a normal hepatic ultrasound, a liver biopsy is not needed.

HELLP (Hemolysis, Elevated Liver enzymes, and Low Platelets) syndrome presents during the third trimester and is an advanced complication of preeclampsia. HELLP syndrome typically presents with abdominal pain, new-onset nausea and vomiting, pruritus, and jaundice. A peripheral blood smear will reveal schistocytes. This patient is not anemic and does not have thrombocytopenia or hypertension; therefore, a peripheral blood smear to support the diagnosis of HELLP syndrome is not needed.

Pruritic urticarial papules and plaques of pregnancy (PUPPP) is the most common specific dermatosis of pregnancy. PUPPP is a clinical diagnosis confirmed by the appearance late in the third trimester of erythematous plaques in the distribution of striae. Persistent and bothersome pruritus is a symptomatic hallmark of the condition. It is not associated with jaundice or elevated transaminase levels. The condition usually resolves shortly after delivery. The first-line option for therapy is usually topical glucocorticoids of low to mid potency. Topical glucocorticoids are of no value in intrahepatic cholestasis of pregnancy.

KEY POINT

- The mainstay of therapy for intrahepatic cholestasis of pregnancy is ursodeoxycholic acid, which is associated with alleviated symptoms, improved fetal outcomes, and improved liver test abnormalities.

Bibliography

Bacq Y, le Besco M, Lecuyer AI, Gendrot C, Potin J, Andres CR, et al. Ursodeoxycholic acid therapy in intrahepatic cholestasis of pregnancy: results in real-world conditions and factors predictive of response to treatment. Dig Liver Dis. 2017;49:63-69. [PMID: 27825922] doi:10.1016/j.dld.2016.10.006

Item 61   Answer: A

Educational Objective: Evaluate isolated right-colon ischemia.

CT angiography is the best next test for this patient, whose clinical presentation with the sudden onset of right-sided, cramping abdominal pain followed by a bloody bowel movement is typical of isolated right-colon ischemia. A CT scan showing thickening of the ascending colon and the colonoscopy

features are helpful in confirming this diagnosis. The most common cause of colon ischemia is a nonocclusive low-flow state in the colonic microvasculature. Most cases of colonic ischemia involve the left colon, which is supplied by the inferior mesenteric artery; as with ischemia involving the right colon, the diagnosis is clinical and supported by CT and colonoscopy. Patients with left-sided colonic ischemia tend to heal well with conservative therapy alone, whereas isolated right-colon ischemia can be the harbinger of acute mesenteric ischemia caused by a focal thrombus or embolus of the superior mesenteric artery. This artery supplies both the small intestine and right colon, and the consequences of acute mesenteric ischemia involving the small bowel are severe, with mortality rates that can approach 60%. For this reason, patients with isolated right-colon ischemia require urgent, noninvasive imaging of the mesenteric vasculature to assess the extent of ischemia and nature of the intervention. CT angiography is the recommended method of imaging for diagnosing acute mesenteric ischemia because it can be obtained rapidly. CT angiography visualizes the origins and length of the vessels, characterizes the extent of occlusion, and aids in planning revascularization.

Doppler ultrasonography of the mesenteric vessels is an effective, low-cost tool that can assess the proximal visceral vessels but has limited ability to visualize distal vessels. It is best reserved for the evaluation of patients with chronic mesenteric ischemia, which typically presents with postprandial abdominal pain, sitophobia, and weight loss.

MR angiography provides information about mesenteric arterial flow and avoids the potential harms of radiation and use of contrast that are associated with CT angiography; however, MR angiography takes longer to perform, lacks the required resolution to identify arterial occlusion, and can overestimate the severity of stenosis.

Selective catheter angiography was the standard method for diagnosing mesenteric ischemia; however, it is now used after a revascularization plan has been chosen because CT angiography can be obtained rapidly and is noninvasive.

KEY POINT

- Isolated right-colon ischemia may be a warning sign of acute mesenteric ischemia caused by embolism or thrombosis of the superior mesenteric artery and should be evaluated using CT angiography.

Bibliography

Clair DG, Beach JM. Mesenteric ischemia. N Engl J Med. 2016;374:959-68. [PMID: 26962730] doi:10.1056/NEJMra1503884

Item 62   Answer: B

Educational Objective: Diagnose medication-induced enteropathy.

Discontinuing olmesartan, an angiotensin II receptor blocker, is the most appropriate next step in the management of this patient. The patient's presentation is most consistent with drug-associated enteropathy related to

CONT.

olmesartan. In 2013, the FDA issued a warning that olmesartan medoxomil can cause intestinal symptoms known as sprue-like enteropathy and approved labeling changes to include this concern. The enteropathy may develop months to years after starting olmesartan. Drug-associated enteropathy can mimic refractory celiac disease with findings of villous atrophy and increased intraepithelial lymphocytes in the first part of the duodenum. The clinical presentation can include severe diarrhea, weight loss, and dehydration requiring hospitalization. Most of the reported cases of drug-associated enteropathy are caused by olmesartan, although other angiotensin-receptor blocking drugs have been implicated. In addition to adequate fluid resuscitation, the offending medication should be discontinued. In most cases of drug-associated enteropathy, symptoms and pathological changes resolve when the drug is stopped.

Other medications, such as NSAIDs, proton pump inhibitors, antibiotics, colchicine, metformin, and cholesterol-lowering drugs (such as statins), can cause diarrhea and should be considered when evaluating a patient with symptoms of chronic diarrhea (>4 weeks' duration). However, because of the severity of the patient's presentation, the diarrhea is unlikely to be caused by atorvastatin. Additionally, atorvastatin and other statins are not linked to villous atrophy.

A gluten-free diet is the mainstay of treatment for celiac disease. Given the patient's normal celiac serology testing, his symptoms are unlikely to be caused by celiac disease and a gluten-free diet is not indicated. Villous atrophy and increased intraepithelial lymphocytes are not specific for celiac disease.

Other causes of villous atrophy, such as refractory celiac disease, Crohn disease, and autoimmune enteropathy, are treated with glucocorticoids such as prednisone. This patient's presentation and his older age are not consistent with these causes of villous atrophy, so glucocorticoids are not indicated.

KEY POINT

- Olmesartan causes medication-induced enteropathy that can mimic refractory celiac disease.

Bibliography
Ianiro G, Bibbò S, Montalto M, Ricci R, Gasbarrini A, Cammarota G. Systematic review: sprue-like enteropathy associated with olmesartan. Aliment Pharmacol Ther. 2014;40:16-23. [PMID: 24805127] doi:10.1111/apt.12780

Item 63   Answer: A

Educational Objective: Manage a patient with Barrett esophagus with low-grade dysplasia.

Endoscopic ablation therapy is the most appropriate next step in the management of this patient's Barrett esophagus with low-grade dysplasia. Barrett esophagus is a consequence of chronic reflux, regardless of the presence of gastroesophageal reflux disease (GERD) symptoms. The damage from GERD causes a change in the normal squamous lining of the distal esophagus to a specialized columnar epithelium

visible on endoscopy. Barrett esophagus can present with no dysplasia, indefinite dysplasia, low-grade dysplasia, or high-grade dysplasia, and in some patients dysplasia progresses to adenocarcinoma of the esophagus. In the past, guidelines recommended a surveillance endoscopy in 6 months for patients with low-grade dysplasia. However, more recent guidelines recommend that patients with minimal comorbidities undergo endoscopic ablation therapy for permanent eradication of Barrett esophagus. Endoscopic ablation should be considered after confirmation of dysplasia by a second expert pathologist. If a patient is ineligible for or unwilling to undergo ablation therapy, annual surveillance endoscopy is recommended as an alternative. If two consecutive surveillance endoscopies show no dysplasia, the surveillance interval is changed every 3 to 5 years, the same interval used in patients with Barrett esophagus with no dysplasia. Patients with Barrett esophagus with high-grade dysplasia are also treated with endoscopic ablation.

Esophagectomy is reserved for patients in whom ablation does not result in eradication of the dysplasia or who have esophageal cancer.

Surgical treatments for GERD consist of laparoscopic fundoplication, an endoscopic procedure that does not cure Barrett esophagus or reduce the risk for progression of dysplasia or cancer, and bariatric surgery (for obese patients). Indications for surgery include patient preference to stop taking medication, medication side effects, large hiatal hernia, and refractory symptoms despite maximal medical therapy (although patients with medically refractory symptoms may be less likely to benefit from surgery). Approximately one third of patients require resumption of PPI therapy within 5 to 10 years after surgery. Postoperative complications include dysphagia, diarrhea, and inability to belch because of a tight fundoplication.

Guidelines recommend that patients with Barrett esophagus undergo surveillance only after adequate counseling regarding the risks and benefits of surveillance. Patients with nondysplastic Barrett esophagus should undergo endoscopic surveillance no more frequently than every 3 to 5 years.

KEY POINT

- Barrett esophagus with low-grade dysplasia should be treated with endoscopic ablation therapy in patients without significant comorbidities.

Bibliography
Shaheen NJ, Falk GW, Iyer PG, Gerson LB; American College of Gastroenterology. ACG Clinical guideline: diagnosis and management of Barrett's esophagus. Am J Gastroenterol. 2016;111:30-50; quiz 51. [PMID: 26526079] doi:10.1038/ajg.2015.322

Item 64   Answer: D

Educational Objective: Diagnose *Giardia lamblia* infection.

Stool testing for *Giardia* infection is the most appropriate next step in the management of this patient. The patient presents with persistent diarrhea, defined as lasting between

2 and 4 weeks, and because of his occupational exposure, the most likely cause is *Giardia lamblia* (also known as *Giardia intestinalis*). Transmission is waterborne or through the fecal-oral route. It occurs most commonly among children (especially in developing countries), child care workers, and backpackers or campers who drink untreated water from lakes, rivers, or wells. *Giardia* is a noninvasive organism that infects the small intestine and causes diarrhea associated with nausea, bloating, and foul-smelling gas due to malabsorption. Because *Giardia* cysts are intermittently shed, stool microscopy is less sensitive than stool antigen testing, and the recommended test is a stool enzyme-linked immunosorbent assay. Treatment options include tinidazole, metronidazole, and nitazoxanide. Treatment of giardiasis with metronidazole is curative in more than 85% of patients.

A colonoscopy is not indicated because this patient's diarrhea is not associated with weight loss, abdominal pain, or blood in the stool, making inflammatory bowel disease an unlikely diagnosis. Microscopic colitis would be an unlikely diagnosis in a 45-year-old man who is not taking any medications known to be associated with microscopic colitis, such as NSAIDs.

A CT scan of the abdomen and pelvis would be unlikely to suggest a cause for watery diarrhea of 4 weeks' duration. The patient's symptoms and occupation suggest a parasitic cause of diarrhea that would not be diagnosed with an imaging study.

A 24-hour 5-hydroxyindoleacetic acid measurement is used to evaluate for carcinoid tumors. Up to 85% of patients with gastrointestinal carcinoid syndrome experience intermittent flushing. In addition to flushing, diarrhea is prominent in most patients and is related to rapid intestinal transit time. Approximately 40% of patients also have right-sided valvular heart disease. This patient has no flushing or evidence of a heart murmur, making carcinoid syndrome unlikely and measurement of 5-hydroxyindoleacetic unnecessary.

KEY POINT

- *Giardia lamblia* infection is a common parasitic infection that occurs most often among children, child care workers, and backpackers or campers who drink untreated water from lakes, rivers, or wells.

Bibliography
DuPont HL. Persistent diarrhea: a clinical review. JAMA. 2016;315:2712-23. [PMID: 27357241] doi:10.1001/jama.2016.7833

Item 65   Answer: A

Educational Objective: Diagnose gastroparesis.

Gastric emptying scintigraphy is the most appropriate next step in management. The diagnosis of gastroparesis requires: (1) the presence of specific symptoms; (2) the absence of mechanical outlet obstruction; and (3) objective evidence of delay in gastric emptying into the duodenum. Commonly reported symptoms include early satiety, postprandial fullness, nausea, vomiting, upper abdominal pain, bloating, and weight loss, but these symptoms correlate poorly with the findings on objective gastric emptying tests. Various other upper gastrointestinal disorders can present with similar symptoms. Exclusion of other upper gastrointestinal disorders, objective documentation of delayed gastric emptying, and an attempt to identify the cause of the gastroparesis are essential before treatment. Retained food in the stomach during upper endoscopy is not objective evidence of delayed gastric emptying. The three tests to objectively demonstrate delayed gastric emptying are gastric scintigraphy, wireless motility capsule, and the gastric emptying breath test. If scintigraphy is pursued, the 4-hour study is preferred over 90- or 120-minute studies due to increased diagnostic accuracy.

A 24-hour pH probe may be considered when heartburn symptoms do not respond to a higher dose of acid suppression therapy, such as twice-daily proton pump inhibitor therapy or a proton pump inhibitor plus a histamine receptor antagonist. This patient's medical therapy for heartburn symptoms should be optimized before further testing is pursued, and this test will not explain the patient's predominant symptoms of nausea, bloating, and epigastric pain.

Both metoclopramide and domperidone are effective in the treatment of gastroparesis. Metoclopramide is the only FDA-approved agent for the treatment of gastroparesis. Domperidone can be used under a special program administered by the FDA. The side effects of metoclopramide include dystonia, Parkinson-type movements, and tardive dyskinesia. Domperidone can prolong the QT interval on electrocardiography, potentially leading to cardiac arrhythmia. Before initiating treatment for gastroparesis, it is necessary to confirm the diagnosis.

KEY POINT

- The diagnosis of gastroparesis requires the presence of specific symptoms, absence of mechanical outlet obstruction, and objective evidence of delay in gastric emptying into the duodenum.

Bibliography
Camilleri M, Parkman HP, Shafi MA, Abell TL, Gerson L; American College of Gastroenterology. Clinical guideline: management of gastroparesis. Am J Gastroenterol. 2013;108:18-37; quiz 38. [PMID: 23147521] doi:10.1038/ajg.2012.373

Item 66   Answer: B

Educational Objective: Treat bleeding esophageal varices.

Ciprofloxacin for 7 days is the most appropriate next treatment for this patient with variceal bleeding. Variceal bleeding is a life-threatening complication of portal hypertension. Risk factors for variceal hemorrhage are Child-Turcotte-Pugh class B and C cirrhosis, large varices (>5 mm), and the endoscopic finding of red markings on varices. Approximately 15% to 20% of patients die within 6 weeks of hemorrhage.

The mainstay of therapy for variceal hemorrhage is endoscopic therapy. Antibiotic therapy is an important adjunctive therapy for variceal bleeding because bacterial infection occurs in 30% to 40% of patients within 1 week of variceal bleeding. The most common infections seen are spontaneous bacterial peritonitis as well as bacteremia, urinary tract infections, and pneumonia. Antibiotic therapy after variceal bleeding reduces rates of infection and rebleeding as well as mortality after variceal bleeding. There is also benefit to administering antibiotics for patients with cirrhosis who present with nonvariceal upper gastrointestinal bleeding.

This patient does not require a blood transfusion. Hemodynamically stable patients with acute upper gastrointestinal bleeding, no acute coronary syndrome, and no history of peripheral vascular disease or stroke should be transfused when the hemoglobin level is 7 g/dL (70 g/L) or less. This transfusion threshold is associated with improved clinical outcomes compared to higher transfusion thresholds. The goal of transfusion is a hemoglobin level of 7 g/dL (70 g/L) to 9 g/dL (90 g/L). In the setting of hemodynamic stability, overtransfusion should be avoided because it can cause an increase of portal pressure and thereby precipitate rebleeding.

Platelet transfusion is not warranted because hemostasis has already been achieved. This patient has thrombocytopenia, but a transfusion of platelets also has the potential to cause volume overload leading to an increase in portal hypertension and rebleeding. Patients with thrombocytopenia with clinically significant active bleeding, as well as patients without bleeding in whom nonneuraxial surgery is planned, should be transfused to a target platelet count of 50,000 to 100,000/µL (50-100 × 10^9/L) depending on the clinical circumstances.

Transjugular intrahepatic portosystemic shunt (TIPS) placement is useful in the 10% to 20% of patients with variceal bleeding in whom hemostasis is unable to be achieved by endoscopic therapy. In this patient in whom endoscopic therapy was successful, TIPS placement is not indicated.

KEY POINT

- The mainstay of therapy for variceal hemorrhage is endoscopic therapy, and adjunctive therapies such as antibiotic therapy improve outcomes.

Bibliography
Satapathy SK, Sanyal AJ. Nonendoscopic management strategies for acute esophagogastric variceal bleeding. Gastroenterol Clin North Am. 2014;43:819-33. [PMID: 25440928] doi:10.1016/j.gtc.2014.08.011

Item 67 Answer: D
Educational Objective: Manage hepatic encephalopathy.

Discontinuing alprazolam is the most appropriate next step in the management of this patient. Hepatic encephalopathy is a significant, potentially reversible, complication of cirrhosis, with cognitive impairment ranging from mild personality changes to overt coma. Hepatic encephalopathy is a clinical diagnosis and should be suspected in patients with cirrhosis who have changes in mental status, mood, or behavior. Hepatic encephalopathy can be seen in the setting of acute liver failure as well as cirrhosis. The initial management of hepatic encephalopathy centers on identifying and mitigating a precipitating factor. Up to 80% of patients have a precipitating factor, most commonly infection or gastrointestinal bleeding. Other precipitants include opioids, benzodiazepines, electrolyte abnormalities, hypoglycemia, hypoxia, transjugular intrahepatic portosystemic shunt placement, inappropriate lactulose dosing, and dehydration. In this patient who uses a benzodiazepine, alprazolam therapy should be discontinued and alternative means of managing anxiety must be sought. Tapering is likely unnecessary in this patient because the medication was initiated recently. All patients with overt episodic hepatic encephalopathy should undergo screening for infections, including diagnostic paracentesis when ascites is present.

CT of the head can be a useful study in patients with altered mental status of unknown cause, but in patients with hepatic encephalopathy without a history of head trauma or a focal neurological examination, head CT is unnecessary.

Early concerns regarding dietary protein consumption as a precipitant of hepatic encephalopathy have been largely debunked, and outside of rare circumstances, dietary protein restriction should not be undertaken, even in the setting of acute hepatic encephalopathy. Furthermore, due to the high risk for protein-calorie malnutrition in patients with cirrhosis, dietary protein restriction can result in worsened clinical outcomes.

Lactulose is first-line treatment and should be titrated to produce three stools per day. Rifaximin is added to lactulose for prevention of recurrent episodes after a second episode of hepatic encephalopathy. Due to its expense, it is not a first-line therapy for hepatic encephalopathy.

KEY POINT

- Up to 80% of patients with hepatic encephalopathy have a precipitating factor, most commonly infection or gastrointestinal bleeding.

Bibliography
Vilstrup H, Amodio P, Bajaj J, Cordoba J, Ferenci P, Mullen KD, et al. Hepatic encephalopathy in chronic liver disease: 2014 practice guideline by the American Association for the Study of Liver Diseases and the European Association for the Study of the Liver. Hepatology. 2014;60:715-35. [PMID: 25042402] doi:10.1002/hep.27210

Item 68 Answer: B
Educational Objective: Screen for colorectal cancer in a high-risk individual.

This patient should undergo his first screening colonoscopy at age 40 years. Based on the patient's family history, he is at increased risk for colon cancer. Individuals with a first-degree relative with colon cancer or an advanced adenoma diagnosed at an age younger than 60 years, or two or more first-degree relatives with colon cancer or advanced adenoma diagnosed at any age, should begin colon cancer screening at age 40 years (or 10 years earlier than the youngest age at which colon cancer was diagnosed in a first-degree relative, whichever is first). Colonoscopy, rather than imaging or stool-based testing, is the recommended screening modality. If colonoscopy is performed and findings are normal, the recommended interval for repeat screening is 5 years if the first-degree relative was younger than age 60 years at the time of diagnosis and 10 years if the first-degree relative was age 60 years or older at the time of diagnosis.

Although age 42 years is 10 years earlier than the age at which his father was diagnosed with colon cancer, guidelines recommend starting colon cancer screening at age 40 years or 10 years earlier than the family member's diagnosis, whichever comes first. Therefore, age 40 years is the appropriate age at which to begin screening in this patient.

In average-risk patients, 50 years is the recommended age to begin screening for colon cancer. Because of this patient's family history, waiting until age 50 years to begin screening for colon cancer is not appropriate.

KEY POINT

- Individuals with a first-degree relative with colon cancer or an advanced adenoma diagnosed at an age younger than 60 years, or two or more first-degree relatives with colon cancer or advanced adenoma diagnosed at any age, should begin colon cancer screening at age 40 years (or 10 years earlier than the youngest age at which colon cancer was diagnosed in a first-degree relative, whichever is first).

Bibliography

Lieberman DA, Rex DK, Winawer SJ, Giardiello FM, Johnson DA, Levin TR; United States Multi-Society Task Force on Colorectal Cancer. Guidelines for colonoscopy surveillance after screening and polypectomy: a consensus update by the US Multi-Society Task Force on Colorectal Cancer. Gastroenterology. 2012;143:844-57. [PMID: 22763141] doi:10.1053/j.gastro.2012.06.001

Item 69   Answer: B

Educational Objective: **Treat hepatocellular carcinoma with liver transplantation.**

Referral for liver transplantation is the most appropriate next step in management for this patient. A diagnosis of hepatocellular carcinoma can be made in a patient with cirrhosis in the presence of lesions larger than 1 cm that enhance in the arterial phase and have washout of contrast in the venous phase. This patient meets the Milan criteria (up to three hepatocellular carcinoma tumors ≤3 cm or one tumor ≤5 cm) for liver transplantation. Patients who meet the Milan criteria and have a tumor 2 cm or larger with arterial enhancement and venous washout on CT or MRI are eligible to receive Model for End-Stage Liver Disease exception points, placing them at a higher priority for liver transplantation.

Liver transplantation is the only curative therapy for hepatocellular carcinoma and for end-stage liver disease.

Patients meeting the Milan criteria have excellent 5-year survival rates after liver transplantation.

Biopsy of the lesion is not indicated in this patient. In the context of cirrhosis, a lesion larger than 1 cm with contrast enhancement in the arterial phase and portal venous washout meets radiologic criteria for hepatocellular carcinoma and, therefore, does not require a lesion biopsy. Additionally, there is potential for harm from a lesion biopsy due to coagulopathy or the very small risk for tumor seeding.

Sorafenib is a multikinase inhibitor that is reserved for patients with advanced hepatocellular carcinoma with vascular invasion or extrahepatic spread that is not amenable to surgery, liver transplantation, or locoregional therapies. Treatment of these patients with sorafenib confers a survival benefit. This patient is not a candidate for resection and should be evaluated for liver transplantation; sorafenib is not indicated.

Surgical resection would be dangerous for this patient, given the evidence of portal hypertension, which confers increased risk for intraoperative bleeding as well as risk for postoperative liver failure.

KEY POINT

- Patients with cirrhosis and who meet the Milan criteria (up to three hepatocellular carcinoma tumors ≤3 cm or one tumor ≤5 cm) are best treated with liver transplantation and have excellent 5-year survival rates.

Bibliography

Heimbach J, Kulik LM, Finn R, Sirlin CB, Abecassis M, Roberts LR, et al. AASLD guidelines for the treatment of hepatocellular carcinoma. Hepatology. 2017. [PMID: 28130846] doi:10.1002/hep.29086

Item 70   Answer: C

Educational Objective: **Diagnose eosinophilic esophagitis.**

Eosinophilic esophagitis is the most likely diagnosis in this patient. Defined as esophageal squamous mucosal inflammation caused by eosinophilic infiltration, eosinophilic esophagitis is commonly seen in young men presenting with symptoms of dysphagia. It often co-occurs in patients with food allergies, asthma, and eczema. Rings and furrows in the esophagus are common findings on upper endoscopy. The diagnosis is confirmed with biopsies of the esophagus showing more than 15 eosinophils/hpf. Treatment begins with a trial of a proton pump inhibitor (PPI) for a period of 2 months. Clinical improvement with a PPI indicates gastroesophageal reflux disease–associated eosinophilia rather than eosinophilic esophagitis. In this case, repeat upper endoscopy with biopsies should be considered; if esophageal eosinophilia is still present, the diagnosis of eosinophilic esophagitis is confirmed. For patients with confirmed eosinophilic esophagitis, treatment includes restriction of dietary elements (elemental diet or targeted elimination diet) and swallowed aerosolized topical glucocorticoids. Patients should also be counseled that the condition may recur.

This patient's endoscopic findings are not consistent with a diagnosis of achalasia. In patients with achalasia, endoscopy often shows a dilated esophageal body with resistance at the gastroesophageal junction. A manometry test confirms the diagnosis of achalasia. The most effective treatment options include pneumatic dilation and surgical myotomy.

Candida esophagitis rarely occurs in immunocompetent patients but is seen more often in patients with HIV and other immunocompromised patients. The most common symptom is odynophagia rather than dysphagia. Oral thrush may also be present, but its absence does not exclude esophageal involvement. Endoscopic findings in patients with *Candida* esophagitis are small, raised, white plaques. It is treated with oral fluconazole and management of the immunocompromised state.

Because this patient takes only a multivitamin and has no ulcers seen on endoscopy, pill-induced esophagitis is unlikely. Pill-induced esophagitis has been observed with medications including alendronate, quinidine, tetracycline, doxycycline, potassium chloride, ferrous sulfate, and mexiletine. Pills typically cause local injury at sites of anatomic narrowing of the esophagus. Clinical symptoms include chest pain, dysphagia, and odynophagia. Symptoms may begin hours to days after starting therapy, and stopping the medication often leads to symptom relief.

KEY POINT

- Eosinophilic esophagitis typically presents in young men with symptoms of dysphagia and in patients with a history of food allergies, eczema, and asthma.

Bibliography

Dellon ES, Gonsalves N, Hirano I, Furuta GT, Liacouras CA, Katzka DA; American College of Gastroenterology. ACG clinical guideline: evidenced based approach to the diagnosis and management of esophageal eosinophilia and eosinophilic esophagitis (EoE). Am J Gastroenterol. 2013;108:679-92; quiz 693. [PMID: 23567357] doi:10.1038/ajg.2013.71

Item 71   Answer: D

Educational Objective: Manage asymptomatic gallstones.

This patient's asymptomatic gallstone disease requires no further intervention at this time but should be managed as symptoms arise. Gallstone disease is a common finding in up to 15% of patients in Western countries. Gallstones that are found incidentally during abdominal imaging performed for another reason do not usually require intervention. Stones that produce symptoms typical of biliary colic or cause symptoms due to passage of the stone into the common bile duct require intervention. This patient has no symptoms potentially attributable to gallstones, and the ultrasonographic findings do not suggest any complications of gallstones. Because there are no complications, no intervention is necessary at this time and clinical observation is the appropriate management.

Eighty percent of patients with asymptomatic gallstones remain asymptomatic over a 15-year period, and most seri-ous complications of gallstone disease are preceded by an episode of biliary colic; therefore, cholecystectomy is not generally advised in asymptomatic patients. Indications for cholecystectomy include symptomatic disease such as biliary colic or cholecystitis. Prophylactic cholecystectomy is recommended for patients with an anomalous pancreaticobiliary duct junction, gallbladder polyps 1 cm or larger, gallbladder polyp(s) with concomitant gallstones, or polyps of any size in the setting of primary sclerosing cholangitis. Prophylactic cholecystectomy can also be considered in patients with a porcelain gallbladder or with gallstones larger than 3 cm. These patients are at increased risk for gallbladder cancer. In this patient with small, asymptomatic gallstones, there is no indication for surgical intervention.

Referral for endoscopic retrograde cholangiopancreatography (ERCP) is not warranted in this setting because the patient is asymptomatic. Patients with gallstones in the common bile duct or patients who are not candidates for cholecystectomy may benefit from ERCP with sphincterotomy to reduce the risk for recurrent bouts of cholangitis.

Serial abdominal imaging, such as ultrasonography, to monitor asymptomatic gallstones is not warranted. Patients with gallbladder polyps may benefit from monitoring with serial gallbladder ultrasound because gallbladder polyps are a risk factor for gallbladder cancer. Diagnosis at a late stage contributes to the poor prognosis of gallbladder cancer.

KEY POINT

- Incidentally found gallstones with no associated symptoms and no complications require no further intervention.

Bibliography

Warttig S, Ward S, Rogers G; Guideline Development Group. Diagnosis and management of gallstone disease: summary of NICE guidance. BMJ. 2014;349:g6241. [PMID: 25360037] doi:10.1136/bmj.g6241

Item 72   Answer: A   🅗

Educational Objective: Diagnose aortoenteric fistula.

A CT scan with intravenous contrast is the most appropriate next test for this patient. The patient presents with the classic "herald bleed" of aortoenteric fistula: a brisk bleed associated with hypotension that stops spontaneously and then is followed later by massive gastrointestinal hemorrhage. An aortoenteric fistula is a communication between the aorta and the gastrointestinal tract, most commonly located in the distal duodenum, especially the third portion, because the duodenum is fixed and located just anterior to the aorta. The possibility of an aortoenteric fistula must be considered in a patient with previous aortic graft surgery who presents with gastrointestinal bleeding. It is a life-threatening condition, with a mortality rate of 50% even with surgical intervention. In this setting, the aortoenteric fistula is most commonly due to graft infection, and associated fever and leukocytosis occurs. When there is a high degree of suspicion for aortoenteric fistula, CT with intravenous contrast should be performed before other

CONT.

types of gastrointestinal evaluation because CT can be performed promptly and is noninvasive. CT can reveal evidence of graft infection, such as perigraft soft-tissue thickening or loss of tissue planes, and its reported sensitivity for aortoenteric fistula is 80% or greater.

Mesenteric angiogram can detect bleeding rates as slow as 1 mL/min compared with 0.2 mL/min for tagged red blood cell scintigraphy; however, given the intermittent nature of bleeding from an aortoenteric fistula, mesenteric angiogram and tagged red blood cell scintigraphy are rarely helpful in the diagnosis of this condition.

Upper endoscopy may be performed to rule out other more common sources of bleeding, but in this patient, the presence of fever, leukocytosis, and bleeding points to aortoenteric fistula as the most likely diagnosis, and CT angiogram is the most urgently needed test.

KEY POINT

- Gastrointestinal bleeding occurring in patients following aortic graft surgery should raise the possibility of aortoenteric fistula; CT with contrast is the initial test in appropriate patients.

Bibliography

Singh M, Koyfman A, Martinez JP. Abdominal vascular catastrophes. Emerg Med Clin North Am. 2016;34:327-39. [PMID: 27133247] doi:10.1016/j.emc.2015.12.014

 Item 73   Answer: C

Educational Objective: Manage lower gastrointestinal bleeding.

Colonoscopy within 24 hours with adequate bowel preparation is the most appropriate next step in management. Almost 80% of lower gastrointestinal bleeding (LGIB) is due to diverticulosis, colitis, hemorrhoids, or postpolypectomy bleeding. LGIB typically stops within 24 hours. Colonoscopy is the recommended initial diagnostic test after hemodynamic resuscitation in most patients with significant LGIB. LGIB typically occurs in older individuals and presents as acute bright red blood per rectum or red- or maroon-colored stool (hematochezia). Colonoscopy is able to identify the source of bleeding in two thirds of patients. The American College of Gastroenterology's 2016 guidelines for LGIB recommend oral bowel preparation to increase colonoscopy's diagnostic yield. Randomized controlled trials have not shown a benefit in clinical outcomes or cost with rapid bowel preparation and colonoscopy within 8 to 12 hours compared with a standard oral bowel preparation and colonoscopy within 24 hours for patients with LGIB.

For patients who continue to bleed and have failed endoscopic hemostasis treatments (for example, electrocoagulation, hemoclips, submucosal epinephrine injection), the next therapeutic step is arterial embolization of the bleeding source. Major complications include contrast dye reactions, acute kidney injury, transient ischemic attack, bowel ischemia, hematoma formation, and femoral artery

thrombosis. This patient should be evaluated first with colonoscopy before using a more invasive treatment strategy.

Radiographic techniques such as tagged red cell scintigraphy may be useful in evaluating overt gastrointestinal bleeding from an unknown source. Nuclear scans can identify only a general area where bleeding is occurring; they cannot offer accuracy or intervention. Follow-up studies after a positive scan can include repeat endoscopy or angiography; both can offer more accurate localization and therapy. Nuclear scans are often done before angiography.

Transfusion strategies specifically for patients with LGIB have not been developed. Data extrapolated from patients with upper gastrointestinal bleeding found that a restrictive transfusion strategy with a transfusion threshold of hemoglobin less than 7 g/dL (70 g/L) improved survival and decreased rebleeding when compared with a threshold of 9 g/dL (90 g/L). Patients with massive bleeding, acute coronary syndrome, symptomatic peripheral vascular disease, or a history of cerebrovascular disease were excluded from these studies and may benefit from a more lenient transfusion strategy.

KEY POINT

- Colonoscopy is the recommended initial diagnostic test after hemodynamic resuscitation in most patients with significant lower gastrointestinal bleeding.

Bibliography

Strate LL, Gralnek IM. ACG clinical guideline: management of patients with acute lower gastrointestinal bleeding. Am J Gastroenterol. 2016;111:459-74. [PMID: 26925883] doi:10.1038/ajg.2016.41

Item 74   Answer: C

Educational Objective: Treat uncomplicated diverticulitis.

The patient has uncomplicated diverticulitis that can be managed with oral antibiotics. Approximately 5% of patients with diverticula will experience an episode of diverticulitis. Symptoms include abdominal pain, fever, and altered bowel habits. Physical examination findings include fever, left-lower-quadrant tenderness, and/or a lower abdominal or rectal mass. If clinical features are highly suggestive of diverticulitis, imaging studies are unnecessary. If the diagnosis is not clear or if an abscess is suspected (severe pain, high fever, palpable mass), CT imaging is indicated. Although the use of a 7-day course of oral antibiotics does not shorten the clinical course of diverticulitis, it may prevent complications from diverticulitis, such as an abscess, and may help prevent a future episode of diverticulitis. The antimicrobial agents used should cover colonic organisms and include anaerobic coverage (such as ciprofloxacin and metronidazole). Treatment can be done on an outpatient basis with close monitoring, and the patient should adhere to a liquid diet for 2 to 3 days, then advance the diet as tolerated. The routine use of antibiotics in uncomplicated diverticulitis has been questioned because of overuse of antibiotics.

CONT.

Colonoscopy should not be done during acute diverticulitis due to the risk for perforation. In patients who have not undergone screening colonoscopy within the past 3 years, colonoscopy should be done 4 to 8 weeks after resolution of symptoms to exclude colon malignancy.

Intravenous antibiotics are appropriate in patients who cannot take oral medications or who have complicated diverticulitis, such as abscess or fistula formation. Fistulas may form between the colon and other adjacent structures including the bladder, vagina, skin, or peritoneum. CT-guided percutaneous drainage of abscesses is preferred.

Surgery is required for diverticulitis complicated by peritonitis and may be lifesaving. Patients with recurrent diverticulitis may also benefit from surgical resection of the affected area of the colon.

KEY POINT

- Patients with uncomplicated diverticulitis should be treated conservatively with oral antibiotics.

Bibliography

Strate LL, Peery AF, Neumann I. American Gastroenterological Association Institute technical review on the management of acute diverticulitis. Gastroenterology. 2015;149:1950-1976.e12. [PMID: 26453776] doi: 10.1053/j.gastro.2015.10.001

Item 75 Answer: C

Educational Objective: Manage a patient with Barrett esophagus that is indefinite for dysplasia.

The most appropriate next step in managing this patient is to optimize medical therapy and then repeat upper endoscopy. This patient's Barrett esophagus is indefinite for dysplasia, which falls between nondysplastic Barrett esophagus and low-grade dysplasia. In patients whose Barrett esophagus is indefinite for dysplasia, medical therapy for gastroesophageal reflux disease (GERD) should be optimized (in this patient, proton pump inhibitor therapy would increase to twice daily) and then the patient should receive a repeat upper endoscopy. Guidelines do not specify a time for repeating the endoscopy; 6 months to 1 year after antisecretory therapy is optimized would be reasonable. If the repeat endoscopy still shows Barrett esophagus that is indefinite for dysplasia, the patient should continue medical therapy and undergo a repeat endoscopy in 1 year. If the endoscopy is normal at 1 year, a surveillance interval of 3 to 5 years can be resumed.

The patient has a history of GERD, which can lead to Barrett esophagus. Other risk factors for Barrett esophagus include male gender, age, current or past smoking, central obesity, and white race. Barrett esophagus is a precancerous condition that is classified with five levels of histologic findings, from no dysplasia to esophageal cancer. It may progress from intestinal metaplasia to low-grade dysplasia to high-grade dysplasia to invasive adenocarcinoma.

Endoscopic ablation therapy is indicated for patients with Barrett esophagus with low-grade or high-grade dysplasia, although continued endoscopic surveillance is also acceptable for patients with low-grade dysplasia. Because this patient's Barrett esophagus is indefinite for dysplasia, endoscopic ablation therapy is inappropriate.

Esophagectomy is considered for patients with a diagnosis of esophageal cancer.

A repeat endoscopy at 1 year without optimizing medical therapy for GERD is not recommended by current guidelines. Patients with nondysplastic Barrett esophagus should undergo a repeat surveillance endoscopy in 3 to 5 years. Patients with Barrett esophagus with low-grade dysplasia should undergo surveillance endoscopy in 6 to 12 months to detect prevalent dysplasia, and dysplasia should be confirmed by an expert pathologist.

KEY POINT

- Patients whose Barrett esophagus is indefinite for dysplasia should begin optimized antisecretory medical therapy and undergo a repeat endoscopy.

Bibliography

Shaheen NJ, Falk GW, Iyer PG, Gerson LB; American College of Gastroenterology. ACG Clinical Guideline: Diagnosis and Management of Barrett's Esophagus. Am J Gastroenterol. 2016;111:30-50; quiz 51. [PMID: 26526079]

Item 76 Answer: A

Educational Objective: Evaluate fecal incontinence in an elderly patient.

An abdominal radiograph is the most appropriate next step in management of this patient. Fecal incontinence is the involuntary loss of stool. Prevalence increases with age and is 16% in adults older than 70 years. Urge fecal incontinence is the inability to postpone defecation. This patient's explosive diarrhea is the likely source of her urge fecal incontinence. Before treating the diarrhea, it is essential to determine whether the diarrhea is due to overflow from fecal loading (excess stool in the colon). An abdominal radiograph is a simple, safe, and inexpensive diagnostic test. Fecal loading with resultant overflow diarrhea is a common cause of fecal incontinence in elderly patients, particularly those who are hospitalized or have degenerative neurologic disorders. This patient has several risk factors for developing fecal loading, including Alzheimer dementia, history of constipation, and use of constipating medications (memantine and calcium).

Anorectal manometry is useful in the diagnostic evaluation of fecal incontinence to help assess for anal sphincter weakness, rectal hypersensitivity, and/or dyssynergic defecation. Due to its limited availability, cost, and logistical considerations for the patient, its use is reserved for patients with rectal findings suggestive of anal sphincter weakness or dyssynergia, or patients with a lack of response to initial treatment measures.

A trial of loperamide may alleviate this patient's diarrhea in the short term; however, loperamide use will add to the underlying fecal loading, causing her diarrhea and fecal incontinence to worsen over time.

Use of psyllium is unlikely to alleviate the patient's symptoms and would add stool bulk to an already overloaded colon, which would likely worsen her urgency, explosive diarrhea, and fecal incontinence. Furthermore, the patient is likely to experience bloating and abdominal distention caused by the fermentation of the psyllium in the gastrointestinal tract.

KEY POINT

- Fecal loading (excess stool in the colon) with resultant overflow diarrhea is a common cause of fecal incontinence in elderly patients, particularly those who are hospitalized or have degenerative neurologic disorders.

Bibliography

Yu SW, Rao SS. Anorectal physiology and pathophysiology in the elderly. Clin Geriatr Med. 2014;30:95-106. [PMID: 24267605] doi:10.1016/j.cger.2013.10.003

Item 77   Answer: D

Educational Objective: Diagnose ischemic colitis.

Ischemic colitis is the most likely diagnosis in this patient. The patient initially presented in septic shock from a urinary tract infection. He was hypotensive and required intravenous fluids and vasopressor support, which are risk factors for ischemic colitis in elderly patients. Ischemic colitis is a low-flow state of the colon occurring most frequently in the left colon. Conditions that can alter circulation include hypotension, dehydration, strenuous physical activity, medications and illicit drugs, thrombophilia, aortic or cardiac bypass, vasculitis, or an obstructing colon lesion. Diarrhea with rectal bleeding is common. Colonoscopy may show sharply demarcated pale mucosa with petechial bleeding, as it does in this patient. Left colon inflammatory changes may be detected by colonoscopy or abdominal CT. Treatment is supportive care with normalization of blood pressure.

Acute mesenteric ischemia (AMI) is an uncommon vascular emergency. Embolism to the mesenteric arteries causes 50% of cases of AMI. Most emboli are from cardiac sources. Patients typically present in the seventh decade of life and often have associated cardiovascular comorbidities. The classic presentation of early AMI is central abdominal pain out of proportion to the physical examination findings. This patient's gradual onset of left-sided, moderate-intensity abdominal pain is not typical of AMI.

Diverticula represent herniation of mucosa or submucosa through the muscular layers of the colon, typically at the entry site of vasa recta (small arteries), which are a source for bleeding. Diverticular bleeding is usually painless with passage of large-volume red- to maroon-colored blood per rectum. It occurs spontaneously without associated infection or other illness, making it unlikely in this patient.

The most common initial symptoms of enterohemorrhagic *Escherichia coli* are bloody diarrhea and abdominal tenderness, without fever. The timing of this patient's development of gastrointestinal symptoms, 1 day after presentation with hypotension secondary to urosepsis, makes the diagnosis of ischemic colitis more likely.

KEY POINT

- Ischemic colitis is a low-flow state of the colon occurring most frequently in the left colon and characterized by moderate, left-sided, cramping abdominal pain followed by bloody diarrhea.

Bibliography

Trotter JM, Hunt L, Peter MB. Ischaemic colitis. BMJ. 2016;355:i6600. [PMID: 28007701] doi:10.1136/bmj.i6600

Item 78   Answer: B

Educational Objective: Treat ileal Crohn disease.

Infliximab is the most appropriate treatment for this patient. This patient has moderate to severe ileal Crohn disease that has required multiple courses of tapering prednisone for flares of disease over the last year, despite treatment with the immunomodulator azathioprine. Infliximab is an anti–tumor necrosis factor (TNF)-α antagonist effective in inducing and maintaining remission in moderate to severe Crohn disease. Other FDA-approved anti-TNF agents include adalimumab and certolizumab pegol. Evidence indicates that efficacy is better when an anti-TNF agent is used together with an immunomodulator. In addition, the risk for developing antibodies against the anti-TNF agent is lower with combination therapy. Patients whose disease does not respond to one anti-TNF agent are often switched to a second or third anti-TNF agent. Fibrostenosing Crohn disease in the absence of ongoing mucosal inflammation is unlikely to respond to any anti-TNF agent. Patients with no response to or intolerance of anti-TNF agents should be treated with either surgery or a leukocyte trafficking blocker (natalizumab or vedolizumab).

Budesonide is a potent glucocorticoid with high first-pass metabolism in the liver, which limits systemic side effects related to conventional glucocorticoids. Budesonide can be an effective therapy for treating mild flares of ileal Crohn disease, but it is unlikely to induce remission in more severe Crohn disease and cannot be used to maintain remission.

Mesalamine agents are mainly used to treat ulcerative colitis of mild to moderate severity. Mesalamine may have efficacy in treating mild to moderate Crohn colitis, but it is not efficacious in treating small-bowel Crohn disease.

Reinitiating prednisone may induce remission of the patient's current disease flare, but it would not be helpful for maintenance of remission. Because this patient has required three separate tapering doses of glucocorticoids over the last year, she requires a medication such as infliximab that can both induce remission and maintain Crohn disease in remission.

Answers and Critiques

KEY POINT

- Anti–tumor necrosis factor agents such as infliximab are effective in inducing and maintaining remission in moderate to severe Crohn disease.

Bibliography

Lichtenstein GR, Hanauer SB, Sandborn WJ; Practice Parameters Committee of American College of Gastroenterology. Management of Crohn's disease in adults. Am J Gastroenterol. 2009;104:465-83; quiz 464, 484. [PMID: 19174807] doi:10.1038/ajg.2008.168

Item 79   Answer: D

Educational Objective: Manage Lynch syndrome.

This patient should undergo a screening colonoscopy now, and if it is normal, have a repeat colonoscopy every 1 to 2 years until age 40 years, and then yearly thereafter. The patient has Lynch syndrome based on her family history and the identification of a deleterious mutation in the *MSH2* gene. The Amsterdam II criteria (known as the "3-2-1-1-0 rule") can be used to screen for Lynch syndrome; a diagnosis is warranted if the following criteria are met:

- Three family members are affected with a Lynch syndrome–associated cancer
- At least two successive generations are affected
- One affected family member is a first-degree relative of the other two affected family members
- One of the cancers was diagnosed before age 50 years
- Familial adenomatous polyposis has been excluded
- Tumors have been verified histologically

The Amsterdam criteria are specific for Lynch syndrome but lack sensitivity. Additional clinical tools, such as the Bethesda criteria or clinical models such as the PREdiction Model for gene Mutations 5 (PREMM$_5$) (premm.dfci.harvard. edu), may be used to screen for Lynch syndrome.

Lynch syndrome is caused by germline mutation in one of the DNA mismatch repair genes (*MLH1, MSH2, MSH6, PMS2*) or the epithelial cell adhesion molecule (*EPCAM*) gene. The appropriate age to begin screening colonoscopy in patients with Lynch syndrome is between ages 20 and 25 years or 2 to 5 years before the earliest age of colorectal cancer diagnosis in the family, whichever comes first; thus, this patient should undergo a colonoscopy now. The risk for colorectal cancer in patients with Lynch syndrome is elevated significantly compared with the general population and is as high as 80% for some individuals. Women with Lynch syndrome are at increased risk for endometrial cancer. Additional cancers, such as gastric, small intestinal, urothelial, ovarian, and pancreaticobiliary cancers, are also associated with this syndrome.

Colectomy and continued annual endoscopic surveillance of the remaining rectum is the recommended management for patients with Lynch syndrome who are found to have colorectal cancer on screening colonoscopy. Colectomy is not a recommended option for managing patients with Lynch syndrome in the absence of a documented cancer.

Screening starting at age 40 years or 10 years earlier than the youngest age of colon cancer diagnosis in the family is appropriate for individuals with a family history of colon cancer that does not meet criteria for Lynch syndrome.

KEY POINT

- Patients with Lynch syndrome should begin screening colonoscopy between ages 20 and 25 years or 2 to 5 years before the earliest age of colorectal cancer diagnosis in the family, whichever comes first, and colonoscopy should be repeated every 1 to 2 years if the baseline examination is normal.

Bibliography

Rubenstein JH, Enns R, Heidelbaugh J, Barkun A; Clinical Guidelines Committee. American Gastroenterological Association Institute guideline on the diagnosis and management of lynch syndrome. Gastroenterology. 2015;149:777-82; quiz e16-7. [PMID: 26226577] doi:10.1053/j.gastro.2015.07.036

Item 80   Answer: D

Educational Objective: Diagnose hereditary diffuse gastric cancer.

Upper endoscopy is the most appropriate next test for this patient. The patient's presentation is suggestive of gastric cancer, specifically diffuse gastric cancer. Proposed criteria for selection of patients for genetic testing for hereditary diffuse gastric cancer include the following: family members with two or more documented cases of gastric cancer in first- or second-degree relatives, with at least one diffuse gastric cancer diagnosed before age 50 years; family members with multiple lobular breast cancers with or without diffuse gastric cancer in first- or second-degree relatives; and, a personal diagnosis of diffuse gastric cancer before age 35 years from a low-incidence population such as in Canada and the United States. Based on the patient's young age and history of multiple family members with gastric and lobular breast cancer, hereditary diffuse gastric cancer is a likely diagnosis. The best diagnostic test for gastric cancer is an upper endoscopy with multiple biopsies of the stomach. The syndrome of hereditary diffuse gastric cancer is associated with mutations in the *CDH1* gene. The risk for diffuse gastric cancer approaches 80% in carriers of the mutation, and prophylactic gastrectomy is recommended in mutation carriers who have not developed gastric cancer.

A colonoscopy is not indicated as the initial test because the patient has primarily upper gastrointestinal symptoms. Colon polyps and cancer have been associated with hereditary diffuse gastric cancer, and more frequent screening colonoscopy for colon polyps is indicated in mutation carriers.

Delayed gastric emptying can present with abdominal pain and early satiety but is also often accompanied by nausea and vomiting. The patient has no risk factors for gastroparesis, such as diabetes mellitus, so a gastric emptying study is not indicated.

While *Helicobacter pylori* can present with dyspeptic symptoms, serological testing is not the most appropriate next step for this patient because his weight loss and family history raise concern for gastric cancer.

An upper gastrointestinal radiograph series might show thickened gastric folds related to diffuse gastric cancer, but it cannot be used to obtain biopsies to diagnose cancer.

KEY POINT

- A history of multiple family members with gastric cancer, particularly before age 50 years, or multiple family members with lobular breast cancer with or without gastric cancer, suggest the possibility of hereditary diffuse gastric cancer and the need for upper endoscopy and testing for mutations of the *CDH1* gene.

Bibliography

Syngal S, Brand RE, Church JM, Giardiello FM, Hampel HL, Burt RW; American College of Gastroenterology. ACG clinical guideline: genetic testing and management of hereditary gastrointestinal cancer syndromes. Am J Gastroenterol. 2015;110:223–62; quiz 263. [PMID: 25645574] doi:10.1038/ajg.2014.435

Item 81   Answer: D

Educational Objective: Manage drug-induced liver injury.

Continued observation is the most appropriate management of this patient. Drug-induced liver injury is a rare adverse reaction to medication that can result in jaundice, liver failure, and, potentially, death. This patient meets the criteria for diagnosis, which requires a history of drug or supplement exposure within 6 to 12 months, a biochemical pattern that fits the hepatotoxicity profile of the causative agent (in this case, cholestatic for amoxicillin-clavulanate), improvement after drug removal (dechallenge), and the absence of underlying liver or biliary diseases. The most common medications associated with drug-induced liver injury are antibacterial agents (especially amoxicillin-clavulanate) as well as herbal and dietary supplements. In this patient with drug-induced liver injury and well-preserved liver function, the offending medication has already been discontinued, and observation until resolution of symptoms occurs is the best course of action. The prognosis of drug-induced liver injury is generally good, with 70% of patients recovering without needing hospitalization and 90% recovering without developing acute liver failure.

Endoscopic retrograde cholangiography (ERCP) is used to treat biliary obstruction. In this setting, ultrasound has confirmed the absence of biliary dilation, and, therefore, ERCP would not be expected to provide benefit.

A liver biopsy is rarely necessary in patients with drug-induced liver injury but is helpful in cases of uncertainty or suspected drug-induced autoimmune hepatitis. Zone 3 necrosis and eosinophilia are classic histologic findings in drug-induced liver injury, but other findings may

include hepatitis, cholestasis, steatosis, or granulomas. This patient has a classic presentation, and a cholestatic biochemical profile and negative antibody tests make autoimmune hepatitis unlikely.

No specific antidotes are available for idiosyncratic drug-induced liver injury. The administration of glucocorticoids like prednisone is not indicated unless there is suspicion for drug hypersensitivity reaction. The absence of a morbilliform rash, fever, facial swelling, lymphadenopathy, and substantially elevated aminotransferase levels make a hypersensitivity reaction unlikely and prednisone unnecessary in this patient.

KEY POINT

- In patients with well-preserved liver function, drug-induced liver injury should be managed with discontinuation of the offending medication and observation until resolution of symptoms occurs.

Bibliography

Chalasani NP, Hayashi PH, Bonkovsky HL, Navarro VJ, Lee WM, Fontana RJ; Practice Parameters Committee of the American College of Gastroenterology. ACG clinical guideline: the diagnosis and management of idiosyncratic drug-induced liver injury. Am J Gastroenterol. 2014;109:950–66; quiz 967. [PMID: 24935270] doi:10.1038/ajg.2014.131

Item 82   Answer: C

Educational Objective: Treat centrally mediated abdominal pain syndrome.

Cognitive-behavioral therapy is the most appropriate treatment for this patient. She meets the diagnostic criteria for centrally mediated abdominal pain syndrome (CAPS): near-constant abdominal pain lasting longer than 6 months, involving a large anatomic distribution, and without initiating triggers or alarm features. Treatment includes a combination of pharmacologic and/or psychological therapies. She already takes a selective serotonin reuptake inhibitor for depression, but it has not improved her abdominal pain syndrome. Four classes of psychotherapy have shown benefit in patients with CAPS when combined with medical therapy: cognitive-behavioral therapy, psychodynamic-interpersonal therapy, mindfulness- and acceptance-based therapy, and hypnotherapy.

Irritable bowel syndrome (IBS) is a symptom complex characterized by abdominal pain and altered bowel habits. The diagnosis is made by the fulfillment of symptom-based criteria, including the presence of recurrent abdominal pain or discomfort at least 3 days per month in the last 3 months that is associated with two or more of the following: relief with defecation, onset associated with a change in frequency of stool, or onset associated with a change in form of stool. IBS is further subtyped based on the predominant stool pattern as IBS with predominant constipation (IBS-C), IBS with predominant diarrhea (IBS-D), mixed IBS, or IBS unclassified. CAPS differs from IBS in that there are no consistent initiating triggers and symptoms are not alleviated with bowel movements. The patient reports no constipation, and her pain is not relieved with bowel movements, so IBS is an unlikely diagnosis.

Alosetron is a 5-HT$_3$ antagonist available for women with IBS-D whose symptoms have not responded to conventional therapy; however, owing to an increased risk for severe constipation and ischemic colitis with its use, it is restricted by a mandatory prescribing program. Because this patient does not have IBS, alosetron is not indicated.

Budesonide is indicated in patients with inflammatory bowel disease. This patient reports no chronic diarrhea, a hallmark symptom of inflammatory bowel disease, and a colonoscopy earlier this year was normal, showing no inflammation.

Linaclotide is a guanylate cyclase-C activator used in the treatment of IBS-C after fiber supplementation or osmotic and stimulatory laxative therapy fails. It has no role in the treatment of CAPS.

KEY POINT

- Centrally mediated abdominal pain syndrome is characterized by near-constant abdominal pain lasting longer than 6 months, involving a large anatomic distribution, and without initiating triggers or alarm features.

Bibliography

Keefer L, Drossman DA, Guthrie E, Simrén M, Tillisch K, Olden K, et al. Centrally mediated disorders of gastrointestinal pain. Gastroenterology. 2016. [PMID: 27144628] doi:10.1053/j.gastro.2016.02.034

Item 83   Answer: D

Educational Objective: Treat upper gastrointestinal bleeding.

This patient does not require transfusion. For patients with upper gastrointestinal bleeding, initial resuscitation is the first priority and should include stabilization of blood pressure with infusion of sufficient volumes of crystalloid fluid and/or red blood cells. The decision to transfuse red blood cells is based mainly on the presenting hemoglobin level. In hemodynamically stable patients, a restrictive transfusion strategy (transfusion threshold of less than 7 g/dL [70 g/L] with a target hemoglobin level of 7-9 g/dL [70-90 g/L]) is associated with decreased mortality, length of hospital stay, and transfusion-related adverse events compared to a liberal transfusion strategy (transfusion threshold of less than 9 g/dL [90 g/L] with a target hemoglobin level of 9-10 g/dL [90-100 g/L]). This patient is hemodynamically and physiologically stable with no evidence of ongoing overt gastrointestinal blood loss or symptoms of tissue ischemia; therefore, it is appropriate to continue maintenance intravenous fluids because he is at an appropriate target hemoglobin level of 7 to 9 g/dL (70-90 g/L).

A modification of the restrictive transfusion threshold may be considered in specific subpopulations, such as patients with hypotension due to severe bleeding and

patients with cardiovascular disease. It may be reasonable to give transfusions to patients who are hemodynamically unstable before a decline in hemoglobin level to less than 7 g/dL (70 g/L) to prevent complications of tissue underperfusion. There is uncertainty regarding the need for a higher transfusion threshold in patients with cardiovascular disease, but current guidelines recommend considering transfusion when hemoglobin levels decrease below 8 g/dL (80 g/L) or when cardiovascular symptoms develop (for example, chest pain, dyspnea) in patients who are otherwise hemodynamically stable.

KEY POINT

- In patients with upper gastrointestinal bleeding, a restrictive transfusion strategy (transfusion threshold of less than 7 g/dL [70 g/L] with a target hemoglobin level of 7-9 g/dL [70-90 g/L]) is associated with decreased mortality, length of hospital stay, and transfusion-related adverse events compared to a liberal transfusion strategy.

Bibliography

Fortinsky KJ, Bardou M, Barkun AN. Role of medical therapy for nonvariceal upper gastrointestinal bleeding. Gastrointest Endosc Clin N Am. 2015;25:463-78. [PMID: 26142032] doi:10.1016/j.giec.2015.02.003

Item 84   Answer: C

Educational Objective: Screen for duodenal cancer in a patient with familial adenomatous polyposis syndrome.

Upper endoscopy with duodenoscopy is the most appropriate next test for this patient. The adenomatous polyposis syndromes include familial adenomatous polyposis (FAP) and *MutYH*-associated polyposis (MAP). Patients with FAP and MAP should receive genetic counseling and should be offered genetic testing. Although an autosomal dominant disorder, a positive family history is found in only 54% to 78% of patients diagnosed with FAP. Upper endoscopy with duodenoscopy, using both a standard upper scope and a side viewing scope, is indicated to screen for periampullary and duodenal adenomas and adenocarcinoma. At least 50% of patients with FAP develop adenomatous changes of the periampullary region of the duodenum. Upper-endoscopy screening in patients with FAP should begin at the time of onset of colonic polyps or at age 25 to 30 years, whichever comes first. Upper endoscopy with duodenoscopy for surveillance of duodenal cancer is indicated every 1 to 5 years at an interval based on the stage of the duodenal polyposis.

A barium upper gastrointestinal series has a low sensitivity for periampullary and duodenal adenomas, which may be flat or sessile lesions, and it does not allow for tissue biopsy if lesions are found.

Double-balloon enteroscopy allows endoscopy to reach the entire small-bowel lumen and is used in patients with occult gastrointestinal blood loss to look for a source of bleeding and provide therapeutic options. It may also be used to remove small-bowel mucosal lesions such as adenomas

Answers and Critiques

if they are located beyond the reach of a standard esophagogastroduodenoscopy (EGD). Double-balloon enteroscopy requires longer anesthesia time and is higher-risk than standard EGD, and its availability is limited. Therefore, it is not the standard recommended procedure for initial screening for duodenal and periampullary adenomas in patients with FAP.

Patients with FAP should undergo upper endoscopy because there is more than a 50% chance of discovering duodenal adenomas at the first upper endoscopy. Conducting no further tests in this patient would be an inappropriate approach, given the high probability of finding one or more potentially premalignant lesions.

KEY POINT

- Upper-endoscopy screening for duodenal cancer in patients with familial adenomatous polyposis should begin at onset of colonic polyposis or at age 25 to 30 years, whichever comes first.

Bibliography

Syngal S, Brand RE, Church JM, Giardiello FM, Hampel HL, Burt RW; American College of Gastroenterology. ACG clinical guideline: genetic testing and management of hereditary gastrointestinal cancer syndromes. Am J Gastroenterol. 2015;110:223-62; quiz 263. [PMID: 25645574] doi:10.1038/ajg.2014.435

Item 85   Answer: B

Educational Objective: **Manage colonoscopy surveillance following polypectomy.**

This patient should undergo surveillance colonoscopy in 3 years. Current recommendations emphasize that an adequate bowel preparation and a high-quality colonoscopy that reaches and examines the cecum are required for an adequate screening examination. Screening colonoscopy studies demonstrate that polyps are detected in approximately 60% of average-risk individuals. The prevalence of polyps on average-risk screening colonoscopy is 22% to 25% for adenomas, 12% for hyperplastic polyps, and 0.6% for sessile serrated polyps. The degree of dysplasia in a polyp is reported as high or low. Adenomatous polyps are neoplastic lesions and, therefore, have malignant potential; most colorectal cancers arise from adenomatous polyps. Adenomatous polyps are further defined by their glandular architecture: tubular, villous, or a combination of both. The most common pattern is tubular, followed by tubulovillous, with the least common pattern being villous. After neoplastic polyps (adenomas, sessile serrated polyps, or traditional serrated adenomas) are completely resected, postpolypectomy colonoscopy should be performed; the surveillance interval depends on the size, number, and pathology of the polyp. This patient was found to have three tubular adenomas smaller than 1 cm in size. The presence of three or more adenomas, any adenoma greater than or equal to 1 cm in size, or any adenoma with villous features or high-grade dysplasia has been associated with increased risk for metachronous neoplasia (multiple primary tumors developing at different time intervals), warranting a 3-year surveillance interval.

Guidelines recommend screening average-risk individuals beginning at age 50 years. Repeat colonoscopy is based on initial findings. Individuals with no adenomas should have a repeat colonoscopy in 10 years. Individuals who have two or fewer tubular adenomas are also considered low-risk for colon cancer and should repeat screening in 5 to 10 years. Appropriate follow-up recommendations after screening colonoscopy, including avoidance of inappropriate use of colonoscopy after removal of adenomatous polyps, are core gastroenterology quality measures.

High-risk findings include more than 10 polyps on baseline colonoscopic examination, which should prompt consideration for a polyposis syndrome. These individuals should have a follow-up colonoscopy in less than 3 years, depending on polyp burden and polyposis syndrome. Any patient who has a polyp removed piecemeal should return within 3 to 6 months for repeat colonoscopy, especially if there is any concern for incomplete polyp removal.

KEY POINT

- Patients with three or more adenomas on screening colonoscopy should undergo surveillance colonoscopy in 3 years.

Bibliography

Lieberman DA, Rex DK, Winawer SJ, Giardiello FM, Johnson DA, Levin TR; United States Multi-Society Task Force on Colorectal Cancer. Guidelines for colonoscopy surveillance after screening and polypectomy: a consensus update by the US Multi-Society Task Force on Colorectal Cancer. Gastroenterology. 2012;143:844-57. [PMID: 22763141] doi:10.1053/j.gastro.2012.06.001

Item 86   Answer: C

Educational Objective: **Treat functional dyspepsia.**

Starting a trial of a tricyclic antidepressant is the most appropriate next step in the management of this patient. The patient has functional dyspepsia meeting the diagnostic criteria for epigastric pain syndrome: (1) bothersome postprandial fullness; (2) early satiety; (3) epigastric pain; and/or (4) epigastric burning for at least 3 days per week. These criteria should be met for the 3 months leading up to diagnosis, with symptoms starting at least 6 months before diagnosis and with no evidence of structural disease to explain the symptoms. The absence of an underlying organic disease is demonstrated by this patient's normal upper endoscopy, including gastric and small-bowel biopsies, as well as normal laboratory testing and the lack of alarm features such as vomiting, weight loss, or family history of gastrointestinal malignancy. Because she tested negative for *Helicobacter pylori* infection and her symptoms did not respond to a trial of once-daily omeprazole for a minimum of 4 weeks, the recommended next step in the treatment of functional dyspepsia is a trial of a tricyclic antidepressant. In the treatment of functional dyspepsia, this class of antidepressants was found to be more effective than other classes, including selective serotonin reuptake inhibitors or serotonin-norepinephrine reuptake inhibitors.

Given this patient's absence of alarm symptoms and normal laboratory test results, further structural testing with CT imaging or abdominal ultrasonography is likely to be of low yield; therefore, such testing is neither clinically indicated nor cost effective.

A gastric emptying test is used to evaluate suspected gastroparesis. Gastroparesis commonly presents with symptoms of early satiety, postprandial fullness, nausea, vomiting, upper abdominal pain, bloating, and weight loss; this patient's lack of compatible symptoms makes the diagnosis unlikely.

There is no evidence that a higher dose of a proton pump inhibitor performs better in the treatment of functional dyspepsia than once-daily omeprazole, which did not alleviate the patient's symptoms.

KEY POINT

- First-line treatment for functional dyspepsia is once-daily omeprazole for at least 4 weeks; if symptoms do not respond, a tricyclic antidepressant is the next recommended treatment.

Bibliography

Moayyedi PM, Lacy BE, Andrews CN, Enns RA, Howden CW, Vakil N. ACG and CAG clinical guideline: management of dyspepsia. Am J Gastroenterol. 2017;112:988-1013. [PMID: 28631728] doi:10.1038/ajg.2017.154

Item 87   Answer: C

Educational Objective: Treat cryoglobulinemia in a patient with chronic hepatitis C viral infection.

A combination of ledipasvir and sofosbuvir is the most appropriate treatment for this patient. The patient has Meltzer triad–consisting of asthenia, arthralgia, and palpable purpura–which is the classic presentation of type II mixed cryoglobulinemia, a vasculitis that most often arises in the context of chronic hepatitis C virus (HCV) infection. Meltzer triad is seen in less than 30% of patients, but nearly all patients with type II cryoglobulinemia develop cutaneous findings, as seen in this patient. Other findings may include peripheral neuropathy; membranoproliferative glomerulonephritis; and pulmonary, central nervous system, or gastrointestinal vasculitis. Urinalysis may show dysmorphic erythrocytes and proteinuria, which are features of glomerulonephritis, but this patient shows no evidence of kidney involvement or other end-organ damage. The best initial treatment for a mild presentation of mixed cryoglobulinemia arising from chronic HCV infection is to treat and eradicate HCV with sofosbuvir-ledipasvir. Other direct-acting antiviral agents that could be used interchangeably to treat genotype 1 HCV include grazoprevir-elbasvir; paritaprevir-ritonavir, ombitasvir, and dasabuvir; glecaprevir-pibrentasvir; sofosbuvir-daclatasvir; and sofosbuvir-velpatasvir. It is expected that other combinations of direct-acting antivirals will be developed. Treatment of HCV infection with direct-acting antiviral combinations results in a sustained virologic response (cure) in more than 90% of patients, even in those who were previously and unsuccessfully treated with pegylated interferon and ribavirin. In approximately 90% of cases, eradication of HCV leads to resolution of the mixed cryoglobulinemia.

Most of the data pertaining to the treatment of HCV infection in patients with mixed cryoglobulinemia involve treatment with pegylated interferon and ribavirin. However, pegylated interferon and ribavirin are no longer recommended for treatment of HCV infection due to adverse effects and lower efficacy compared to interferon-free, direct-acting antiviral therapy.

For severe end-organ damage from mixed cryoglobulinemia, including kidney failure, gastrointestinal vasculitis, rapidly progressive neuropathy, pulmonary or central nervous system vasculitis, or heart failure, rituximab is a first-line agent and may be used with pulse-dose glucocorticoids. However, this patient has mild manifestations of mixed cryoglobulinemia and, therefore, does not require immunosuppressive therapy with rituximab, cyclophosphamide, or glucocorticoids.

KEY POINT

- Mixed cryoglobulinemia arising from chronic hepatitis C viral infection resolves after treatment and eradication of the virus.

Bibliography

Dammacco F, Sansonno D. Therapy for hepatitis C virus-related cryoglobulinemic vasculitis. N Engl J Med. 2013;369:1035-45. [PMID: 24024840] doi:10.1056/NEJMra1208642

Item 88   Answer: B

Educational Objective: Treat microscopic colitis.

Budesonide is the most appropriate treatment for this patient. Her primary symptom of chronic watery diarrhea, colonoscopy results showing normal-appearing mucosa, and biopsy results revealing lymphocytic infiltration and a subepithelial collagen band are diagnostic for collagenous colitis. Collagenous colitis is a subtype of microscopic colitis. It is a clinicopathologic diagnosis made based on clinical presentation, endoscopy features, and histopathology. The condition occurs more commonly in women than in men and typically presents with abrupt or gradual onset of watery diarrhea that has a relapsing and remitting course over months to years. Mild weight loss may occur. The colonic mucosa is macroscopically normal, and inflammatory changes are only appreciated on histopathologic review of colon biopsy specimens. Several medication classes, including NSAIDs, selective serotonin reuptake inhibitors, and proton pump inhibitors, have been associated with the development of microscopic colitis. The first step in management is to discontinue a potentially causative medication. Supportive treatment with antidiarrheal agents such loperamide can be tried as initial treatment. For patients like this one, whose symptoms do not respond to antidiarrheal medication, the

American Gastroenterological Association (AGA) strongly recommends, based on moderate-quality evidence, the use of budesonide for induction of clinical remission of microscopic colitis because of its favorable harm-benefit profile and convenience of once-daily dosing. The rate of relapse after discontinuation of budesonide is high, and maintenance therapy with the lowest possible dose to maintain remission may be required. Patients treated with budesonide for longer than 6 months should be monitored for corticosteroid-related adverse effects.

Because budesonide is expensive, alternative treatments such as bismuth salicylate may be considered if cost is a determining factor. The AGA conditionally recommends, based on low-quality evidence, bismuth subsalicylate for induction of remission when budesonide therapy is not feasible. Bismuth subsalicylate therapy consists of two to three 262-mg tablets taken orally three to four times daily.

The benefit of mesalamine in achieving clinical remission in microscopic colitis is uncertain, and it is recommended as a potential second-line therapy.

Prednisone should not be used as first-line treatment of microscopic colitis because of its unfavorable side effects, but it may be considered in patients who have microscopic colitis refractory to budesonide.

The AGA conditionally recommends, based on low-quality evidence, against the use of probiotics over no treatment for induction of clinical remission. Various probiotic strains, dosages, and formulations are available, but most have not been evaluated in the treatment of microscopic colitis.

KEY POINT

- The first step in the management of microscopic colitis is to discontinue a potentially causative medication, after which supportive treatment with antidiarrheal agents such loperamide can be tried, with budesonide recommended for patients whose symptoms do not respond.

Bibliography
Pardi DS, Tremaine WJ, Carrasco-Labra A. American Gastroenterological Association Institute technical review on the medical management of microscopic colitis. Gastroenterology. 2016;150:247-274.e11. [PMID: 26584602] doi:10.1053/j.gastro.2015.11.006

Item 89   Answer: A
Educational Objective: Manage hepatic adenoma.

The most appropriate management is to discontinue the oral contraceptive agent. Hepatocellular adenomas are generally seen in women because they can be dependent on estrogen for growth. They may also occur in men, and these adenomas carry a higher risk for malignant transformation. Hepatic adenomas may also be associated with anabolic-steroid use, obesity, and the metabolic syndrome. They are often solitary, ranging in size from 1 to 30 cm. Most patients are asymptomatic, and the adenoma is discovered incidentally during imaging for unrelated problems or because of

right-upper-quadrant abdominal pain. The diagnosis is often based on the characteristic imaging findings in a woman of reproductive age. Histology can confirm the diagnosis, but biopsy is not always needed in cases where imaging findings are characteristic; needle biopsy is avoided because it is associated with bleeding.

Hepatic adenomas may increase in size during pregnancy. Women with adenomas greater than 2 cm who are contemplating pregnancy, or who are pregnant, can be treated with radiofrequency ablation but the decision to treat and the treatment modality must be individualized.

The natural history and prognosis of hepatic adenomas is ill-defined. The risk for malignant transformation of hepatic adenomas is approximately 10%. Adenomas larger than 5 cm in size have an increased risk for bleeding that can occasionally cause hemodynamic compromise. In general terms, surgical resection is typically recommended for any symptomatic hepatic adenoma, adenomas 5 cm or larger, or an adenoma found in a male.

Asymptomatic women who are taking estrogen-containing oral contraceptive agents and who have adenomas smaller than 5 cm in size can be managed conservatively, as the risk for hemorrhage or malignant transformation is relatively low. However, liver imaging should be conducted every 6 months for at least 2 years to ensure that the lesion is not growing. Most adenomas tend to regress or even disappear when oral contraceptive agents are discontinued. Failure to regress, continued growth, or an elevation of the α-fetoprotein level may be an indication for surgical resection.

KEY POINT

- For women with asymptomatic hepatic adenomas smaller than 5 cm in size, estrogen-containing oral contraceptive agents should be discontinued, and follow-up liver imaging is recommended every 6 months for at least 2 years.

Bibliography
Marrero JA, Ahn J, Rajender Reddy K; Americal College of Gastroenterology. ACG clinical guideline: the diagnosis and management of focal liver lesions. Am J Gastroenterol. 2014;109:1328-47; quiz 1348. [PMID: 25135008] doi:10.1038/ajg.2014.213

Item 90   Answer: A
Educational Objective: Evaluate the small bowel for a source of gastrointestinal bleeding.

The most appropriate next step in management of this patient is capsule endoscopy. The patient has occult gastrointestinal bleeding, indicated by unexplained iron deficiency anemia with stool testing positive for occult blood and no source of bleeding identified on repeated endoscopy and colonoscopy. The next step is evaluation for potential small-bowel bleeding. Causes of small-bowel bleeding depend on the patient's age. In older patients, vascular lesions such as angiodysplasia account for up to 40% of cases. Capsule endoscopy is noninvasive and is generally able to visualize the entire small bowel. The main disadvantages are its inability to sample tissue or treat findings. Its overall diagnostic yield ranges from 30% to 70%. Capsule endoscopy is contraindicated in patients with gastroparesis, swallowing difficulty, and partial bowel obstructions, and in any patient who cannot undergo follow-up surgery. Capsule endoscopy has become the first-line test in evaluating the small bowel after a negative endoscopy and colonoscopy in patients with gastrointestinal bleeding of an unknown cause.

CT enterography should be considered for patients presenting with or having a history of small-bowel obstruction where a lesion or mass is suspected. Patients aged 40 years or younger who present with occult small-bowel bleeding are more likely to have tumors (leiomyoma, carcinoid, adenocarcinoma, or lymphoma) as the cause of bleeding.

Push enteroscopy is performed with advancement of the endoscope beyond the ligament of Treitz into the jejunum. The depth of insertion is operator dependent but is also limited because of looping of the scope in the stomach. The diagnostic yield is between 24% and 56%. The primary disadvantage of using push enteroscopy is that the amount of additional small bowel that can be examined is limited compared to capsule endoscopy; however, it does allow for tissue sampling and therapeutic intervention. Studies have shown that sequencing capsule endoscopy followed by push enteroscopy is an effective approach for management of occult small-bowel bleeding.

The diagnostic yield of radiographic imaging with small-bowel follow-through is very low (0%-5%) and, therefore, should not be used in the evaluation of suspected small-bowel bleeding.

KEY POINT

- Capsule endoscopy is the most appropriate test to evaluate patients for causes of small-bowel bleeding after negative upper endoscopy and colonoscopy.

Bibliography
Gerson LB, Fidler JL, Cave DR, Leighton JA. ACG clinical guideline: diagnosis and management of small bowel bleeding. Am J Gastroenterol. 2015;110:1265-87; quiz 1288. [PMID: 26303132] doi:10.1038/ajg.2015.246

Item 91   Answer: D

Educational Objective: Treat chronic hepatitis B viral infection in its immune-active, hepatitis B e antigen–positive phase.

Tenofovir is the most appropriate treatment for this patient. Entecavir would be an equally suitable choice. Chronic hepatitis B virus (HBV) infection is characteristically divided into phases of disease. Not all patients go through each phase. Patients in the hepatitis B e antigen (HBeAg)-positive ("immune-active") or HBeAg-negative ("reactivation") phases have an elevated alanine aminotransferase (ALT) level and an HBV DNA level above 10,000 IU/mL. The patient has chronic HBV infection in the immune-active, HBeAg-positive phase, with ALT and aspartate aminotransferase levels exceeding two times the

upper limit of normal and HBV DNA exceeding 20,000 IU/mL. Treatment is necessary to decrease hepatic inflammation, risk for progression to fibrosis, and eventual cirrhosis that will occur without treatment. In approximately 50% of untreated patients with chronic HBV infection in the United States, HBV infection will contribute to the cause of death (from hepatocellular carcinoma or other complications of end-stage liver disease, such as cirrhosis). Patients who respond to treatment have a decreased risk of liver-related complications of HBV infection. Tenofovir or entecavir is first-line treatment for immune-active HBV infection because of low rates of resistance. Treatment goals for HBV infection in the immune-active, HBeAg-positive phase are loss of HBeAg and anti–hepatitis B e antibody seroconversion. For most patients, chronic treatment is necessary because seroconversion of HBeAg or hepatitis B surface antigen is not commonly achieved.

Adefovir and lamivudine are not preferred antiviral agents given the risk for HBV resistance. Resistance rates at 5 years are approximately 30% for adefovir and 70% for lamivudine.

In this patient, oral antiviral regimens are preferred over pegylated interferon because pegylated interferon may exacerbate psoriasis. Pegylated interferon is most appropriate for patients who have higher ALT levels, low HBV DNA levels, and no cirrhosis.

KEY POINT

- Chronic hepatitis B viral infection in the immune-active, hepatitis B e antigen–positive phase should be treated with tenofovir or entecavir to decrease hepatic inflammation and the risk for progression to fibrosis.

Bibliography
Terrault NA, Bzowej NH, Chang KM, Hwang JP, Jonas MM, Murad MH; American Association for the Study of Liver Diseases. AASLD guidelines for treatment of chronic hepatitis B. Hepatology. 2016;63:261-83. [PMID: 26566064] doi:10.1002/hep.28156

Item 92   Answer: C

Educational Objective: Treat irritable bowel syndrome with predominant constipation.

A trial of polyethylene glycol (PEG) 3350 therapy is the most appropriate next step for this patient. She has abdominal discomfort and a change in bowel habits predominated by constipation; these symptoms fulfill the diagnostic criteria for irritable bowel syndrome with predominant constipation (IBS-C). Given her young age and lack of any alarm features, such as blood in the stool, anemia, or a first-degree family member with colon cancer, a diagnosis of IBS-C can be made and treatment can be initiated. The soluble fiber supplement psyllium has demonstrated limited efficacy in IBS, primarily addressing stool frequency and consistency. Insoluble fiber supplements such as bran appear to worsen IBS-C symptoms. Although various surfactant, osmotic, and stimulant laxatives can be used for the constipation symptoms

Answers and Critiques

associated with IBS-C, only the osmotic laxative PEG has been tested in IBS. PEG 3350 has demonstrated efficacy in IBS, and a trial of it is an appropriate first step in management.

A colonoscopy is not warranted, given this patient's age and the nature of her symptoms. The remote family history of colorectal cancer does not increase her risk enough to require a colonoscopy at this time.

This patient has no risk factors for small intestinal bacterial overgrowth, such as small-bowel disease, previous bowel resection, or a primary/secondary gastrointestinal motility disorder; therefore, a glucose breath test is not indicated. Bloating is commonly reported in patients with IBS. If bloating persists after correction of constipation, then testing for small intestinal bacterial overgrowth could be considered.

Although symptoms of bloating, abdominal pain, and constipation can occur in celiac disease, this patient's symptoms do not warrant serum anti–tissue transglutaminase antibody testing for celiac disease. Testing would be indicated if she had a first-degree relative with celiac disease or if she had symptoms of IBS with predominant diarrhea (IBS-D) or IBS with mixed diarrhea and constipation. Furthermore, results of testing for celiac antibodies such as the anti–tissue transglutaminase may be normal in patients on a gluten-free diet. The patient's response to gluten elimination does not necessarily indicate celiac disease because gluten is a FODMAP (Fermentable Oligosaccharides, Disaccharides, Monosaccharides, And Polyols) carbohydrate, which can cause bloating due to FODMAP intolerance.

KEY POINT

- Polyethylene glycol 3350 is a first-line treatment for patients whose symptoms meet the criteria for irritable bowel syndrome with predominant constipation.

Bibliography
Mearin F, Lacy BE, Chang L, Chey WD, Lembo AJ, Simren M, et al. Bowel disorders. Gastroenterology. 2016. [PMID: 27144627] doi:10.1053/j.gastro.2016.02.031

Item 93   Answer: C

Educational Objective: Treat *Helicobacter pylori* infection persisting after treatment.

Bismuth, metronidazole, omeprazole, and tetracycline for 14 days is the most appropriate treatment regimen for this patient. The salvage therapy regimen should consist of different antibiotics from those used in the initial, unsuccessful regimen. This strategy reduces the likelihood of antibiotic resistance, the major reason for treatment failure.

Additional factors in choosing salvage therapy after initial treatment failure include a history of quinolone antibiotic use and penicillin allergy. If the initial unsuccessful treatment was clarithromycin triple therapy and the patient is allergic to penicillin, the best salvage therapy is a bismuth quadruple therapy (bismuth, metronidazole, omeprazole, and tetracycline). In patients with no penicillin allergy, but

whose history includes quinolone antibiotic use for any reason, salvage therapies could include bismuth quadruple therapy, rifabutin triple therapy (rifabutin, penicillin, and a proton pump inhibitor [PPI] such as omeprazole) or high-dose dual therapy (amoxicillin and a PPI). Disruption of therapy can cause treatment failure, and the likelihood of treatment success diminishes with each successive treatment attempt. It is essential to counsel the patient carefully on the importance of treatment adherence and potential side effects of the therapy.

Treatment with the same regimen (amoxicillin, clarithromycin, and omeprazole) for a longer period of time will be ineffective because the patient's *Helicobacter pylori* infection is likely resistant to clarithromycin and/or penicillin.

The combination of amoxicillin, metronidazole, and omeprazole is not a recognized treatment regimen for *H. pylori* in any setting. Metronidazole is typically used in patients with penicillin allergy.

Using metronidazole rather than amoxicillin is unlikely to result in *H. pylori* eradication because resistance to clarithromycin is also a likely cause of the initial treatment's failure. Furthermore, the regimen of clarithromycin, metronidazole, and omeprazole could lead to the development of metronidazole resistance in the likely event of treatment failure with this regimen.

KEY POINT

- For *Helicobacter pylori* infection that persists after eradication therapy, the salvage therapy regimen should consist of different antibiotics from those used in the initial, unsuccessful regimen.

Bibliography
Chey WD, Leontiadis GI, Howden CW, Moss SF. ACG clinical guideline: treatment of *Helicobacter pylori* infection. Am J Gastroenterol. 2017;112:212-239. [PMID: 28071659] doi:10.1038/ajg.2016.563

Item 94   Answer: C   H

Educational Objective: Diagnose hepatorenal syndrome.

Hepatorenal syndrome is the most likely diagnosis in this patient. In patients with end-stage liver disease and portal hypertension, hepatorenal syndrome is characterized by the development of oliguric kidney failure, bland urine sediment, and marked sodium retention (edema, ascites, low urinary sodium). Two types of hepatorenal syndrome have been recognized. Type 1 is characterized by acute kidney dysfunction and is usually triggered by a precipitating event such as spontaneous bacterial peritonitis, other infections, gastrointestinal hemorrhage, or a major surgical procedure. Type 2 is more common and is characterized by more slowly progressive kidney failure in patients with refractory ascites. Type 1 hepatorenal syndrome is characterized by a rise in serum creatinine of at least 0.3 mg/dL (26 µmol/L) and/or ≥50% from baseline within 48 hours with a bland urinalysis and normal findings on renal ultrasonography. It is also supported by a lack of

CONT.
improvement in kidney function after withdrawal of diuretics and two days of volume expansion with intravenous albumin. Often patients with hepatorenal syndrome also have low urine sodium, low fractional excretion of sodium, and oliguria. In addition, patients should have no evidence of shock, no current or recent use of nephrotoxic drugs, and no evidence of renal parenchymal disease (proteinuria less than 0.5 g/day, no microhematuria, and normal renal ultrasound). The main treatment of hepatorenal syndrome is the removal of drugs that may reduce kidney perfusion and volume expansion. Ultimately, hepatorenal syndrome is a condition for which the only cure is liver transplantation.

Acute interstitial nephritis may be associated with drugs, infection, autoimmune diseases, and malignancy. It should be suspected in a patient who presents with an elevated serum creatinine level and urinalysis showing leukocytes, leukocyte casts, and possibly eosinophiluria; urinary sodium level is typically elevated.

Acute tubular necrosis is most commonly caused by ischemia or toxins (including drugs). Urinalysis typically shows pigmented granular (muddy brown) casts and tubular epithelial cells; urinary sodium is typically elevated.

Membranous glomerulonephritis is associated with the nephrotic syndrome (proteinuria, edema, hypertension, microhematuria) and erythrocytes or erythrocyte casts; urinary sodium can be low.

KEY POINT

- In patients with end-stage liver disease and portal hypertension, hepatorenal syndrome is characterized by the development of oliguric kidney failure, bland urine sediment, and marked sodium retention (edema, ascites, low urinary sodium).

Bibliography
Glass L, Sharma P. Evidence-based therapeutic options for hepatorenal syndrome. Gastroenterology. 2016;150:1031-3. [PMID: 26922867] doi:10.1053/j.gastro.2016.02.050

Item 95   Answer: D

Educational Objective: Manage walled-off necrosis after acute pancreatitis.

The most appropriate management of the fluid collection is observation. Walled-off necrosis of the pancreas is the most likely diagnosis. The pancreatic fluid collection incidentally found during kidney stone–protocol CT corresponds to the location of pancreatic necrosis during his acute gallstone pancreatitis 6 months earlier. By definition, acute necrotic collections are classified as walled-off necrosis after 4 weeks. The necrotic tissue liquifies with time and develops a mature wall as part of the healing process, as seen on imaging. These fluid collections do not require therapy if they are asymptomatic, and as many as 60% may resolve spontaneously within 1 year; fluid-related complications are rare.

Areas of pancreatic necrosis are frequently identified on imaging during an episode of acute pancreatitis. Patients with uninfected pancreatic necrosis do not benefit from antibiotic use during the acute phase of pancreatitis or later, in the resolving stage. Patients whose condition does not improve or deteriorates 7 to 10 days after presentation of acute pancreatitis may have infected necrosis. CT-guided fine-needle aspiration may help guide treatment decisions regarding antibiotic use, drainage, and continued supportive care. Neither CT-guided fine-needle aspiration nor antibiotic therapy is needed in this asymptomatic patient with walled-off necrosis of the pancreas that is likely to resolve spontaneously. The patient's left flank pain is due to passage of a kidney stone, not the pancreatic fluid collection.

Many walled-off necroses of the pancreas resolve spontaneously, but some persist, enlarge, have a mass effect, and/or cause symptoms. Symptomatic collections may require decompression or debridement. However, this patient is asymptomatic and no intervention is required at this time.

KEY POINT

- Asymptomatic patients with walled-off necrosis of the pancreas require no intervention.

Bibliography
Tyberg A, Karia K, Gabr M, Desai A, Doshi R, Gaidhane M, et al. Management of pancreatic fluid collections: a comprehensive review of the literature. World J Gastroenterol. 2016;22:2256-70. [PMID: 26900288] doi:10.3748/wjg.v22.i7.2256

Item 96   Answer: C

Educational Objective: Screen for hepatocellular carcinoma in a patient with cirrhosis.

The most appropriate management for this patient is ultrasonography screening for hepatocellular carcinoma every 6 months. Liver diseases associated with the highest risk for hepatocellular carcinoma are hepatitis B virus (HBV) and hepatitis C virus (HCV) infections and hemochromatosis. Approximately 80% of hepatocellular carcinoma occurs in patients with cirrhosis, but it can develop in the absence of cirrhosis in patients with HBV infection. All patients with cirrhosis from any cause should undergo liver ultrasonography every 6 months with or without α-fetoprotein measurement. Patients with HCV infection who achieve sustained virologic response (which is synonymous with virologic cure) have a reduced risk for hepatocellular carcinoma. Regardless of virologic response, surveillance is recommended for patients with stage 3 or stage 4 fibrosis (stage 4 fibrosis signifies cirrhosis, as found in this patient).

Liver transplantation evaluation is not indicated for this patient with Child-Turcotte-Pugh Class A cirrhosis and a very low Model for End-Stage Liver Disease (MELD) score. Indications for liver transplantation are a MELD score of at least 15 or decompensated cirrhosis. Virologic cure in patients with compensated cirrhosis prevents decompensation. However, development of hepatocellular carcinoma would be a reason for referral for liver transplantation evaluation.

Measuring HCV RNA again in 12 weeks is not indicated because this patient has achieved virologic cure with undetectable HCV RNA at week 12 after completing treatment for HCV infection. Large studies have demonstrated 98% to 99% concordance between sustained virologic response at 12 and at 24 weeks. Therefore, sustained virologic response at 12 weeks is considered to be consistent with virologic cure, and additional testing is unnecessary.

Upper endoscopy is not necessary because the patient had an upper endoscopy 1 year ago. The standard follow-up interval for small varices in a patient who is not taking a nonselective β-blocker is 2 years.

KEY POINT

- Patients with hepatitis C viral infection who achieve sustained virologic response have a reduced risk for hepatocellular carcinoma; regardless of virologic response, ultrasonographic surveillance is recommended for patients with stage 3 or stage 4 fibrosis.

Bibliography
Morgan RL, Baack B, Smith BD, Yartel A, Pitasi M, Falck-Ytter Y. Eradication of hepatitis C virus infection and the development of hepatocellular carcinoma: a meta-analysis of observational studies. Ann Intern Med. 2013;158:329-37. [PMID: 23460056]

Answers and Critiques

Index

Note: Page numbers followed by f and t indicates figure and table respectively. Test questions are indicated by Q.

A

Pantoprazole, for chronic GERD, Q59
Parvovirus B19, 55
Pegylated interferon, for HBV infection, 52–53
Pelvic floor dyssynergia, 35. *See also* Constipation
Pelvic floor muscle training, for fecal incontinence, 42
Penicillin G, for *Amanita* mushroom poisoning, 57
Peptic ulcer disease (PUD), 11–13
    causes of, 11
    complications of, 11
    diagnosis of, 11
    epigastric pain in, 11
    and GI bleeding, 70
    and *Helicobacter pylori* infection, 11–12
    idiopathic, 11
    management of, 12
    and NSAIDs, 11, 12, Q10
    perforated, 11, 12
Perianal disorders, 41–43
    anal cancer, 42–43, 43f
    anal fissures, 42, 42f
    fecal incontinence, 42
    hemorrhoids, 41–42, 41f
Peripancreatic fluid collections, acute, 21
Peroral endoscopic myotomy, for achalasia, 7
Peutz-Jeghers syndrome (PJS), 48, 49f
Pharyngoesophageal (Zenker) diverticulum, 2, Q7
Phenytoin, and liver injury, 56
Pill-induced esophagitis, 6
Plecanatide, for constipation, 36t
Pneumatic dilation, for achalasia, 7
Pneumatosis intestinalis, 39
Polyartheritis nodosa, Q25
Polyethylene glycol 3350, for constipation, 36t, Q92
Polymerase proofreading-associated polyposis (PPAP), 48
Porcelain gallbladder, 67
Portal hypertensive gastropathy, 60–61
Portal vein thrombosis, 66–67
Portal venous gas, 39
Portopulmonary hypertension, 63
Postpolypectomy bleeding, 74. *See also* Gastrointestinal bleeding, lower
Postprandial distress syndrome, 10. *See also* Dyspepsia
    Rome 4 diagnostic criteria for, 10t
PPI. *See* Proton pump inhibitor (PPI)
Prednisone
    for autoimmune hepatitis, 55
    for autoimmune pancreatitis, 24
    in pregnancy, 66
Pregnancy
    acute fatty liver of, 66
    intrahepatic cholestasis of, 66, Q60
    liver disease in, 66
Primary biliary cholangitis (PBC), 58–59
    liver chemistry studies in, 50t
Primary sclerosing cholangitis (PSC), 32, 34, 59, Q43
    liver chemistry studies in, 50t
Probiotics, for IBS-C, 37
Proctitis, 30
Prothrombin time, 49–50
Proton pump inhibitor (PPI), 2
    adverse effects of, 5t
    for Barrett esophagus, 9
    for dyspepsia, 11
    for eosinophilic esophagitis, Q70
    for gastrinomas, 25
    for gastroesophageal reflux disease, 4–5, Q44, Q59
    for NSAID-induced injury, 15–16
    for peptic ulcer disease, 12
    for upper GI bleeding, 71
Prucalopride, for constipation, 36t
Pseudoachalasia, 6, Q5
Psychotherapy, for centrally mediated abdominal pain syndrome, 38
PTEN hamartoma syndrome (PJS), 48
Pyridoxin, for hyperemesis gravidarum, 66

R
Rectal bleeding, Q22
Refractory celiac disease, 29
Regorafenib, for hepatocellular carcinoma, 65
Regurgitation, in gastroesophageal reflux disease, 3–4
Reynold pentad, 69
Rifaximin
    for chronic diarrhea, 28

for hepatic encephalopathy, 61
for IBS-D, 37
Rituximab, for autoimmune pancreatitis, 24

S
Schatzki ring, 2, 2f
Screening
    for Barrett esophagus, 8
    for colorectal cancer, 44–45, 45t
Secretagogues, 36t
Serologic testing
    for *Helicobacter pylori* infection, 13
Serotonergic agent, for constipation, 36t
Serrated polyposis syndrome, 44, 48
Serrated polyps, 44, 44f, Q11
Serum ceruloplasmin measurement, for Wilson disease, Q55
Short bowel syndrome, 29–30
Sitophobia, in chronic mesenteric ischemia, 40
Small and large bowel, disorders of
    anorectal disorders, 41–43
    carbohydrate malabsorption, 30
    celiac disease, 28–29
    centrally mediated abdominal pain syndrome, 38
    constipation, 35–37
    diarrhea, 26–28
    diverticular disease, 38–39
    inflammatory bowel disease, 30–35
    irritable bowel syndrome, 37–38
    ischemic bowel disease, 39–41
    nonceliac gluten sensitivity, 29
    short bowel syndrome, 29–30
    small intestinal bacterial overgrowth, 29
Small-bowel bleeding, 70, 75–77
    angiodysplasia and, 75, 75f
    causes of, 75, 75f, 75t
    evaluation of, 75–77
    management of, 77
    occult, 75
    overt, 75
Small intestinal bacterial overgrowth (SIBO), 29
Somatostatin analogs, for gastrinomas, 25
Sorafenib, for hepatocellular carcinoma, 65
Spontaneous bacterial peritonitis (SBP), 61–62, Q27
    diagnosis of, 62
    treatment for, 62
Steatorrhea, 26t, 27
Stimulant laxatives, 36t
Stool antigen testing, for *Helicobacter pylori*, 13, Q52
Stool enzyme–linked immunosorbent assay, for *Giardia* infection, 26
Stool softeners, 36t
Strictures, in Crohn disease, 31

T
Technetium-labeled nuclear scan, for small-bowel bleeding, 76
Teduglutide, for short bowel syndrome, 30
Telbivudine
    for HBV infection, 52
    in pregnancy, 66
Tenesmus, in ulcerative colitis, 30
Tenofovir
    for HBV infection, 52, Q30, Q91
    in pregnancy, 66
Thalidomide, 77
Thiopurines, for inflammatory bowel disease, 33
Toxic megacolon, Q14
Transabdominal ultrasonography, for acute pancreatitis, 20
Transfer dysphagia. *See* Oropharyngeal dysphagia
Transjugular intrahepatic portosystemic shunt (TIPS), for gastric varices, 61
Transoral incisionless fundoplication, 5
Tricyclic antidepressants
    for functional dyspepsia, Q86
    for IBS-D, 38
Trientine, 58
Tumor necrosis factor (TNF)-α, 33

U
Ulcerative colitis, 30, Q54. *See also* Inflammatory bowel disease (IBD)
    clinical presentation of, 30, 31t
    left-sided, Q51
    therapy for, 33, 33f
Ultrasonography
    for acalculous cholecystitis, 68

A — NAME AND ADDRESS (Please complete.)

Last Name   First Name   Middle Initial

Address

Address cont.

City   State   ZIP Code

Country

Email address

ACP®
American College of Physicians
Leading Internal Medicine, Improving Lives

Medical Knowledge Self-Assessment Program® 18

TO EARN *CME Credits and/or MOC Points* YOU MUST:

1. Answer all questions.
2. Score a minimum of 50% correct.

TO EARN *FREE* INSTANTANEOUS *CME Credits and/or MOC Points* ONLINE:

1. Answer all of your questions.
2. Go to **mksap.acponline.org** and enter your ACP Online username and password to access an online answer sheet.
3. Enter your answers.
4. You can also enter your answers directly at **mksap.acponline.org** without first using this answer sheet.

To Submit Your Answer Sheet by Mail or FAX for a $20 Administrative Fee per Answer Sheet:

1. Answer all of your questions and calculate your score.
2. Complete boxes A–H.
3. Complete payment information.
4. Send the answer sheet and payment information to ACP, using the FAX number/address listed below.

B — Order Number

(Use the 10-digit Order Number on your MKSAP materials packing slip.)

C — ACP ID Number

(Refer to packing slip in your MKSAP materials for your 8-digit ACP ID Number.)

D — Required Submission Information if Applying for MOC

Birth Month and Day   M M   D D

ABIM Candidate Number

COMPLETE FORM BELOW ONLY IF YOU SUBMIT BY MAIL OR FAX

Last Name   First Name   MI

Payment Information. Must remit in US funds, drawn on a US bank.
The processing fee for each paper answer sheet is $20.

☐ Check, made payable to ACP, enclosed

Charge to   ☐ **VISA**   ☐ **MasterCard**   ☐ **AMERICAN EXPRESS**   ☐ **DISCOVER**

Card Number _____

Expiration Date _____ / _____
     MM   YY

Security code (3 or 4 digit #s) _____

Signature _____

Fax to: 215-351-2799

Mail to:
Member and Customer Service
American College of Physicians
190 N. Independence Mall West
Philadelphia, PA 19106–1572

E

TEST TYPE

	Maximum Number of CME Credits
○ Cardiovascular Medicine	30
○ Dermatology	16
○ Gastroenterology and Hepatology	22
○ Hematology and Oncology	33
○ Neurology	22
○ Rheumatology	22
○ Endocrinology and Metabolism	19
○ General Internal Medicine	36
○ Infectious Disease	25
○ Nephrology	25
○ Pulmonary and Critical Care Medicine	25

F

CREDITS OR POINTS CLAIMED ON SECTION
1 hour = 1 credit or 1 point

Enter the number of credits earned on the test to the nearest quarter hour. Physicians should claim only the credit commensurate with the extent of their participation in the activity.

G

Enter your score here.

Instructions for calculating your own score are found in front of the self-assessment test in each book. You must receive a minimum score of 50% correct.

_____ %

Credit Submission Date:_____

H

☐ I want to submit for CME credits

☐ I want to submit for CME credits and MOC points.

1 Ⓐ Ⓑ Ⓒ Ⓓ Ⓔ
2 Ⓐ Ⓑ Ⓒ Ⓓ Ⓔ
3 Ⓐ Ⓑ Ⓒ Ⓓ Ⓔ
4 Ⓐ Ⓑ Ⓒ Ⓓ Ⓔ
5 Ⓐ Ⓑ Ⓒ Ⓓ Ⓔ

6 Ⓐ Ⓑ Ⓒ Ⓓ Ⓔ
7 Ⓐ Ⓑ Ⓒ Ⓓ Ⓔ
8 Ⓐ Ⓑ Ⓒ Ⓓ Ⓔ
9 Ⓐ Ⓑ Ⓒ Ⓓ Ⓔ
10 Ⓐ Ⓑ Ⓒ Ⓓ Ⓔ

11 Ⓐ Ⓑ Ⓒ Ⓓ Ⓔ
12 Ⓐ Ⓑ Ⓒ Ⓓ Ⓔ
13 Ⓐ Ⓑ Ⓒ Ⓓ Ⓔ
14 Ⓐ Ⓑ Ⓒ Ⓓ Ⓔ
15 Ⓐ Ⓑ Ⓒ Ⓓ Ⓔ

16 Ⓐ Ⓑ Ⓒ Ⓓ Ⓔ
17 Ⓐ Ⓑ Ⓒ Ⓓ Ⓔ
18 Ⓐ Ⓑ Ⓒ Ⓓ Ⓔ
19 Ⓐ Ⓑ Ⓒ Ⓓ Ⓔ
20 Ⓐ Ⓑ Ⓒ Ⓓ Ⓔ

21 Ⓐ Ⓑ Ⓒ Ⓓ Ⓔ
22 Ⓐ Ⓑ Ⓒ Ⓓ Ⓔ
23 Ⓐ Ⓑ Ⓒ Ⓓ Ⓔ
24 Ⓐ Ⓑ Ⓒ Ⓓ Ⓔ
25 Ⓐ Ⓑ Ⓒ Ⓓ Ⓔ

26 Ⓐ Ⓑ Ⓒ Ⓓ Ⓔ
27 Ⓐ Ⓑ Ⓒ Ⓓ Ⓔ
28 Ⓐ Ⓑ Ⓒ Ⓓ Ⓔ
29 Ⓐ Ⓑ Ⓒ Ⓓ Ⓔ
30 Ⓐ Ⓑ Ⓒ Ⓓ Ⓔ

31 Ⓐ Ⓑ Ⓒ Ⓓ Ⓔ
32 Ⓐ Ⓑ Ⓒ Ⓓ Ⓔ
33 Ⓐ Ⓑ Ⓒ Ⓓ Ⓔ
34 Ⓐ Ⓑ Ⓒ Ⓓ Ⓔ
35 Ⓐ Ⓑ Ⓒ Ⓓ Ⓔ

36 Ⓐ Ⓑ Ⓒ Ⓓ Ⓔ
37 Ⓐ Ⓑ Ⓒ Ⓓ Ⓔ
38 Ⓐ Ⓑ Ⓒ Ⓓ Ⓔ
39 Ⓐ Ⓑ Ⓒ Ⓓ Ⓔ
40 Ⓐ Ⓑ Ⓒ Ⓓ Ⓔ

41 Ⓐ Ⓑ Ⓒ Ⓓ Ⓔ
42 Ⓐ Ⓑ Ⓒ Ⓓ Ⓔ
43 Ⓐ Ⓑ Ⓒ Ⓓ Ⓔ
44 Ⓐ Ⓑ Ⓒ Ⓓ Ⓔ
45 Ⓐ Ⓑ Ⓒ Ⓓ Ⓔ

46 Ⓐ Ⓑ Ⓒ Ⓓ Ⓔ
47 Ⓐ Ⓑ Ⓒ Ⓓ Ⓔ
48 Ⓐ Ⓑ Ⓒ Ⓓ Ⓔ
49 Ⓐ Ⓑ Ⓒ Ⓓ Ⓔ
50 Ⓐ Ⓑ Ⓒ Ⓓ Ⓔ

51 Ⓐ Ⓑ Ⓒ Ⓓ Ⓔ
52 Ⓐ Ⓑ Ⓒ Ⓓ Ⓔ
53 Ⓐ Ⓑ Ⓒ Ⓓ Ⓔ
54 Ⓐ Ⓑ Ⓒ Ⓓ Ⓔ
55 Ⓐ Ⓑ Ⓒ Ⓓ Ⓔ

56 Ⓐ Ⓑ Ⓒ Ⓓ Ⓔ
57 Ⓐ Ⓑ Ⓒ Ⓓ Ⓔ
58 Ⓐ Ⓑ Ⓒ Ⓓ Ⓔ
59 Ⓐ Ⓑ Ⓒ Ⓓ Ⓔ
60 Ⓐ Ⓑ Ⓒ Ⓓ Ⓔ

61 Ⓐ Ⓑ Ⓒ Ⓓ Ⓔ
62 Ⓐ Ⓑ Ⓒ Ⓓ Ⓔ
63 Ⓐ Ⓑ Ⓒ Ⓓ Ⓔ
64 Ⓐ Ⓑ Ⓒ Ⓓ Ⓔ
65 Ⓐ Ⓑ Ⓒ Ⓓ Ⓔ

66 Ⓐ Ⓑ Ⓒ Ⓓ Ⓔ
67 Ⓐ Ⓑ Ⓒ Ⓓ Ⓔ
68 Ⓐ Ⓑ Ⓒ Ⓓ Ⓔ
69 Ⓐ Ⓑ Ⓒ Ⓓ Ⓔ
70 Ⓐ Ⓑ Ⓒ Ⓓ Ⓔ

71 Ⓐ Ⓑ Ⓒ Ⓓ Ⓔ
72 Ⓐ Ⓑ Ⓒ Ⓓ Ⓔ
73 Ⓐ Ⓑ Ⓒ Ⓓ Ⓔ
74 Ⓐ Ⓑ Ⓒ Ⓓ Ⓔ
75 Ⓐ Ⓑ Ⓒ Ⓓ Ⓔ

76 Ⓐ Ⓑ Ⓒ Ⓓ Ⓔ
77 Ⓐ Ⓑ Ⓒ Ⓓ Ⓔ
78 Ⓐ Ⓑ Ⓒ Ⓓ Ⓔ
79 Ⓐ Ⓑ Ⓒ Ⓓ Ⓔ
80 Ⓐ Ⓑ Ⓒ Ⓓ Ⓔ

81 Ⓐ Ⓑ Ⓒ Ⓓ Ⓔ
82 Ⓐ Ⓑ Ⓒ Ⓓ Ⓔ
83 Ⓐ Ⓑ Ⓒ Ⓓ Ⓔ
84 Ⓐ Ⓑ Ⓒ Ⓓ Ⓔ
85 Ⓐ Ⓑ Ⓒ Ⓓ Ⓔ

86 Ⓐ Ⓑ Ⓒ Ⓓ Ⓔ
87 Ⓐ Ⓑ Ⓒ Ⓓ Ⓔ
88 Ⓐ Ⓑ Ⓒ Ⓓ Ⓔ
89 Ⓐ Ⓑ Ⓒ Ⓓ Ⓔ
90 Ⓐ Ⓑ Ⓒ Ⓓ Ⓔ

91 Ⓐ Ⓑ Ⓒ Ⓓ Ⓔ
92 Ⓐ Ⓑ Ⓒ Ⓓ Ⓔ
93 Ⓐ Ⓑ Ⓒ Ⓓ Ⓔ
94 Ⓐ Ⓑ Ⓒ Ⓓ Ⓔ
95 Ⓐ Ⓑ Ⓒ Ⓓ Ⓔ

96 Ⓐ Ⓑ Ⓒ Ⓓ Ⓔ
97 Ⓐ Ⓑ Ⓒ Ⓓ Ⓔ
98 Ⓐ Ⓑ Ⓒ Ⓓ Ⓔ
99 Ⓐ Ⓑ Ⓒ Ⓓ Ⓔ
100 Ⓐ Ⓑ Ⓒ Ⓓ Ⓔ

101 Ⓐ Ⓑ Ⓒ Ⓓ Ⓔ
102 Ⓐ Ⓑ Ⓒ Ⓓ Ⓔ
103 Ⓐ Ⓑ Ⓒ Ⓓ Ⓔ
104 Ⓐ Ⓑ Ⓒ Ⓓ Ⓔ
105 Ⓐ Ⓑ Ⓒ Ⓓ Ⓔ

106 Ⓐ Ⓑ Ⓒ Ⓓ Ⓔ
107 Ⓐ Ⓑ Ⓒ Ⓓ Ⓔ
108 Ⓐ Ⓑ Ⓒ Ⓓ Ⓔ
109 Ⓐ Ⓑ Ⓒ Ⓓ Ⓔ
110 Ⓐ Ⓑ Ⓒ Ⓓ Ⓔ

111 Ⓐ Ⓑ Ⓒ Ⓓ Ⓔ
112 Ⓐ Ⓑ Ⓒ Ⓓ Ⓔ
113 Ⓐ Ⓑ Ⓒ Ⓓ Ⓔ
114 Ⓐ Ⓑ Ⓒ Ⓓ Ⓔ
115 Ⓐ Ⓑ Ⓒ Ⓓ Ⓔ

116 Ⓐ Ⓑ Ⓒ Ⓓ Ⓔ
117 Ⓐ Ⓑ Ⓒ Ⓓ Ⓔ
118 Ⓐ Ⓑ Ⓒ Ⓓ Ⓔ
119 Ⓐ Ⓑ Ⓒ Ⓓ Ⓔ
120 Ⓐ Ⓑ Ⓒ Ⓓ Ⓔ

121 Ⓐ Ⓑ Ⓒ Ⓓ Ⓔ
122 Ⓐ Ⓑ Ⓒ Ⓓ Ⓔ
123 Ⓐ Ⓑ Ⓒ Ⓓ Ⓔ
124 Ⓐ Ⓑ Ⓒ Ⓓ Ⓔ
125 Ⓐ Ⓑ Ⓒ Ⓓ Ⓔ

126 Ⓐ Ⓑ Ⓒ Ⓓ Ⓔ
127 Ⓐ Ⓑ Ⓒ Ⓓ Ⓔ
128 Ⓐ Ⓑ Ⓒ Ⓓ Ⓔ
129 Ⓐ Ⓑ Ⓒ Ⓓ Ⓔ
130 Ⓐ Ⓑ Ⓒ Ⓓ Ⓔ

131 Ⓐ Ⓑ Ⓒ Ⓓ Ⓔ
132 Ⓐ Ⓑ Ⓒ Ⓓ Ⓔ
133 Ⓐ Ⓑ Ⓒ Ⓓ Ⓔ
134 Ⓐ Ⓑ Ⓒ Ⓓ Ⓔ
135 Ⓐ Ⓑ Ⓒ Ⓓ Ⓔ

136 Ⓐ Ⓑ Ⓒ Ⓓ Ⓔ
137 Ⓐ Ⓑ Ⓒ Ⓓ Ⓔ
138 Ⓐ Ⓑ Ⓒ Ⓓ Ⓔ
139 Ⓐ Ⓑ Ⓒ Ⓓ Ⓔ
140 Ⓐ Ⓑ Ⓒ Ⓓ Ⓔ

141 Ⓐ Ⓑ Ⓒ Ⓓ Ⓔ
142 Ⓐ Ⓑ Ⓒ Ⓓ Ⓔ
143 Ⓐ Ⓑ Ⓒ Ⓓ Ⓔ
144 Ⓐ Ⓑ Ⓒ Ⓓ Ⓔ
145 Ⓐ Ⓑ Ⓒ Ⓓ Ⓔ

146 Ⓐ Ⓑ Ⓒ Ⓓ Ⓔ
147 Ⓐ Ⓑ Ⓒ Ⓓ Ⓔ
148 Ⓐ Ⓑ Ⓒ Ⓓ Ⓔ
149 Ⓐ Ⓑ Ⓒ Ⓓ Ⓔ
150 Ⓐ Ⓑ Ⓒ Ⓓ Ⓔ

151 Ⓐ Ⓑ Ⓒ Ⓓ Ⓔ
152 Ⓐ Ⓑ Ⓒ Ⓓ Ⓔ
153 Ⓐ Ⓑ Ⓒ Ⓓ Ⓔ
154 Ⓐ Ⓑ Ⓒ Ⓓ Ⓔ
155 Ⓐ Ⓑ Ⓒ Ⓓ Ⓔ

156 Ⓐ Ⓑ Ⓒ Ⓓ Ⓔ
157 Ⓐ Ⓑ Ⓒ Ⓓ Ⓔ
158 Ⓐ Ⓑ Ⓒ Ⓓ Ⓔ
159 Ⓐ Ⓑ Ⓒ Ⓓ Ⓔ
160 Ⓐ Ⓑ Ⓒ Ⓓ Ⓔ

161 Ⓐ Ⓑ Ⓒ Ⓓ Ⓔ
162 Ⓐ Ⓑ Ⓒ Ⓓ Ⓔ
163 Ⓐ Ⓑ Ⓒ Ⓓ Ⓔ
164 Ⓐ Ⓑ Ⓒ Ⓓ Ⓔ
165 Ⓐ Ⓑ Ⓒ Ⓓ Ⓔ

166 Ⓐ Ⓑ Ⓒ Ⓓ Ⓔ
167 Ⓐ Ⓑ Ⓒ Ⓓ Ⓔ
168 Ⓐ Ⓑ Ⓒ Ⓓ Ⓔ
169 Ⓐ Ⓑ Ⓒ Ⓓ Ⓔ
170 Ⓐ Ⓑ Ⓒ Ⓓ Ⓔ

171 Ⓐ Ⓑ Ⓒ Ⓓ Ⓔ
172 Ⓐ Ⓑ Ⓒ Ⓓ Ⓔ
173 Ⓐ Ⓑ Ⓒ Ⓓ Ⓔ
174 Ⓐ Ⓑ Ⓒ Ⓓ Ⓔ
175 Ⓐ Ⓑ Ⓒ Ⓓ Ⓔ

176 Ⓐ Ⓑ Ⓒ Ⓓ Ⓔ
177 Ⓐ Ⓑ Ⓒ Ⓓ Ⓔ
178 Ⓐ Ⓑ Ⓒ Ⓓ Ⓔ
179 Ⓐ Ⓑ Ⓒ Ⓓ Ⓔ
180 Ⓐ Ⓑ Ⓒ Ⓓ Ⓔ

MK7010-23